Textbook of
Pediatric Neurology

TOPICS IN PEDIATRICS
Series Editor: Gerald S. Golden, M.D.

TEXTBOOK OF PEDIATRIC NEUROLOGY
Gerald S. Golden, M.D.

Textbook of
Pediatric Neurology

Gerald S. Golden, M.D.

Director, Child Development Center
Shainberg Professor of Pediatrics
Professor and Acting Chairman, Department of Neurology
The Health Science Center
University of Tennessee, Memphis
Memphis, Tennessee

Plenum Medical Book Company • New York and London

Library of Congress Cataloging in Publication Data

Golden, Gerald S.
    Textbook of pediatric neurology.

    (Topics in pediatrics)
    Includes bibliographies and index.
    1. Pediatric neurology. I. Title. II. Series: Topics in pediatrics (New York, N.Y.)
[DNLM: 1. Nervous System Diseases—in infancy & childhood. WS 340 G619t]
RJ486.G65   1987   618.928   86-30432
ISBN 0-306-42359-6

© 1987 Plenum Publishing Corporation
233 Spring Street, New York, N.Y. 10013

Plenum Medical Book Company is an imprint of Plenum Publishing Corporation

Printed in the United States of America

To the Memory of D. A. G.,
always an advocate for what is right

Preface

Neurological signs or symptoms are present in approximately 20% of all children admitted to the hospital. These may be the reason for admission or may be part of preexisting and often unrelated problems. In ambulatory practice, acute neurological disease is not seen as frequently, but issues relating to normal and abnormal development are constantly being faced. For these reasons, familiarity with the progress of normal development and factors interfering with it, as well as knowledge of the major acute and chronic disorders of the nervous and neuromuscular systems, is important for any practitioner, specialist, or generalist who cares for children.

The pathophysiology of neurological disorders in childhood is based on the same principles of the organization, structure, and function of the nervous system as apply to adults. Two pitfalls are present for the student, however. First, the abnormalities are superimposed on a changing, developing brain, not a rather static, mature organ. The manifestations of the disease may vary, therefore, in seemingly unpredictable fashion depending on the rate of progression of the disorder and the rate and adequacy of the ongoing developmental changes in the nervous system. The second problem is the large number of unfamiliar conditions, many of which have no counterpart in adult neurology or medicine. These include developmental malformations, disorders specific to the neonatal period, and many hereditary and metabolic diseases.

In order to provide the necessary background and tools for neurological diagnosis in children, the first section of this book reviews the development of the central nervous system. This provides a framework for the neurological and developmental examinations at different ages. Discussion of the major disease categories follows. In each chapter a similar format is used when appropriate. Essential basic science background is presented, and this is used to formulate a general approach to the disorders in this group. Each major disease is then discussed following the traditional outline of symptoms, signs, diagnosis, course, treatment, and prognosis. The final two sections are devoted to specific symptoms that cut across a number of disease categories and to neurological aspects of systemic disease.

This text is written primarily for medical students and house officers, but will fill the needs of practicing neurologists, pediatricians, and primary-care providers in many disciplines. It is structured to form a bridge between pocket manuals, which may provide an approach but are necessarily limited in scope, and the more encyclopedic standard texts.

Emphasis is on an approach to diagnosis, and an attempt is made to provide coverage of all of the major neurological disorders of childhood. Rare conditions are included only if they illustrate important points or pathophysiological concepts. The references and additional readings are not meant to be comprehensive, but include important general reference sources and "classic" articles, both new and old.

The author hopes that this text will introduce the student to the fascinating and exciting world of pediatric neurology. Few events in human biology are as exciting as those of normal development, few as trying for families and physicians as disorders that disturb this process. A logical approach to these conditions and an understanding of their diagnosis, course, therapy, and prognosis will ease the way for both.

Gerald S. Golden

Memphis

Contents

III. Specific Symptoms

IV. Neurological Complications

I

Developmental Neurology

1

The Developing Nervous System

Growth and development of the nervous system involve a complex series of biologically determined and environmentally influenced events. A full understanding of normal and abnormal physical, cognitive, and behavioral development requires knowledge of these events and of the timetable on which they take place.

The task, at first glance, seems overwhelming. Starting with a fertilized ovum, the eventual outcome is a brain that contains from 10 to 100 billion neurons, each of which makes and receives synaptic connections with, on the average, 10 thousand others. All of the supporting structures of the brain must develop, as must the body's other organs, a complex system destined mainly to provide a stable internal environment for brain function. This neural structure is capable of learning, processing extraordinary amounts of complex data, and communicating with similar structures in other individuals. The major principles needed for understanding this development will be outlined in this chapter.

Two related terms will be used throughout this text. *Growth* refers only to an increase in size or mass. *Development* has several interrelated meanings, but the unifying principle is one of increasing complexity and differentiation. Thus, one can speak of development of the nervous system in terms of an increasingly complex and differentiated structure. Cognitive development implies an increase in complexity and differentiation of cognitive abilities.

STRUCTURAL GROWTH AND DEVELOPMENT

The neural plate, from which the central nervous system will develop, is one of the first clearly defined landmarks recognizable in the embryo. It is present 18 days postfertilization in the human. The neural groove forms as a depression in the center of the plate, and closure over the groove produces the neural tube (Figure 1-1). This closure initially takes place in the thoracic region and moves in caudad and cephalad directions. The last portion to close at each end is the

3

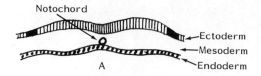

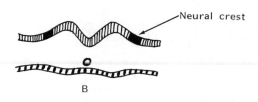

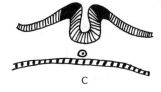

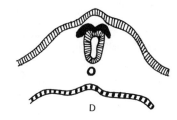

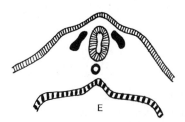

FIGURE 1-1. Development of neural tube. Cross-section of embryo. A, 18 days; B, 20 days; C, 21 days; D, 23 days; E, 24 days.

neuropore. The anterior neuropore closes by 24 days, and a fully closed tube is achieved by 26 days.

By the time the tube is complete, it becomes obvious that the cephalic end is wider, and expansions, or vesicles, are seen. These enlarge and form the embryonic forebrain, midbrain, and hindbrain. The differential expansion of the vesicles and development of flexures in the cervical and midbrain regions give the brain its mature shape. The portion of the neural tube caudal to the brain forms the spinal cord.

The expanding forebrain does not completely cover the deeper structures at 3 months. At 6 months, the basic brain structure is clearly recognizable, although the sylvian fissure is open and the insula can be seen. Sulci first appear at 5 months, and all of the main sulci and convolutions are apparent by 7 months. The development of secondary and tertiary sulci will continue through the first few years of life.

Anatomical differences between the hemispheres may be related to functional differences. The superior surface of the temporal lobe (planum temporale) has a larger area in the left hemisphere in most people. It has been hypothesized that this is related to the left hemisphere's dominance for language. This difference is apparent by 31 weeks of fetal life.[1] There is also asymmetrical development of the transverse temporal gyri. The right superior frontal and superior temporal gyri appear 1–2 weeks before their counterparts in the left hemisphere.

Attempts have been made to find sexual dimorphism in brain structure. The only consistent difference is in the shape of the splenium of the corpus callosum.[2] One speculation is that the larger number of fibers in this area in the female explains the relative lack of hemispheric specialization for visuospatial functions in women.

The rate of brain growth is greatest during the fetal period. At the time of birth, the brain weighs 350 g, one-quarter of its adult weight. The brain weighs 800 g at 1 year and 1200 g at 4 years of age. The adult human brain weighs 1200–1450 g.

Fetal and early postnatal brain growth appear to be on a rather inflexible time schedule. There is only limited capacity for catchup growth if there is interference with the normal flow of events. In addition, all developmental events are closely integrated, with each step dependent on successful completion of the last. For these reasons, insults to the brain during early stages of development have a devastating impact on the final structure and function. The pattern of abnormalities provides a strong clue to the timing of the destructive process.

Growth and development of the peripheral and autonomic nervous systems are interlocked with that of the central nervous system. While the neural groove is closing to form the neural tube, a group of cells differentiates along the line of fusion. This is clearly visible by 22 days and then becomes detached from the neural tube. This *neural crest* separates into two halves, which migrate laterally. Segmentation takes place, and the spinal ganglia are formed. These give rise to peripheral and autonomic neurons. Ganglia of the cranial nerves develop from the analogous structure in the cephalic region.

CELLULAR GROWTH AND DEVELOPMENT

As the neural tube becomes complete, a number of zones can be differentiated in its walls. The mantle (subependymal) layer, that closest to the central canal, becomes the site of rapid cell division. It is in this highly cellular layer, the germinal matrix, that neurons are formed. In the seventh fetal week these cells begin to migrate peripherally. They come to rest under the outermost (marginal) layer. A plate of cells forms and increases in thickness, becoming the embryonic cerebral cortex. During this migration, the axons form and are left traversing through the fiber-rich intermediate zone.

A second stage of neuronal migration from the subependymal area occurs after the eleventh week. These cells eventually occupy a more superficial position in the cortex and form the smaller neurons. The cells from the original migratory wave produce deeper and larger neurons. The mechanisms responsible for this cell movement are not clear, but neurons appear to follow radially oriented glial fibers as their guides.

Late fetal and early postnatal development are concerned with organization of the layers and columns seen in the mature cortex. Cell division is virtually complete at birth, except in the cerebellum. The germinal matrix in the subependymal layer is largely gone by the end of gestation. It is present in the small premature infant, however, and is the major site of subependymal hemorrhage. Remodeling of the cortex involves neuronal loss, which is rapid and continues postnatally.

AXONAL GROWTH AND DEVELOPMENT

In order for the brain to function, it is necessary for each neuronal system to be organized properly and for the interconnections between systems to be correct. It is clear that axons grow outward from the cell body, but the factors guiding them to their final destination are less well understood. There are three possible strategies that could be used. The first is to have sufficient information available within the cell to guide each axon toward a discrete, preprogrammed, point-to-point connection. This seems to occur in lower organisms, but in more complex animals would require tremendous amounts of information and would be quite inflexible. Small perturbations in developmental sequences would have disastrous effects.

The second possibility is that a large number of axons are guided to a general terminus. At that point, specific features of the chemical environment initiate a proper pattern of synaptogenesis.

The third possibility allows formation of connections with only a minimal amount of specific guidance, but requires validation for the maintenance of these synapses. This validation could either be internal and programmed by chemical or physiological messages, or external and dependent on environmental experiences. Both types of validation seem to be used in varying proportions, depending on the system under study.

An important feature of early brain development is the selective dropout of neurons. This, and evidence obtained from animal experimentation, suggests that the growth of axons is, in fact, programmed in only general fashion and that validation of synaptic connections is required for most brain systems. This approach is much more flexible and requires significantly less information than the other approaches.

A related issue is remodeling of connections after they are formed. The possible role of environmental factors in changes following injury is discussed in subsequent sections.

SYNAPTIC GROWTH AND DEVELOPMENT

Brain function is dependent on intercellular communication through synapses. Synaptogenesis is a relatively new area for experimental study, and information is limited. Major developmental processes appear to include the formation of new synapses, changes in the morphology of synaptic spines on dendrites, and remodeling of existing synapses.

Synapses differentiate biochemically before morphological development is complete.[3] The hypothesis that a neuron's specific neurotransmitter is important in programming synaptic connections is appealing, but there is little support from experimental studies.

One of the most exciting issues in neurobiology is the determination of the extent to which synaptic growth and remodeling are dependent on environmental experiences. There is some evidence, in experimental animals, that an enriched environment can enhance these processes.

GROWTH AND DEVELOPMENT OF MYELIN

Myelination of axons increases the speed and efficiency of information processing and transfer in the nervous system. Not only is the velocity of action potentials along the axon increased, but the myelin also prevents cross-talk with neighboring axons. The earliest identifiable traces of myelin are found by electron microscopy in the spinal cord between 11 and 14 weeks of gestational age. Myelin is not visible by light microscopy in the brain until approximately 4½ months of gestation, at which time it is present in the medial lemniscus and the cochlear and vestibular tracts.

At the time of birth, gross inspection of the brain reveals myelination in the median longitudinal fasciculus, correlating with the fact that the infant has well-coordinated conjugate eye movements. Some is seen in the pyramidal tract. Myelin development is predominantly a postnatal event and correlates well with the increasing functional skills of the child. It is impossible to determine when myelination is complete, but it probably continues through most of childhood and is one factor responsible for the slow increase in brain weight that occurs until adulthood is reached.

FUNCTIONAL DEVELOPMENT

A large portion of the functional development of the brain is, almost certainly, biologically programmed. Early motor development is an example of such a phenomenon. Other developmental features depend entirely on the interaction of the environment and the neural substrate. Language development, for instance, will not occur without exposure to a specific language; its rates and limits, however, are set by the capabilities of the individual's brain.

The nature–nurture controversy raises two major issues. The first is the degree of impact of each of the two when examining any specific success or failure in development. The second is the role, if any, of a critical period. The concept of a critical period states that there is a specific time frame during which a given developmental event must occur or will never be achieved. This event may be dependent on a previous developmental stage or on a defined environmental interaction.

Examination of the role of nutrition in brain development illustrates these principles. Studies carried out on rats show that early, severe malnutrition reduces the total number of brain cells and produces permanent deficits in functional ability. Malnutrition after cell division is complete will cause reduced brain weight, but nutritional rehabilitation is possible. The problem with broad interpretation of these results is that cell division is largely prenatal in the human, whereas active neuronal proliferation continues postnatally in the rat.

Detailed studies have been carried out on children whose mothers were pregnant during the severe famine of 1944–1945 in the Netherlands.[4] When the subjects were studied at 19 years of age, there was no correlation between mental retardation and either conception or gestation during the famine.

Korean orphans who were adopted by families in this country also demonstrate that nutritional rehabilitation is possible.[5] The children were all taken into care by 2 years of age and followed for at least 6 years. Comparing those who were malnourished, moderately nourished, or well nourished at the time of their arrival in the United States, each group when evaluated at follow-up had normal weights, heights, and IQ and academic achievement test scores. The IQ scores of the malnourished children were lower than those of the well-nourished group (mean 102 compared to 112). These were still within the normal range, however, and approximately 40 points higher than had previously been reported for a similar group returned to their original home environment. The malnourished children had achievement test scores slightly lower than the others, but still well within the normal range.

These findings confirm a large amount of information obtained from previous studies.[6] The environment to which the child returns after treatment of the malnutrition is a major factor determining the ultimate outcome. Whether or not the child becomes handicapped depends as much on the socioeconomic status of the home as it does on the severity of the nutritional insult.

The critical-period concept is also illustrated by studies of the visual system of cats. If one eyelid of a kitten is sutured closed at birth, and that eye deprived of vision for 3–4 months, the animal will be deficient in any task requiring the use of vision, especially if pattern or form recognition is required. Neurophysiological studies have shown that few neurons in the visual cortex respond normally to stimulation of that eye.

New findings indicate that even in this experiment the critical period may not be absolute, however. If the normal eye is then continuously occluded, some visual abilities will return to the amblyopic eye. This recovery will be even more striking if the normal eye is removed.[7]

Whether or not an enriched environment can enhance the brain development of children with normal or damaged central nervous systems has become a question of major importance. Large amounts of money are being spent on early-childhood-intervention programs and "schools" for normal infants and young children. Experimental studies show that animals exposed to enriched environments have increased brain weight and may have increased complexity of synaptic connections.[8] Short-term improvement in cognitive skills can be demonstrated in preschool children provided with special experiences. There is, however, little documentation that these gains are sustained unless the enrichment programs continue. This area is in great need of well-designed studies.

REGENERATION

One of the classic dicta of neurobiology is that the central nervous system is incapable of regeneration. This is true if regeneration is defined as the formation of new neurons to replace those which have been lost. It is clearly not true if examined in the context of the reappearance of functional abilities that have been lost.

Clinical observation shows that children under 4 years of age who suffer damage to the dominant hemisphere and become aphasic will make a rapid and, for all practical purposes, complete recovery of language function. If the insult occurs between 4 and 8 years of age, recovery is slower and residual deficits are frequently found. By age 12 years, recovery seems to follow the same rules as for the adult. This *plasticity* is not shared by the motor system, as the associated hemiparesis will probably not make as striking a recovery, regardless of the age at which the damage was acquired.

To what extent the recovery of language skills is a result of anatomical changes, and to what extent it is due to functional reprogramming, is not known. The latter mechanism is probably the major one, as even complete removal of the damaged hemisphere does not modify the pattern of recovery. How this reprogramming is carried out is unknown.

If central nervous system axons are cut, there is sprouting from the proximal end.[9] This has been demonstrated in a number of neuronal systems, although whether or not these neurites establish functional connections is not clear. Anatomical remodeling also takes place through another mechanism. If a given nucleus within the central nervous system receives inputs from two sources, and the axons of one are cut, intact axons from the other will sprout and fill the vacant synaptic sites. Whether the functional result is positive, negative, or neutral depends on the specific circumstances.

Axonal sprouting and development of new synapses have been demonstrated in animals following the administration of drugs that block synaptic transmission.[10] If these changes are not reversible, they may represent the anatomical substrate for such disorders as tardive dyskinesia. This phenomenon also has important theoretical implications for the use of such drugs in young children who have rapidly developing brains.

DEVELOPMENT OF ASSOCIATED STRUCTURES

There is an obvious interrelationship between the development of the brain and spinal cord and that of the meninges, overlying bony structures, muscle, and skin. This is most apparent when examining children with developmental malformations such as myelomeningocele.

The earliest evidence of meninges is found between the neural tube and the vertebrae at 35 days of gestation. It is a loose matrix with few cells. The dura, which is of mesodermal origin, first becomes identifiable in the cervical and thoracic regions at 45 days. It surrounds the entire neural tube by 50 days. The falx cerebri and tentorium cerebelli are formed by dural reflections. They can first be identified at 50 days and are complete by 90 days.

The arachnoid is also of mesodermal origin and appears to develop from the inner surface of the dura. Separation from the dura, with formation of a subarachnoid space, begins at 140 days but is probably not complete until the seventh month of gestation.

The pia is primarily mesodermal in origin and can first be visualized at 35 days. There is some evidence that neural crest cells are also found in the pia.

The meninges do not appear to play a primary role in the formation of structural anomalies of the central nervous system. They probably are affected passively.

The bones of the base of the *skull* are of endochondral origin, whereas those of the cranial vault are membranous. The sutures are areas of nonossified connective tissues lying between the bones. Growth of the skull is dependent on brain growth. This is clearly seen in microcephaly. The situation is somewhat more complicated in the case of hydranencephaly, however. The growth of the head in the absence of most of the brain tissue is probably a response to increased intracranial pressure. Skull defects in anomalies such as encephalocele are secondary to the brain defect.

Developing *vertebral bodies* are not congruent with the embryonic somites; each vertebra is formed from the caudal half of one somite fused with the cranial half of the next. Chondrification begins in the bodies at 40 days and in the posterior arches at 45 days. Ossification centers appear at 55 days. There are multiple centers with a good deal of individual variation in the pattern. Formation of bone is rapid, but continues into early childhood. As is the case with the meninges and skull, defects in the bony structures of the spinal column appear to be secondary to the underlying abnormality of the nervous system.

There are three mechanisms of *muscle development:*

1. Branchiomeric musculature arises from the branchial arches and is innervated by the cranial nerves.
2. Myotomic muscles develop in the fetal somites and are innervated by spinal nerves.
3. Limb muscles, in most cases, develop *in situ* from mesenchyme. They are also innervated by spinal nerves.

Muscle histogenesis begins at 4 weeks of gestation with the formation of myoblasts in the mesenchyme. Myotubes form and become syncytial. Myofibrils are first evident at 5 weeks and become more prominent as development continues. The typical striated appearance of skeletal muscle can be defined at 5 months. At that time, nuclei move from the center of the fiber to a more peripheral position. It is obvious that muscle growth continues into adulthood. This is due to both the formation of new muscle fibers and an increase in the size of individual fibers.

There is a good deal of remodeling of individual muscles. The major processes include fusion, splitting, and migration. The majority of muscles have their final form and location by 8 weeks of gestation.

Muscle tendons arise from lateral-plate, rather than myotomic, mesoderm, and their presence is required for muscle development. A hierarchy of preferred sites for muscle attachment has been developed by the study of abnormal fetuses.[11] The preferential point of attachment is the bone that normally receives the tendon insertion. If this is not available, the tendon arises from the next closest bone, other tendons, or the fascia of another muscle, in that order. A muscle does not develop if there is no connective tissue attachment site.

The muscle appears to have a primary role in programming the pattern of innervation. The nerve is attracted to the muscle and remains attached even during migration. The development of these connections seems to only be a function of the proximity of the muscle to the nerve and is not as tightly programmed as are pathways within the central nervous system.

Cerebral vasculature is first seen very early in fetal life with the development of a plexus of undifferentiated endothelial-lined channels. These then differentiate into arteries and veins, and cerebral circulation begins at 27–28 days of gestation. The major blood vessels are present by 45 days. A good approximation of the adult arterial pattern is found at 60 days; the venous pattern can be discerned by 80 days.

REFERENCES

1. Chi, J. G., Dooling, E. C., and Gilles, F. H., 1977, Gyral development of the human brain, *Ann. Neurol.* **1:**86–93.

2. Lacoste-Utamsing, C., and Holloway, R. L., 1982, Sexual dimorphism in the human corpus callosum, *Science* **216:**1431–1432.
3. Golden, G. S., 1982, A review of the neuroembryology of monoamine systems, *Brain Res. Bull.* **9:**553–558.
4. Stein, Z., Susser, M., Saenger, G., and Marolla, F., 1972, Nutrition and mental performance, *Science* **178:**708–713.
5. Winnick, M., Katchadurian, K., and Harris, R. C., 1975, Malnutrition and environmental enrichment by early adoption, *Science* **190:**1173–1175.
6. Richardson, S. A., 1976, The relation of severe malnutrition in infancy to the intelligence of school children with differing life histories, *Pediatr. Res.* **10:**57–61.
7. Smith, D. C., 1981, Functional restoration of vision in the cat after long-term monocular deprivation, *Science* **213:**1137–1139.
8. Greenough, W. T., 1975, Experiential modifications of the developing brain, *Am. Sci.* **63:**37–46.
9. Raisman, G., 1978, What hope for repair of the brain? *Ann Neurol* **3:**101–106.
10. Benes, F. M., Paskevich, P. A., and Domesick, V. B., 1983, Haloperidol-induced plasticity of axon terminals in rat substantia nigra, *Science* **221:**969–971.
11. Graham, J. M., Stephens, T. D., Siebert, J. R., and Smith, D. W., 1982, Determinants in the morphogenesis of muscle tendon insertions, *J. Pediatr.* **101:**825–831.

ADDITIONAL READING

Crelin, E. S., 1981, *Development of the Musculoskeletal System,* Ciba Pharmaceutical Co., Summit, NJ.
Lemire, R. J., Loeser, J. D., Leech, R. W., and Alvord, E. C., 1975, *Normal and Abnormal Development of the Human Nervous System,* Harper and Row, Hagerstown, MD.
Rodier, P. M., 1980, Chronology of neuron development: Animal studies and their clinical implications, *Dev. Med. Child. Neurol.* **22:**525–545.
Stein, D. C., Rosen, J. J., and Butters, N. (eds.), 1974, *Plasticity and Recovery of Function in the Central Nervous System,* Academic Press, New York.

2

The Neurological History

The neurological history and examination are complementary. The first provides the information on which hypotheses concerning the general classification and course of the disorder are built; the second, the localizing anatomy of the lesion or lesions. In some conditions the history is so typical that virtually the entire diagnosis can be based on this information. A systematic approach to obtaining the history will permit data acquisition with the greatest efficiency and with the least possibility of omitting important facts (Table 2-1).

INFORMANT

The primary source of information is usually the child's parents. In some cases, however, the parent may not be the primary caretaker and so will not be able to provide the most detailed information. In these instances, the most useful historian may well be a grandparent, other relative, babysitter, teacher, or worker in a child care center. It is important to be certain that one of the individuals present is the child's legal guardian or has the guardian's written permission to bring the child for evaluation. Failure to do so can lead to unpleasant legal entanglements.

CHIEF COMPLAINT

The reason for seeking consultation should be recorded in the historian's own words. An attempt should also be made to ascertain who referred the child, why consultation was sought at that time, and what specific questions the parent or referral source would like answered. This allows the history and examination to be appropriately structured and ensures that all relevant concerns are met. If the child was sent by another physician, it is also important to determine whether the referral was made to obtain another opinion or to relinquish the child's care.

TABLE 2-1
Important Components of History

Identifying data	Family history
Informant	Three-generation pedigree
Chief complaint	Social and environmental history
Present illness	Family structure
Mode of onset	Family employment and income
Specific features	Parental relationships
Precipitating event	Parent–child interaction
Anatomical location	Behavior problems and management
Character or quality	Past medical history
Severity	Health maintenance
Frequency	Growth
Methods of relief	Illnesses
Factors causing worsening	Accidents
Associated features	Operations
Course	Immunizations and reactions
Pregnancy and perinatal period (Table 2-4)	Review of systems
Developmental history (Table 2-5)	

PRESENT ILLNESS

There are four major components to this section of the history: mode of onset, specific features, associated features, and course.

The mode of onset is generally characterized as being acute, subacute, or insidious. Table 2-2 lists the categories of disease represented by each pattern. Some, such as metabolic disorders, can manifest any mode of presentation. At times, a slowly progressive disorder appears to have an acute onset when the parents suddenly become aware of the symptoms. The child may have become progressively impaired, but this is often not noticed until the symptoms rise to the threshold of clinical recognition. This is frequently the case with slow loss of vision or hearing. A critical retrospective search of the history will clarify the issues.

TABLE 2-2
Patterns of Onset of Neurological Diseases

Acute	Subacute	Insidious
Trauma	Infection	Metabolic
Infection	Metabolic	Toxic
Vascular	Toxic	Neoplastic
Toxic	Neoplastic	Degenerative
Metabolic	Degenerative	Congenital
Seizures		
Demyelinating		
Postinfectious		

A detailed description of the specific features of the illness should be obtained. This includes symptoms about which the child complains and signs observed by the parents. Important to note are the loss of preexisting functional abilities and the occurence of new phenomena such as adventitious movements. An accurate chronology of the illness is vital and provides an efficient framework for the written narrative. The historian's words should be used whenever possible. Although the physician will eventually have to formulate hypotheses based on the information obtained, the history of the present illness is not the place for interpretative statements.

Associated features can be viewed as a neurological review of symptoms. No matter what the complaint, it is important to inquire specifically about seizures, headaches, problems with vision and hearing, motor deficits, abnormal sensory phenomena, changes in cognitive function, and behavioral abnormalities. This section of the history should also document the response of the child and family to the illness, coping mechanisms being used, their conceptions of the problem, and their underlying concerns.

The course of the illness also requires detailed assessment and critical analysis. When the mode of onset and course of illness are considered together, certain overall patterns emerge. These are listed in Table 2-3. The written history should be organized to allow the definition of one of these patterns.

Although students are taught to ask nondirective questions when taking a history, and this is a most useful technique, it must be supplemented with more directed questions when children are involved. If the child is not old enough to be the primary historian, the physician is obtaining interpretative information from the parents or other caretakers. They may not understand the value of some of their observations without prompting. In addition, they have not been trained in the subtleties of neurological disease and may not be sure what the questioner needs to know or what information is relevant.

It should be obvious that the child must be questioned directly. Children as young as 3 or 4 years of age can provide valuable historical information. It is not uncommon, however, to have the parents of a 10- or 12-year-old give the entire history in the patient's presence, while the child sits quietly and is referred to in the third person.

TABLE 2-3
Course of Illness

Acute onset	Subacute onset	Insidious onset
Single attack	Resolution of process	Resolution of process
Complete recovery	Complete recovery	Complete recovery
Static impairment	Static impairment	Static impairment
Repeated attacks	Progressive impairment	Progressive impairment
Complete recovery		Static congenital condition
Progressive impairment		

PREGNANCY AND PERINATAL PERIOD

Detailed information should always be obtained, as the assumption that the condition being evaluated has had recent origins may be incorrect and it may, in fact, have originated prenatally or perinatally. Table 2-4 lists major factors to be sought in the history of the pregnancy, delivery, and neonatal period.

In any specific instance, it may be difficult to correlate these risk factors with outcome. This is especially true in the case of prenatal events. Features of labor and delivery associated with serious motor and mental handicaps are the lowest fetal heart rate in the second stage of labor, arrested progress of labor, and the use of midforceps. Neonatal problems found more frequently in children with a poor outcome are difficulty in initiating and maintaining respiration, low birth weight and small head circumference, lowest hemoglobin or hematocrit, overall neurological status, intracranial hemorrhage, and neonatal seizures. The last two factors are the strongest independent discriminators.[1]

The Apgar score is traditionally recorded 1 and 5 min after the birth of the infant. It has been found that similar measurements at 10 and 20 min, if significantly depressed, have higher predictive value for static neurological disease.[2]

Perinatal risk factors are most strongly correlated with the subsequent development of cerebral palsy.[3] The same events are associated with mental retardation when accompanied by cerebral palsy, but not with mental retardation alone. Epilepsy also appears to result from perinatal difficulties only if it is associated with mental retardation and cerebral palsy.

It is essential to inquire about previous pregnancies and abortions, both spontaneous and induced. A history of fetal wastage or poor reproductive efficiency is often the forerunner of the birth of a child with congenital abnormalities, either with or without an associated chromosomal defect.

It is also important not to overinterpret data from this portion of the history, as many children will have one or more risk factors and still have normal development and neurological function. These features must be evaluated in

TABLE 2-4
Important Historical Features

Prenatal	Perinatal	Neonatal
Prior obstetrical history	Premature rupture of	Infection
Difficulty conceiving	membranes	Cyanosis
Abortions, spontaneous or	Duration and quality of labor	Jaundice
induced	Fetal distress	Feeding problems
Relatives with repeated	Presentation and forceps	Lethargy or irritability
spontaneous abortions	Anesthesia	Need for special care
Illnesses, hypertension, edema,	Resuscitation	
fever		
Medications		
Drugs, alcohol, smoking		
Diet, weight gain		

conjunction with the course of the child in the nursery and subsequent developmental progress.

DEVELOPMENTAL HISTORY

This should also be documented in detail, especially if the condition under investigation is congenital or has its origin early in life (Table 2-5). Repeated examinations are important in the investigation of suspected degenerative disorders to demonstrate slowing in the rate of development and, eventually, loss of preexisting developmental achievements. The developmental assessment is discussed in detail in Chapter 7.

FAMILY HISTORY

A detailed family history should be obtained in all cases, as many of the neurological disorders of childhood have a genetic basis. This information is needed for diagnostic purposes, as well as for genetic counseling. It should be noted, in passing, that every family is concerned about possible genetic implications of the illness, even if it is clearly an acquired condition. The family history should, whenever possible, be presented as a complete three-generation pedigree. The general health and presence or absence of neurological conditions should be ascertained for each individual. Although this is time consuming, there is great variability in the expressivity of many hereditary neurological disorders, and important clues to the nature of the condition will only come from painstaking attention to detail. Here again, this section of the history represents data accumulation, and the terminology of the family should be used. Data interpretation will come later.

SOCIAL AND ENVIRONMENTAL HISTORY

This also needs detailed assessment for a number of reasons. Etiological factors may be found. These could include such features of the history as residence in an old house with peeling paint (lead encephalopathy), living on a farm (exposure to organophosphate insecticides), and living downwind of a smelter (lead or mercury toxicity). The resources of the family, financial, educational, and psychosocial, will have an impact on their ability to seek care, follow through with management plans, and purchase expensive drugs and equipment. Expectations placed on the child and acceptance of disability will also vary greatly with personal and cultural factors. Knowledge of the support systems available to the family will modify the types of management strategies that are appropriate.

Although family and psychosocial data are important, there is now a great tendency to overuse and misuse the information. Just as with the biological por-

TABLE 2-5
Developmental History

Developmental skill	Expected age (months)
Motor development	
Clears face when prone	1
Head bobbingly erect sitting	2
Elevates head and chest prone, face horizontal	3
Elevates head and chest prone, face forward	4
Midline hand play	4
Rolls from prone to supine	5
Sits leaning on hands	7
Sits steadily indefinitely	8
Creeps on hands and knees	9
Pulls to stand	9
Walks with hands held	12
Walks independently (few steps)	15
Toddler gait, seldom falls	18
Climbs stairs	18
Squats in play	21
Runs well	24
Walks up and down stairs alone	24
Alternates feet going up stairs	36
Pedals tricycle	36
Throws overhand	48
Hops on one foot well	54
Skips, alternating feet	60
Adaptive development	
Regards rattle in line of vision	1
Attends to sound, activity diminishes	1
Holds object placed in hand	3
Looks at object placed in hand	4
Removes cloth covering face	5
Reaches and grasps with one hand	6
Reaches and grasps with two hands	7
Transfers object from one hand to the other	7
Reaches for toys out of reach	8
Plays with two objects at a time	8
Picks up crumbs and threads	9
Takes things out of a container (does not dump)	14
Piles objects	15
Pulls toy	18
Scribbles spontaneously	18
Tower of six to seven blocks	24
Tower of nine blocks	36
Makes circular stroke spontaneously	36
Names own drawing	36
Draws two-part man	48
Points and counts to 4	54
Points and counts to 10	60

TABLE 2-5
(Continued)

Developmental skill	Expected age (months)
Personal–social development	
Regards examiner's face	1
Follows with eyes	2
Smiles spontaneously	4
Smiles at mirror	4
Discriminates strangers	6
Feeds self cookie or cracker	8
Imitates nursery trick	10
Holds out object, does not let go	11
Cooperates in dressing	12
Indicates wants by pointing and vocalizing	15
Starts to feed self with spoon	18
Uses cup well	21
Pulls to show something	21
Asks to go to toilet	21
Domestic mimicry	24
Feeds self fairly neatly	36
Understands taking turns	36
Washes face when asked	42
Dresses and undresses with supervision	48
Can carry out simple errands	48
Dresses and undresses without assistance	60
Ties shoes	72
Language development	
Coos	3
Talks back when talked to	3
Laughs out loud	4
High-pitched squeal	4
Imitates social conversation	6
Imitates sounds	8
Knows name	8
Says "mama" and "dada" with meaning	9
Plays nursery trick on verbal request	9
Gives objects on requests	12
Recognizes objects by name	13
Uses jargon	15
Recognizes pictures by pointing	18
Combines two words	21
Uses pronouns	24
Makes three-word sentences	24
Tells first and last names	30
Tells use of objects	30
Tells action in picture	36
Knows at least one color	48
Names coins correctly	60
Knows major colors	60

tion of the formulation, hypotheses should not be developed without adequate and accurate information. This may require consultation with a social worker or with social agencies that already know the family. A home visit by the social worker, another professional such as an occupational or physical therapist, or the physician can be invaluable.

PAST MEDICAL HISTORY

This section follows the standard format used with any pediatric patient (Table 2-1). Illnesses preceding the condition under investigation should be recorded in detail. Even mild, common childhood illnesses should be documented. Repeated episodes of otitis media, for example, are possibly associated with delayed language development.

The child with major illnesses should be carefully evaluated. The illnesses may have etiological significance (streptococcal pharyngitis and chorea), may partially result from the neurological impairment (repeated pneumonia and Werdnig-Hoffman disease), or may be part of an underlying condition that has caused both (immune deficiency and fungal meningitis).

Immunization history is also useful. Serious neurological disease resulting from immunizations is rare, and it is clear that these procedures prevent a number of devastating conditions. These include poliomyelitis, tetanus, and post-measles encephalitis.

OUTSIDE RECORDS

Documentation of history and clarification of developmental progress can be assisted by the use of outside records such as the "baby books" kept by many families. Photographs of the child may allow the physician to determine the presence or absence of previous disability and can provide clues as to the time of onset of the condition. Many families now also have movies or videotapes of the child playing, at parties, or at family functions. These can provide a tremendous amount of information, allowing parts of the neurological examination to be performed in the past. If a genetic condition is suspected, photographs of other family members can also be valuable. Family records can assist in the development of a complete pedigree.

Physician and hospital records should be obtained whenever they are available. Here again, the family may have incomplete information or not fully understand the details of what they had been told. This is especially true of obstetrical and other perinatal records, as the mother may have been sedated for the delivery, and if the child was in a special-care nursery, the parents' access to the infant was probably limited. Parental consent should always be obtained before requesting or releasing records.

School records are another important source of data. They will reflect cognitive skills, academic achievement, and behavioral issues. The child's grades and achievement test scores, as well as the results of standardized psychological and diagnostic testing, provide quantitative data. Declining performance is an important clue to an evolving neurological disorder. If the disease is progressive, this will also provide a tool to follow loss of function.

PARENT CHECKLISTS

A number of self-administered checklists are available and provide a structured way of obtaining information about the child. This can be historical data, parental perceptions about the child, and information concerning the parents. Some of these instruments only provide a framework of information that is used as the takeoff point for a more detailed history-taking session. Others allow the development of scores or profiles which characterize certain aspects of the child's behavior or parental perceptions. These must be scored in standardized fashion, or a good deal of misleading information will be obtained. They should not be used in any other way and do not replace a detailed narrative history.

REFERENCES

1. Nelson, K. B., and Broman, S. H., 1977, Perinatal risk factors in children with serious motor and mental handicaps, *Ann. Neurol.* **2:**371–377.
2. Nelson, K. B., and Ellenberg, J. H., 1981, Apgar scores as predictors of chronic neurologic disability, *Pediatrics* **68:**36–44.
3. Freeman, J. M. (ed.), 1985, *Prenatal and Perinatal Factors associated with Brain Disorders*, US Department of Health and Human Services, Bethesda, MD.

ADDITIONAL READING

Swaiman, K. F., 1982, Neurologic history in childhood, in: *The Practice of Pediatric Neurology*, (K. F. Swaiman and F. S. Wright, eds.), C.V. Mosby Co., St. Louis, pp. 3–8.

3

Examination of the Premature Infant

The definition of prematurity has changed over the last 10–15 years with the realization that not all small infants are born significantly early. It is clear that birth weight and gestational age are usually closely correlated, but in individual cases they may be discrepant. This has given rise to the concept of a child having appropriate weight for gestational age (AGA), being small for gestational age (SGA), or being large for gestional age (LGA). Each of these states has implications for specific underlying problems, common complications, and prognosis[1] (Table 3-1). They are defined by plotting the child's gestational age against birth weight and determining whether or not the weight is outside of acceptable limits, generally set at two or more standard deviations from the mean (Figure 3-1).

These criteria obviously require accurate determination of gestational age. The most useful technique is that described by Dubowitz and Dubowitz.[2] A score is given on the basis of 11 physical findings and a number of characteristics of the neurological examination. The score correlates with gestational age with an error of less than 2 weeks. This method appears to be valid when compared to historical information, maturation of the electroencephalogram, and a number of other independent criteria.

Following this assessment, infants are classified as premature (less than 37 weeks of gestation), low birth weight (less than 2500 g), and very low birth weight (less than 1500 g). They are also described as AGA, SGA, or LGA.

APPROACH TO THE PATIENT

The first step in the evaluation of a low-birth-weight infant is a careful history, searching for factors that could explain the abnormality in weight and/or gestational age.[3] The most common are listed in Table 3-2.

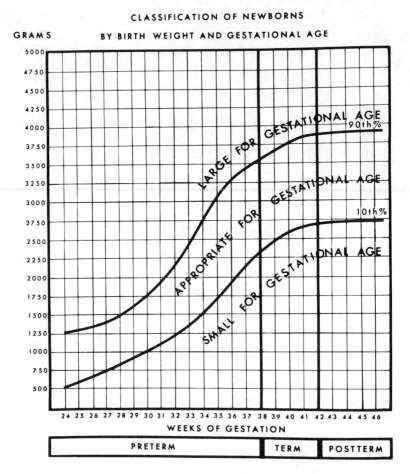

CLASSIFICATION OF NEWBORNS
BY BIRTH WEIGHT AND GESTATIONAL AGE

FIGURE 3-1. Relationship of birth weight and gestational age. (Reprinted with permission from Lubchenko,[1] p. 4.)

History of the labor and delivery are also of great value. The infant's course in the nursery must be assessed in detail, looking for any sudden and unexpected change in status. This may be the only clinical sign of a serious problem such as an intraventricular hemorrhage, sepsis, or a metabolic disorder. Neurological status can also be evaluated by examining the child's ability to maintain homeostasis. This includes unassisted respiration, maintenance of body temperature, and the ability to feed successfully. These functions are sensitive to neurological damage.

NEUROLOGICAL EXAMINATION

Low-birth-weight infants, especially if they have associated medical complications, do not tolerate excessive amounts of handling. A good deal of infor-

TABLE 3-1
Common Problems Related to Birth Weight and Gestational Age[a,b]

Premature	Term
SGA	SGA
Placental insufficiency	Microcephaly
Discordant twin	Congenital anomalies
Chronic hypertension	Chromosomal abnormality
Intrauterine infections	Intrauterine infection
AGA	Smoking
Immaturity of all systems	Twin Pregnancy
Toxemia	Maternal undernutrition
Twin pregnancy	LGA
LGA	Term infant of diabetic mother
Preterm infant of diabetic mother	Postterm
	SGA
	Congenital anomalies
	Placental insufficiency
	AGA
	Maternal undernutrition
	LGA
	Large postterm infant

[a]Modified from Lubchenko.[1]
[b]SGA, small for gestational age; AGA, average for gestational age; LGA, large for gestational age.

mation can be obtained from observation; this mode of evaluation is also often necessitated by the large number of support systems connected to the baby. It is important to remember that any illness or abnormality in physiological status, such as hypothermia, will dramatically alter the findings on neurological examination. No prognostic statements should be made concerning the integrity of the child's central nervous system until an optimal medical status is achieved.

The infant's state (Chapter 4) should noted. This may not be clearly defined in very immature children, and the examination does not change as dramatically between waking and sleep as it does with the full-term infant. Observations of the respiratory pattern, apneic spells, and tremulousness also should be

TABLE 3-2
Factors Associated with Low Birth Weight[a]

Early interference with fetal growth
    Chromosomal abnormalities
    Fetal infection
    Maternal drugs
Chronic intrauterine malnutrition
    Inadequate intrauterine space
    Placental insufficiency
    Maternal malnutrition
Late intrauterine malnutrition
    Placental infarction or fibrosis
    Maternal hypoxemia

[a]From Gaston.[3]

recorded. Seizures are a common problem in this group, but may be difficult to observe clinically. They can be manifested as sudden quieting, a few repetitive movements of one limb, or a transient change in the respiratory pattern.

Growth in weight, length, and head circumference should be followed closely. Norms are available to allow plotting as a function of gestational age (Table 3-3).[4] It is important to remember that systemic illness can cause head growth to come to a virtual standstill. When the infant's medical status improves, dramatic catchup growth of head circumference is possible. The rate may be so rapid that there is a period of separation of the suture lines of the skull.

Assessment of vision and hearing usually requires repeated examinations. These functions can be tested by using reflex responses such as blinking to a bright light or loud sound. More mature behavior, such as visual following or localizing a sound, would not be expected. If serious concerns remain, procedures that do not require a behavioral response can be used. These techniques, such as auditory and visual evoked potentials, measure physiological changes. It is not always clear how the integrity of the pathways translates into functional abilities, however, and a good deal of additional research needs to be done.

Much of the motor examination is incorporated as part of the Dubowitz staging of gestational age.[2] It predominantly evalutes muscle tone and joint mobility, and there are few other motor abilities that can be measured.

Certain primitive reflexes are present even in infants of very low birth weight. The Moro reflex is the first to mature. Its beginnings are present at 28 weeks of gestational age, and it is complete by 32 to 34 weeks. Between 28 and

TABLE 3-3
Intrauterine Head Growth[a]

Gestational age (weeks)	Percentiles		
	10th	50th	90th
26	22.4	25.2	28.5
27	23.2	25.8	28.9
28	24.3	26.7	29.4
29	25.3	27.6	30.2
30	26.2	28.6	31.1
31	26.9	29.6	31.9
32	27.6	30.4	32.7
33	28.4	31.2	33.4
34	29.2	31.9	34.0
35	30.0	32.5	34.5
36	30.6	32.9	34.9
37	31.1	33.2	35.2
38	31.4	33.4	35.4
39	31.6	33.7	35.7
40	31.8	34.0	35.9
41	32.0	34.2	36.0
42	32.1	34.3	36.2

[a]From Lubchenko et al.[4]

30 weeks of gestation, weak sucking and grasp responses can be elicited. Sucking becomes stronger and better coordinated by 32–34 weeks and should be fully developed by 36 weeks. Grasp is stronger at 34–36 weeks and very good at 38 weeks. The traction and stepping responses are first seen at 32 weeks and are fully developed by 40 weeks.

The sensory examination is of little use as part of the routine examination. On occasion, it will help document the presence of a sensory level if a spinal cord lesion is suspected.

When premature infants reach their expected date of birth, the neurological examination is not the same as that of a normal, full-term neonate. The premature infants have weaker responses and more asymmetrical responses.[5] The presence of these abnormalities correlates more closely with low birth weight at a given gestational age than with gestational age as an independent variable.

COMMON ABNORMALITIES

The major neurological complication of low-birth-weight infants is intraventricular hemorrhage. This is discussed in Chapter 15; spastic diplegia, the most frequently associated form of cerebral palsy, is discussed in Chapter 9.

There have been many attempts to define risk factors in this group of infants, so that prognostic statements can be made early and selection criteria used for appropriate referral of children to various types of therapeutic intervention programs. A multitude of interrelated factors makes this task difficult. The most important seem to be gestational age and whether or not birth weight is appropriate, the presence or absence of perinatal asphyxia, and the severity of intraventricular hemorrhage. It is sometimes not clear whether a complicated course in the nursery causes brain damage or is merely an indicator of preexisting problems. Other factors, as diverse as socioeconomic status and educational level of the parents, also seem to modify the final neurological and developmental outcome when these are studied in detail.

The work of Nelson and Ellenberg[6] is of particular interest as it derives from a careful analysis of the outcome of the pregnancies of 54,000 women. The children were followed until age 7 years. Children with birth weight below 1500 g had a risk of developing cerebral palsy 30 times that of infants weighing over 2500 g. SGA babies with a gestational age of 36 weeks or less were at higher risk than children of the same weight born closer to term.

Low Apgar scores at 1 min were not a good predictor of subsequent cerebral palsy. The risk increased with depressed scores at 5 min and was extremely high if low scores were still present at 10 and 20 min. One of the strongest prognostic factors was the physician's global statement at the time of nursery discharge that the child was abnormal neurologically.

Head circumference measuring below the tenth percentile at the time of birth is associated with poor postnatal growth, neurological abnormalities, reduced IQ, and microcephaly.[7] These children also have intrauterine growth retardation and low Apgar scores. There is an overrepresentation in this group of children from families of low socioeconomic status.

Advances in critical care of very-low-birth-weight infants have now improved survival of this group. Although mortality is as high as 80% for those with birth weights less than 800 g, a recent study showed that 81% of the survivors did not have signs of major neurological abnormalities at age 6 months to 3 years.[8] Apgar scores were important predictive tools. The infants with a good outcome were notable in that the majority had no major medical complications and specifically did not have symptomatic intracranial hemorrhage, seizures, or meningitis. It will be important to follow this group into school age so that cognitive abilities can be carefully assessed. There is some evidence that they have an increased incidence of perceptual and visual–motor problems.[9]

Bilirubin encephalopathy (kernicterus) is now a rare condition both clinically and at autopsy. This is a result of aggressive treatment of hyperbilirubinemia; correction of factors that increase the risk, such as acidosis and hypoxemia; and avoidance of drugs, such as sulfonamides, that can contribute. Most new cases of athetoid cerebral palsy have a mixture of spastic and athetoid components and are due to perinatal asphyxia rather than kernicterus.

Retrolental fibroplasia, by contrast, still exists, especially in children of very low birth weight. It appears that there is no completely safe level of oxygen as far as the immature retina is concerned, and retrolental fibroplasia has been reported in infants who received no supplemental oxygen therapy.

Apnea, defined as cessation of respirations for at least 10–20 sec, is a sign of potentially serious disease in the small infant. This must be differentiated from periodic breathing and from the brief apneic spells that are associated with the irregular respirations found during active sleep.

Treatment of an individual episode is easily carried out in many cases by use of a positive-pressure mask. If the spells are frequent or do not respond promptly to resuscitation, other measures must be taken. Continuous positive airway pressure is useful with some children. Maintenance treatment with theophylline or caffeine has also been successful.

Intracranial hemorrhage is one important cause of apnea and should be suspected when a child appears to be doing well and suddenly becomes apneic. These children usually require ventilatory assistance.

REFERENCES

1. Lubchenko, L. O., 1976, *The High Risk Infant,* W.B. Saunders, Philadelphia.
2. Dubowitz, L., and Dubowitz, V., 1977, *Gestational Age of the Newborn,* Addison-Wesley, Reading, MA.
3. Gaston, A. H., 1977, Small for gestational age (SGA) infants, in: *Pediatrics,* 16th ed. (A. M. Rudolph, ed.), Appleton-Century-Crofts, New York.
4. Lubchenko, L. O., Hansman, C., and Boyd, E., 1956, Intrauterine growth in length and head circumference as estimated from live births at gestational ages 26 to 42 weeks, *Pediatrics* **37**:403–408.
5. Howard, J., Parmalee, A. H., Kopp, C. B., and Littman, B., 1976, A neurological comparison of pre-term and full-term infants at term conceptual age, *J. Pediatr.* **88**:995–1002.

6. Nelson, K. B., and Ellenberg, J. H., 1979, Neonatal signs as predictors of cerebral palsy, *Pediatrics* **64:**225–232.
7. Gross, S. J., Kosmetatos, N., Grimes, C. T., and Williams, M. L., 1978, Newborn head size and neurological status, *Am. J. Dis. Child.* **132:**753–756.
8. Bennett, F. C., Robinson, N. M., and Sells, C. J., 1983, Growth and development of infants weighing less than 800 grams at birth, *Pediatrics* **71:**319–323.
9. Klein, N., Hack, M., Gallagher, J., and Fanaroff, A. A., 1985, Performance of children with normal intelligence who were very low-birth-weight infants, *Pediatrics* **75:**531–537.

4

Examination of the Neonate

The examination of the newborn infant relies mainly on observation and the elicitation of responses to manipulation. There are three important rules to keep in mind:

1. The neurological examination will be abnormal if the child is ill for any reason.
2. The findings can be expected to vary daily, especially if the infant was the product of a difficult labor or delivery.
3. The findings are highly dependent on the infant's state at the time of the examination.

The concept of *state* is crucial to understanding the variability in the infant's responses at any given point in time. Five states can be defined[1]: quiet sleep, REM sleep, quiet wakefulness, active wakefulness, and crying.

These states occur in cyclical fashion and depend on many factors, such as the time since the last feeding. The most useful examination is performed with the child in quiet wakefulness. It is important to record the infant's state, and if it interferes with complete assessment, to return and repeat the evaluation.

The examination then proceeds, moving from observation at rest to observation in a number of other positions and finally to gentle manipulation. Intrusive procedures that are likely to upset the infant are reserved until the end of the session.

SUPINE POSITION

The infant is gently uncovered and placed in the supine position. The major characteristic of the baby's posture is symmetrical flexion of the arms and legs. The child may or may not have many spontaneous movements; the presence of abnormal movements such as tremulousness should be noted. If the limbs are gently straightened, they promptly recoil to their previous position. It is difficult

31

to provide a quantitative scale for the amount of flexor tone that should be present, but the examiner will develop reasonable standards by evaluating large numbers of children.

Examination of the head includes observation for symmetry and the presence of any areas of swelling. Palpation confirms these abnormalities and allows ascertainment of suture separation and the size of the fontanelles. Sutures may be separated or overlap as a result of molding of the head during the birth process. As a general rule, the squamosal suture, which lies between the squamous and petrous portions of the temporal bone, should never be separated. The head circumference is measured, recorded, and plotted on an appropriate graph. Auscultation of the head for bruits is also routinely performed.

The face should be symmetrical, both at rest and when the infant cries. It the eyes are not swollen shut and can be seen, there should be no consistent ocular deviation or spontaneous nystagmus. The child may appear to briefly fix his gaze on the examiner's face. The pupils are round and equal in size and react briskly to light. A bright light will cause the child to blink.

When the head is turned gently to one side, the eyes initially do not turn with the head but then come over to the neutral position. Turning the head in the opposite direction gives similar results. This doll's-eye reflex can also be elicited in the vertical plane. This is an extremely important reflex. If it is present, it provides evidence for normal function of the vestibular apparatus, the oculomotor system, and the median longitudinal fasciculus which connects them, running from the medulla to the mesencephalon. This reflex is abnormal or lost with structural damage to the brain stem or general depresssion of central nervous system function from any cause.

The child should blink when a loud noise is presented or appear to become alert if a bell is rung near the ears. It is often difficult to be sure of this reponse without repeating the stimulus a number of times. There is rapid habituation, however, so the attempts should be scattered throughout the examination.

PRONE POSITION

The child is then gently turned over and placed face down on the mattress. A normal infant is able to turn his head and clear his nose. Flexion and symmetry also characterize the prone position. The legs and arms are flexed and drawn up under the body. Some children will briefly lift their head, but if this is exaggerated or sustained, it may be an early sign of spasticity of the extensor muscles of the spine. Crawling movements are sometimes present if the child is awake and active.

PRONE SUSPENSION

The child is lifted in the prone position, lying on the examiner's hand. Some flexion of the limbs remains, and the infant should partially lift his head. Gently scratching the paraspinous region causes the infant to swing the pelvis toward the side of the stimulus (Galant response). Stroking upward over the spine provokes lifting of the head and pelvis (Perez response).

VERTICAL SUSPENSION

The child is supported around the trunk and held vertically. There should be sufficient tone in the shoulder girdle to prevent the infant from "falling through" the examiner's hands. The legs will be held in a semiflexed posture. When the baby's feet are placed on a firm surface, there is a transient weight-supporting response, and the legs then collapse. Gently touching the soles of the feet to a horizontal surface and rotating the child slightly from side to side induces stepping movements. When the dorsum of the foot is brought into contact with the edge of a table, the child steps up onto the surface, the placing response. Doll's-eye movements in all four positions of gaze can also be elicited in vertical suspension.

These responses are usually present in all but the most severely damaged infants. Children with early signs of spasticity frequently have an exaggerated weight-supporting response. Asymmetrical reactions are most often seen with neuromuscular or orthopedic, rather than central nervous system, abnormalities.

INFANTILE RESPONSES

A number of responses or reflexes can be elicited in the normal neonate. They should be easily obtained, although they are highly responsive to the child's state. For example, an infant who is in quiet sleep will have a poor traction response, and one who has just been fed will not have a vigorous suck. These responses may be tested individually at any point during the examination, or they can be grouped together. It is important not to agitate the baby, however, and some maneuvers, such as the Moro response, are best left to the end.

These responses are regularly present in normal neonates. Their absence, especially if documented on repeated examinations, implies a serious abnormality of cerebral function. This can be structural, metabolic, or a response to serious systemic illness or drugs. Asymmetrical responses are rarely due to abnormalities of the central nervous system, but usually indicate damage to peripheral nerves, muscles, or bones.

Root and Suck

Touching the border of the lips causes the child's mouth to open; the head is turned in the direction of the stimulus. When the examiner's finger is placed in the infant's mouth, there should be well-coordinated sucking movements and obvious suction. Biting or chewing is abnormal. The Babkin hand–mouth reflex is elicited by squeezing the infant's hands. The child opens his mouth widely.

Traction and Head Control

Although clearly related, these reflexes should be graded separately. The infant is pulled upward by the hands. This should cause him to respond by flexing the elbows and stabilizing the shoulder joints. There should be some attempt by the infant to actively flex the neck and lift the head toward the examiner. When the child reaches the upright sitting position, the head should be held erect for several seconds.

Palmar and Plantar Grasp

Placing one's finger on the infant's palm will cause a strong, sustained grasp. This is so strong in some children that they can then be lifted from the mattress, although this is not a recommended procedure. Pressing the balls of the feet elicits strong flexion movements of the toes. This reaction is sometimes so strong that a *Babinski* response cannot be obtained. This problem can be avoided by keeping the stimulus well lateral on the sole of the foot and not bringing it across the ball of the foot. A Babinski response is normally present and only of significance if it is consistently asymmetrical.

Moro Response

There are as many ways of eliciting the Moro response as there are examiners. Some, such as striking the bed sharply, confuse the issue by adding an auditory startle response. The child should be held lying supine on the examiner's forearm with the head supported. This allows the movement of arms and legs to be evaluated. The head is suddenly allowed to drop back several centimeters. The full response is abduction at the shoulder, extension at the elbow, and extension of the fingers. This is followed by adduction at the shoulder and flexion at the elbow. The legs may also flex. The extension phase is almost always complete in a vigorous infant, but the flexion phase may be somewhat inconsistent.

OTHER PROCEDURES

Tendon Reflexes

The knee jerk and biceps jerk reflexes are easily elicited and should be symmetrical. The reflexes may be exaggerated if the child is crying, but clonus is not usually present. The ankle jerk is often difficult to obtain.

Sensory Examination

This is of little value in the neonate, and lack of a vigorous response to painful stimuli is more often a result of the infant's state or generalized depression than an indicator of a specific sensory deficit. In the rare instance of spinal cord damage, sometimes found after a traumatic breech delivery, there is often reflex withdrawal of the lower extremities following a painful stimulus, although this will not be accompanied by crying.

The one clinical condition in which sensory testing may be useful is myelomeningocele. It is helpful to determine both a motor and a sensory level. The anal "wink" response assists in ascertaining the integrity of sacral reflex loops, which are important for bowel and bladder function. Scratching the skin near the anus will cause brisk contraction of the anal sphincter.

Funduscopic Examination

The ocular fundi can be examined in the infant, although it takes a good deal of perseverance. The child should be in a dark room, lying quietly on an assistant's lap with the head toward the examiner. A bottle or pacifier will quiet the child, and this often produces spontaneous eye opening. Attempts at forcefully separating the child's eyelids should be avoided, if possible. A red reflex should be present. Its absence suggests corneal opacity, cataracts, or a mass or large hemorrhage within the globe. The appearance of the fundus is similar to that seen in older children. A few small retinal hemorrhages may be present following a difficult labor and delivery.

Cry

If the examiner has had good fortune, the infant will not have cried up to this point. It is important to stimulate this behavior as the last maneuver in the examination. Gently striking the soles of the feet with the fingers will usually produce crying. The quality, intensity, and duration of the cry should be noted. If crying is sustained, the infant's response to attempts at consolation should also be recorded. This can be done by picking the child up or offering a bottle or pacifier.

INTERPRETATION OF THE EXAMINATION

Two types of information are usually sought from the neurological examination of a neonate. The first is the presence of any specific neurological abnormalities; the second, the prognostic significance of these abnormalities. The first task is relatively simple. An Erb palsy should be obvious, as should the functional deficits associated with myelomeningocele.

A major unsolved issue is the prognostic value of the examination. A normal examination is not a guarantee of normal neurological and cognitive development in the future.[2] As discussed in the section on cerebral palsy (Chapter 9), the motor deficit is usually not clinically apparent until 6–18 months of age. Abnormalities detected by the neurological examination, on the other hand, may resolve and later development may progress normally.[3] It is not clear whether these findings represent functional, rather than structural, abnormalities, or whether the positive outcome results from the phenomena of plasticity and regeneration.

Attempts to define a constellation of findings associated with a poor outcome have been made by a number of investigators. The best predictor seems to be a global judgment that the child is abnormal at the time of discharge from the nursery. The role of some of the newer diagnostic techniques, such as ultrasonography, computerized tomography, magnetic resonance imaging, and sensory evoked potentials, for strengthening this clinical impression is not yet clear.

COMMON ABNORMALITIES

The major neurological disorders found in the neonate are discussed in other sections of this text. A number of minor abnormalities may be found on examination which are not of major significance but often raise concern.

Molding is one of the mechanisms that allows the head to conform to the dimensions of the birth canal. The presenting part is usually the occiput, and so the deformation is typically in that direction. The cranial bones may overlap or be separated in almost any combination, but in most cases the skull shape becomes normal within several days, and the sutures become apposed. The premature infant and the child born by cesarean section without a trial of labor will have little or no molding.

Caput succedaneum is edema of the scalp over the portion of the skull that was the presenting part during delivery. There is a soft, boggy feel to the tissue, and the involved area crosses suture lines. Resolution is prompt, and no specific treatment is required.

A *cephalohematoma* differs in that its margins respect suture lines. The most constant location is over one or both parietal bones. This is due to hemorrhage under the periosteum of the bone, most often caused by a shearing force from forceps or the pressure of the head against the bony pelvis during delivery. The presence of a cephalohematoma does not imply damage to underlying neural structures, even if it is associated with a small linear fracture. In rare instances the hematoma will involve the occipital squama and present as an occipital mass which can be mistaken for an encephalocele. The majority of cephalohematomas are best left untreated, as infection can be introduced if an attempt is made to aspirate the contents. During the healing phase a calcified mass may develop, but this will remodel and become part of the skull with growth of the head.

Another abnormality produced by the trauma of birth, with or without forceps, is a *ping-pong fracture* of the skull. The elasticity of the skull of the neonate allows the formation of a depression in bone without an obvious fracture. If the inner table of the skull is depressed more than 0.5 cm, the bone should be surgically elevated.

Asymmetrical crying face should be suspected if the face is symmetrical at rest but there is obvious pulling down of the mouth on one side when the infant cries. The abnormal side is the one that does *not* pull down. This syndrome is due to absence of the depressor anguli oris muscle. The most frequent error is making a diagnosis of facial nerve palsy on the drooping (normal) side. If seventh-nerve weakness is present, there should also be weakness of eye closure on the affected side. Central facial paralysis is rarely seen in the neonate. The cosmetic defect improves as the child gets older, but there is an increased incidence of congenital heart disease with this syndrome, and so the child should be thoroughly evaluated.

The *tremulous infant* (jittery baby) presents a diagnostic problem, although a cause is rarely found. It is most unusual to find associated hypoglycemia and hypocalcemia, but these should be investigated. Many of the children have suffered perinatal complications.[4] Maternal narcotics addiction and neonatal withdrawal syndrome should also be suspected. Although the predictive value of neurological abnormalities at this age is not good, the combination of tremulousness, poor suck, and depressed Moro response raises great concern.

REFERENCES

1. Prechtl, H. F. R., 1977, *The Neurological Examination of the Full Term Newborn Infant.*, J. B. Lippincott Co., Philadelphia.
2. Njiokiktjien, C., and Kurver, P., 1980, Predictive value of neonatal neurological examination for cerebral function in infancy, *Dev. Med. Child. Neurol.* **22:**736–747.
3. Nelson, K. B., and Ellenberg, J. H., 1982, Children who "outgrew" cerebral palsy, *Pediatrics* **69:**529–536.
4. Rosman, N. F., Donelly, J. H., and Braun, M. A., 1984, The jittery newborn and infant: A review, *Dev. Behav. Pediatr.* **5:**263–273.

5

Examination of the Infant and Toddler

There is no single examination format that is appropriate for all children in the age group 1 month–3 years. Certain general approaches will assist in obtaining useful results, however.

1. Observation of the child at play provides more information than attempts to attack the child with diagnostic instruments.
2. The bulk of the examination can be performed with the child sitting on the parent's lap.
3. The child will interact with the parents better than with the examiner and is more likely to accept toys and test objects from them.
4. The intrusive parts of the examination, such as funduscopy, otoscopy, and testing the gag reflex, should be done at the end of the session. If the child's further cooperation will be needed, as for developmental testing, these procedures should be postponed until later in the day.

These points help define the structure of the examination. Basically, it moves from careful observation to interactions that help confirm these observations and then to procedures that are no longer considered by the child to be a game. With many toddlers their active participation and cooperation can be elicited, but only on their terms and after they have been allowed to develop a bond of trust with the examiner. Other children become so refractory to the entire process that no meaningful information, beyond that which can be obtained through observation, is available.

MEASUREMENTS

Height, weight, and head circumference must be measured and plotted on an appropriate graph. Every attempt should be made to get previous anthropometric data. These are plotted on the same graph. The child's current position relative to age-specific norms is assessed, and any movement of measurements across percentile lines noted. This is often the first indicator of serious disease. For example, the sudden cessation of weight gain and linear growth, with measurements falling through percentiles, suggests the possibility of a suprasellar tumor.

Head circumference should be evaluated as a function of age-specific norms (Table 5-1), not only relative to the child's weight and height.[1] If head circumference is more than two standard deviations below the norm for age, the child is at high risk for intellectual retardation and academic failure. This is true whether or not the other measurements are also below this level, although there are modifying factors to consider. There can be a familial trend toward both large and small head size, and so parental measurements should also be obtained.

A sick premature infant or a malnourished infant may also show inadequate head growth, although catchup growth is possible when conditions improve. The child with hypopituitary dwarfism may have a small head circumference and normal intelligence.

TABLE 5-1
Head Circumference[a]

Age	Boys			Girls		
	−2 SD	Mean	+2 SD	−2 SD	Mean	+2 SD
7 days	32.4	35.0	37.6	32.5	34.9	37.3
1 month	34.5	37.1	39.7	34.0	36.6	39.2
2 months	35.8	39.2	42.6	34.3	38.6	42.9
4 months	38.1	41.8	45.5	37.5	40.6	43.7
6 months	39.7	43.7	47.7	40.4	42.7	45.0
9 months	41.3	45.4	49.5	41.4	44.7	48.0
12 months	44.6	47.2	49.8	43.5	46.5	49.5
18 months	45.3	48.4	51.5	44.1	47.2	50.3
2 years	46.4	49.4	52.4	44.6	48.3	52.0
3 years	48.0	51.0	53.4	46.5	49.2	52.2
4 years	48.3	51.3	54.3	47.4	50.0	52.6
5 years	48.6	51.5	54.4	47.6	50.7	53.8
6 years	49.4	52.0	54.6	49.4	50.8	54.2
7–8 years	49.8	52.6	55.4	49.5	51.8	55.1
9–10 years	50.8	53.3	55.8	49.6	52.5	55.4
11–12 years	51.2	54.0	56.8	50.0	53.3	56.5
13–14 years	52.1	54.9	57.7	51.2	54.0	56.8
15–16 years	52.5	55.7	58.5	51.4	54.2	57.0
17–18 years	53.5	56.1	58.7	51.9	54.3	57.0

[a]Modified from Dekaban.[1]

BASIC EXAMINATION

Initial assessment of the *mental status* of a young child is obtained by noting the state of alertness, interaction with the environment, and appropriateness of behavioral responses. Differentiation of parents from strangers and anxiety when faced with procedures or physical restraint reflect appropriate behavior. Some children, especially during long hospitalizations, will become overwhelmed and appear passive, withdrawn, and unresponsive. This should not be misinterpreted as representing an abnormality in the level of consciousness, orientation, or intelligence.

Older children should demonstrate awareness of the fact that the setting is a hospital or doctor's office. They should also be able to state the names of their siblings and family pets. The toddler should not be expected to know the family's home address or to have any good conception of time, date, or even season of the year.

Screening examination of the *special senses* is a mandatory part of the neurological examination. *Vision* is tested by having the child demonstrate the ability to visually track an object and to see small objects at a distance. Visual fields are assessed by bringing an object into the peripheral field from behind the child's head. The usual response is to turn toward the object.

The use of a variety of noise-making objects (clickers, bells, tuning forks) is required to test *hearing*. Response to sound and the ability to localize the source of the sound are both noted. The child often responds once or twice to a novel stimulus, but then ignores it. For this reason, a number of different sounds must be used.

If there is any doubt concerning vision or hearing, more formal evaluation should be obtained. Newer techniques, both subjective and objective, are available. Conditioning the child to respond to visual and auditory stimuli gives surprisingly accurate results. Tympanometry and testing of the stapedius reflex in response to sound require no cooperation on the part of the child. Computer-averaged visual and auditory evoked responses to light and sound are highly reproducible, and norms are now becoming available. The meaning of abnormal responses of various types is not clear at this time, however. These techniques will probably be of more value in the near future as our understanding increases.

Tendon reflexes are elicited in the same fashion as in older individuals, and abnormalities have the same significance. Areflexia suggests pathology in the motor unit, primarily the anterior horn cell and peripheral nerve, and less typically the myoneural junction and muscle. Hyperreflexia is associated with suprasegmental abnormalities, involving spinal cord, brain stem, or brain. Following an acute injury to the central nervous system, reflexes are usually decreased, and spasticity then develops over a period of weeks or months.

The *Babinski sign* is a constant source of debate. It is normally present in the young child, although a strong plantar grasp response can mask it in the infant. The age of disappearance is generally stated to be 12–18 months, or when the child is walking independently. In fact, it is quite variable and unpredictable. The most important concept is that it should not be asymmetrically present at any age.

The *sensory examination* remains of little or no value in this age group, and attempts to pursue it will probably lead to premature termination of the session. The most important use is to determine the level of a lesion if an abnormality of spinal cord function is suspected. There is no need to make this part of the routine neurological examination under most circumstances. Even if cooperation is not lost, the interpretation of the stimulus by the child is too subjective to be of much value, and the examiner is then applying subjective criteria to grade the patient's responses.

MOTOR EXAMINATION

The major part of the examination of the infant and toddler is directed toward analysis of motor function. As will be discussed in Chapter 7, development of motor skills is a result of a complex interaction between three phenomena: the loss of infantile reflexes, the development of automatic responses, and the development of the voluntary motor skills. As an example of this interplay, the events that must precede the ability to sit independently, take a raisin, and place it in one's mouth can be traced. The child must lose the flexor tone characteristic of the neonate, learn to turn over, and achieve a sitting position. Balance while sitting comes slowly. The child first leans on the hands in a "tripod" position. Lateral, forward, and backward propping responses then allow upright sitting and prevent falling. Finally, balance is easily maintained so that the hands and arms are no longer tied up by the propping responses.

Concurrent with these developmental events, the child must gain independent control of the arms and hands. This first requires loss of flexor tone, the Moro response, and the asymmetrical tonic neck reflex. Stability and control are obtained at the shoulder and then the elbow. The child loses the reflex grasp response and begins to reach for and voluntarily grasp objects. The raisin is initially approached with a crude raking movement using the ulnar side of the hand, and later, a radial raking movement. As skill develops, the object is pushed with one finger and attempts are made to pick it up with a three-fingered chuck grasp. An inferior pincer grasp with the thumb apposed to the side of the index finger is replaced by a mature pincer grasp, the pad of the thumb against the pad of the index finger. The raisin can now be efficiently grasped and brought to the mouth. Finally, it must be voluntarily released to be eaten. It should be no surprise that this basic skill takes 9 or 10 months to achieve.

The critical developmental landmarks and major principles are discussed in more detail in Chapter 7. This chapter will concentrate on the more traditional portions of the examination. It must be remembered that there are no standards that are applicable across all age groups, and that there is considerable variation at each age. Unfortunately, each examiner must internalize an individual set of norms, which can only be achieved by interacting with many children.

Muscle tone is assessed by observation and manipulation of the child. The hypotonic child lies in a characteristic posture. When supine, the limbs are flat on the bed. The arms are abducted at the shoulders, flexed and pronated at the elbow, and extended at the wrist. The legs are abducted and externally rotated at the hips. The knees are slightly flexed. This has been referred to, somewhat cruelly, as the "pithed frog" posture.

When the hypotonic child walks, the arms are often held up to assist balance. There is a broad-based waddling gait and a tendency for hyperextension at the knees. The same gait is seen with muscle weakness, and this is often associated with hypotonia.

There is decreased resistance to passive movement of the involved joints. If the arm of a normal individual is shaken, the hand will initially passively flap. This is then inhibited and the hand moves as a unit with the forearm. This inhibition is delayed or does not occur in the hypotonic child. Hypotonia of the axial musculature, the neck and spine, usually accompanies limb hypotonia.

The child with increased tone tends to maintain a flexed posture. There is increased resistance to passive movement at joints, and uninhibited flapping of the hand is not seen when the arm is shaken. Forced retroflexion of the neck and spine is an important early sign of increased muscle tone in the infant.

An attempt should be made to differentiate the clasp-knife increase in tone associated with spasticity from lead-pipe rigidity, which is more characteristic of extrapyramidal disease. With clasp-knife rigidity there is increased resistance to passive movement when the limb is first moved, and then a sudden loss of the hypertonia. Tone remains increased through the entire range of movement with lead-pipe rigidity. It may be difficult to make this distinction in any specific case, however.

It is not generally possible to determine *strength* by having the child resist the examiner's efforts to move a joint. Playing with the child on a mat is a good way of obtaining an approximate assessment of strength. The most useful method, however, is observation of the child's functional capacities during play. The pattern of gait, walking, running, and climbing stairs and the use of the hands and arms provide a great deal of information. As already stated, it may be difficult to differentiate abnormalities in tone from those of strength and, in fact, abnormalities of the two frequently go together.

Coordination is also best evaluated by observation of the child at play. The use of toys, blocks, and coloring books allows statements to be made concerning the adequacy of fine motor skills.

REFERENCES

1. Dekaban, A. S., 1977, Tables of cranial and orbital measurements, cranial volume and derived indexes in males and females from 7 days to 20 years of age, *Ann. Neurol.* **2:**485–491.

ADDITIONAL READING

Baird, H. W., and Gordon, E. C., 1983, *Neurological Evaluation of Infants and Children*, J. B. Lippincott Co., Philadelphia.

Brown, S. B., 1982, Neurologic examination during the first two years of life, in: *The Practice of Pediatric Neurology* (K. F. Swaiman and F. S. Wright, eds.), C. V. Mosby Co., St. Louis, pp. 9–22.

6

Examination of the Older Child

As the child approaches school age, the format and content of the neurological examination become more like that used for the adult. It should be obvious that young children cannot carry out complex tasks as easily or with the same skill as older ones, and that age-specific norms must be acquired through the examiner's experience. Anxiety interferes with a child's performance, and every attempt should be made to minimize this factor. Here again, intrusive and uncomfortable procedures should be reserved for the end of the session. Specific details of the basic examination are spelled out in almost all standard texts. An outline of the major areas is presented in Table 6-1.

DEVELOPMENTAL ASPECTS

Strength, gross motor skills, and fine motor coordination obviously increase with age. Cognitive skills, such as right–left orientation, also become more sophisticated with age. Specific skills developing during the first 6 years are outlined in Chapter 7 and graphically displayed by the Denver Developmental Screening Test. For even more complex motor tasks, a general rule is that the majority of these skills begin to mature by age 7, and by age 10 the child should have nearly achieved adult competence.

The concept of *soft signs* has received a good deal of attention in the literature, especially that related to learning and cognitive disabilities. Neurodevelopmental soft signs are defined as inadequate performance in the ability to carry out certain tasks; this is only abnormal as a function of the child's age. This level of performance would not be abnormal for a younger child. For example, a 4-year-old child should not be able to hop on one foot. A failure on this task at age 7, in the absence of obvious weakness or incoordination, would be considered to be a soft sign.

Other authors consider mild asymmetries in the examination to be soft signs. The presence of a Babinski sign on one side, with no other evidence of a hemiparesis, would be such a finding. In some centers, however, any finding

TABLE 6-1
Neurological Examination

Mental status
Height, weight, head circumference (*plot on chart*)
Head, neck, spine, extremities
Cranial nerves
      1. Smell
      2. Vision
  3,4,6. Extraocular movements, pupils
      5. Facial sensation, muscles of mastication
      7. Facial muscles
      8. Hearing, vestibular function
  9,10. Gag, swallowing
   11. Sternocleidomastoid, trapezius
   12. Tongue movements
Motor
  Muscle bulk, symmetry
  Tone
  Strength
  Coordination
  Involuntary movements
Gait and station
Reflexes
  Tendon jerks
  Plantar
Sensation

suggesting localized or lateralized central nervous system pathology would not be considered to be a soft sign.

The significance of soft signs is not clear. When groups of children are studied, some of these signs are found more frequently in those with disorders of higher cognitive function than in those of a control group. No single sign, or constellation of signs, is diagnostic when examining an individual child, however. In addition, investigators often develop their own battery of tests and their own standardization. The most reasonable approach is to consider these findings to be one index of central nervous system dysfunction or immaturity. They have significance only in the context of the entire clinical evaluation.

Occasionally, children will have such great difficulty in the areas of fine motor skills and coordination that they appear to be *dyspraxic*. The label "clumsy child" has been applied. Even though there may or may not be other evidence of cognitive disorders, the motor problems can produce a significant handicap. These children can also be expected to have difficulty with writing, written spelling, and written arithmetic. This syndrome will be developed in more detail in Chapter 23.

MENTAL STATUS

A brief mental status examination should always be part of the general neurological examination. This includes assessment of the state of alertness and orientation to time, place, and person. Younger school-age children may have a poorly developed concept of the exact time, but should be able to differentiate the parts of the day by reference to meals or bedtime.

General knowledge is assessed through conversation with the child. Although an estimate of intelligence can be made, this can be very inaccurate unless there is marked deviation from normal. There are a number of well-standardized screening instruments for school-age children.[1] If accurate information is required, school records should be obtained or the child referred for psychological evaluation.

Affect, maturity, and appropriateness of the child's behavior should also be observed and recorded. These may differ markedly from that expected for either the child's chronological age or mental age and, if so, this raises consideration of emotional or behavioral problems.

REFERENCE

1. Levine, M. D., Meltzer, L. J., Busch, B., Palfrey, J., and Sullivan, M., 1983, The pediatric early elementary examination: Studies of a neurodevelopmental examination for 7- to 9-year-old children, *Pediatrics* **71:**894–903.

ADDITIONAL READING

Brown, S. B., 1982, Neurologic examination of the older child, in: *The Practice of Pediatric Neurology* (K. F. Swaiman and F. S. Wright, eds.), C.V. Mosby Co., St. Louis, pp. 35–51.

7

Developmental Examination

The terms growth and development should not be used indiscriminately to refer to all of the changes taking place in the first few years of a child's life. Growth means only those events resulting in an increase in size. Growth is most rapid in early childhood and is virtually complete at the end of adolescence.

Development has two aspects, the first purely biological. This is the increased complexity, differentiation, and specialization of organ systems. Like growth, this is most rapid in early life and is largely completed at the end of adolescence. Development, as the term is used in this chapter, refers to the second aspect, that is, the increasing complexity, differentiation, and specialization of the child's interactions with the environment, and the increasing capacity to function as an autonomous individual. It should be obvious that these changes are dependent on both the properties of the biological substrate of the developing nervous system and environmental influences.

The role of environmental influences on development is the source of a good deal of research and even more controversy. The interdependence of nature and nurture is easily seen when examining language. Only the human brain has the biological capacity to generate and understand complex languages. The language that a child learns, however, is absolutely dependent on that spoken in the environment in which he is raised.

The controversies have revolved around the degree to which an impoverished environment can impair the development of cognitive skills and an enriched environment can push these skills toward their biological limit. Attempts to explain group differences in IQ, as measured by standard tests and school achievement, show that some of the variance can be accounted for by socioeconomic status and environmental and genetic factors. The majority of the variance, however, is unaccounted for by any of our current theories.

The assumption that environmental enrichment can enhance development provides the conceptual basis for early infant intervention programs for handicapped children and such programs as Head Start. The studies available clearly show gains during the time the child is enrolled in the program. Research on whether or not there are sustained effects is difficult to interpret.

APPROACH TO DEVELOPMENTAL TESTING

A convenient approach to the evaluation of the development of young children derives from the work of Gesell and various colleagues.[1,2] Developmental abilities are divided into four major categories: gross motor, fine motor–adaptive, language, and personal–social.

This conceptual framework is easy to work with when evaluating children, but it is important to realize that the areas are not completely independent. A child with severely delayed gross motor abilities, for example, will not be able to carry out some of the activities defined as personal–social.

A major problem in using the Gesell scales clinically is that the normal range of variation in the achievement of developmental landmarks is not clearly defined. The Denver Developmental Screening Test (DDST) utilizes a similar approach but, in addition, clearly defines the acceptable limits for each test item.[3] The DDST should be referred to during the following discussion of development in the infant and preschool child.

ADMINISTRATION OF THE DDST

If one plans to use the DDST in practice, it is important to refer to the administration manual to assure that each item is presented in standardized fashion.[3] This section will highlight some of the more important points. Each test item is represented by a bar which indicates the ages at which 25%, 50%, 75%, and 90% of children would be expected to have achieved that skill (Figure 7-1). Those items indicated by "R" can be accepted as being passed on the basis of the parent's report. The others must be documented by the examiner. The numbers included in some bars refer to specific instructions on the back of the scoring sheet (Figure 7-2).

The first step is to draw a vertical line at the child's age, correcting for gestational age during the first year of life. Each skill appropriate for the child is tested, as are items that are somewhat above and below the expected level of performance. They are individually scored as "pass" or "fail."

When administration is complete, the following criteria are used to score the entire examination:

1. *Pass.* The child passes the screening if he passes all items lying directly to the left of the age line without touching it. He also passes if he shows one delay but passes any other item through which the age line passes in the same developmental area.
2. *Abnormal.* Two or more areas show two or more delays, or one area has two or more delays and one additional area has one delay and no passed item intersected by the age line.
3. *Questionable.* One area has two or more delays, or one area has one delay and no item intersected by the age line.
4. *Untestable.* The child refuses to cooperate to the extent that if refused

items were scored as failures, the test would be scored as questionable or abnormal.

In any case where the overall test is scored as abnormal, questionable, or untestable, it should be readministered within the next few weeks. If a passing score is not obtained at that time, referral for full evaluation is indicated.

FIRST YEAR OF LIFE

Man, being an altricial animal, is entirely dependent on the care of others for all needs at the time of birth and for a number of additional years. The developmental changes in the first year of life set the stage for later development. This involves increasing functional abilities of the sensorimotor systems and laying the groundwork for language and other cognitive skills.

The order in which skills are obtained can be easily remembered by reference to two principles:

1. Rostrocaudal development. The infant will gain control of the more rostral structures (head and neck) before the more caudal (lower extremities). The order is head, neck, spine, pelvic girdle, legs.
2. Proximodistal development. Control of the proximal musculature (limb girdles) must occur before the distal extremities can be used for skilled activities. The order in the upper extremities is shoulder, elbow, wrist, fingers.

Gross Motor Development

Analysis of gross motor development in the first year of life is complicated somewhat by the superimposition of three interrelated features: integration of infantile reflexes, development of automatic responses, and development of voluntary motor skills.

At birth, the child has a large repertory of reflex responses which can be elicited by the examiner. These are discussed in Chapters 3 and 4. During the normal processes of development, these regularly disappear at specific ages. Conceptually, it is not clear whether they are lost or whether they form the substrate for more mature motor patterns and are "integrated" into them. Abnormalities may be indicated by either the absence of these reflexes at birth or their persistence to a later age than normal.

Automatic responses are not present at birth, but develop later. The Landau reflex occurs in the prone support position. The child extends the head, trunk, and hips. The trunk and hips flex when the head is passively flexed. Lateral propping is elicited by placing the child in a sitting position and tipping him to the side. The arm extends, as if attempting to provide support. This must be present before independent sitting becomes possible. The parachute response is seen when the child is held in a prone position and suddenly tilted head

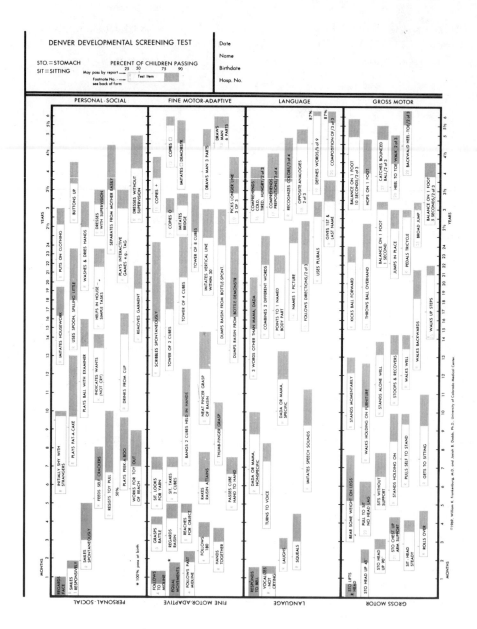

FIGURE 7-1. Denver Developmental Screening Test (front).

1. Try to get child to smile by smiling, talking or waving to him. Do not touch him.
2. When child is playing with toy, pull it away from him. Pass if he resists.
3. Child does not have to be able to tie shoes or button in the back.
4. Move yarn slowly in an arc from one side to the other, about 6" above child's face. Pass if eyes follow 90° to midline. (Past midline; 180°)
5. Pass if child grasps rattle when it is touched to the backs or tips of fingers.
6. Pass if child continues to look where yarn disappeared or tries to see where it went. Yarn should be dropped quickly from sight from tester's hand without arm movement.
7. Pass if child picks up raisin with any part of thumb and a finger.
8. Pass if child picks up raisin with the ends of thumb and index finger using an over hand approach.

9. Pass any enclosed form. Fail continuous round motions.
10. Which line is longer? (Not bigger.) Turn paper upside down and repeat. (3/3 or 5/6)
11. Pass any crossing lines.
12. Have child copy first. If failed, demonstrate

When giving items 9, 11 and 12, do not name the forms. Do not demonstrate 9 and 11.

13. When scoring, each pair (2 arms, 2 legs, etc.) counts as one part.
14. Point to picture and have child name it. (No credit is given for sounds only.)

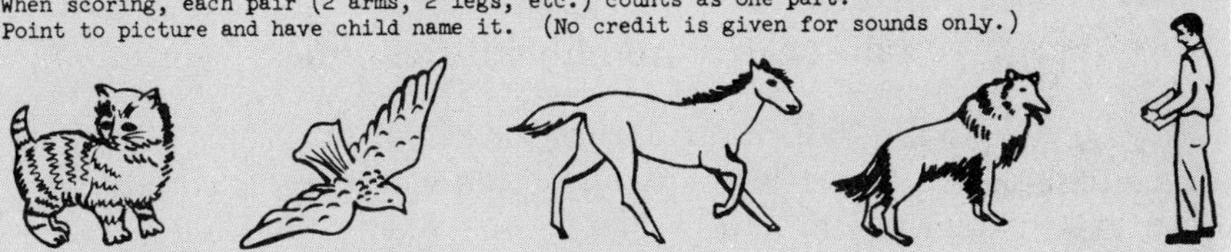

15. Tell child to: Give block to Mommie; put block on table; put block on floor. Pass 2 of 3. (Do not help child by pointing, moving head or eyes.)
16. Ask child: What do you do when you are cold? ..hungry? ..tired? Pass 2 of 3.
17. Tell child to: Put block on table; under table; in front of chair, behind chair. Pass 3 of 4. (Do not help child by pointing, moving head or eyes.)
18. Ask child: If fire is hot, ice is ?; Mother is a woman, Dad is a ?; a horse is big, a mouse is ?. Pass 2 of 3.
19. Ask child: What is a ball? ..lake? ..desk? ..house? ..banana? ..curtain? ..ceiling? ..hedge? ..pavement? Pass if defined in terms of use, shape, what it is made of or general category (such as banana is fruit, not just yellow). Pass 6 of 9.
20. Ask child: What is a spoon made of? ..a shoe made of? ..a door made of? (No other objects may be substituted.) Pass 3 of 3.
21. When placed on stomach, child lifts chest off table with support of forearms and/or hands.
22. When child is on back, grasp his hands and pull him to sitting. Pass if head does not hang back.
23. Child may use wall or rail only, not person. May not crawl.
24. Child must throw ball overhand 3 feet to within arm's reach of tester.
25. Child must perform standing broad jump over width of test sheet. (8-1/2 inches)
26. Tell child to walk forward, ⚬⚬⚬⚬⚬➔ heel within 1 inch of toe. Tester may demonstrate. Child must walk 4 consecutive steps, 2 out of 3 trials.
27. Bounce ball to child who should stand 3 feet away from tester. Child must catch ball with hands, not arms, 2 out of 3 trials.
28. Tell child to walk backward, ◄⚬⚬⚬⚬⚬ toe within 1 inch of heel. Tester may demonstrate. Child must walk 4 consecutive steps, 2 out of 3 trials.

DATE AND BEHAVIORAL OBSERVATIONS (how child feels at time of test, relation to tester, attention span, verbal behavior, self-confidence, etc,):

FIGURE 7-2. Denver Developmental Screening Test (back).

down. Both arms extend over the head with the fingers hyperextended. These responses should always be symmetrical.

The ages of appearance and disappearance of some of the most important responses are listed in Table 7-1. Specific developmental milestones in the first year can be found by reference to the DDST form. These are most easily learned at the bedside by examining children.

TABLE 7-1
Infantile Responses[a]

Response	Appears	Complete	Disappears
Moro	28 weeks	34 weeks	5 months
Suck	30 weeks	36 weeks	4 months
Palmar grasp	30 weeks	38 weeks	3 months
Traction	32 weeks	40 weeks	Persists
Stepping	32 weeks	40 weeks	1.5 months
Tonic neck	Birth	2 months	6 months
Landau	3 months	—	24 months
Lateral propping	6–7 months	—	Persists
Parachute	8–9 months	—	Persists

[a]Weeks refers to gestational age. Months refers to postnatal age.

Fine Motor–Adaptive Development

The proximodistal aspect of normal development is most clearly demonstrated in this area. The child goes from a predominantly flexed position of the upper extremities at birth to the ability to use a fine finger–thumb grasp by age 10–11 months. This has now set the stage for the complex abilities that will develop in the next few years.

Personal–Social Development

In this area the child, during the first year, develops the ability to differentiate familiar individuals from strangers, make basic needs known, and begin to be able to act as an autonomous human being, albeit in a limited number of areas, such as independent feeding.

Language Development

The basic tools for verbal and nonverbal communication also develop during the first year of life. It is important to fully understand language development and to carefully evaluate its progress every time the child is seen. Language skills are probably more closely related to later cognitive function than any of the other developmental abilities tested in the infant. They are also largely independent of gross motor abilities, providing an excellent index of intellectual development in children with motor handicaps. It is important to remember, however, that estimates of infant intelligence correlate very poorly with the well-standardized intelligence tests that can be administered to older children.[4]

PRESCHOOL YEARS

Development in the second through fourth years of life involves an increase of skills in all areas, built on the foundation laid in the first year. There is an increase in the complexity of behavior and in problem-solving skills, and an overall movement toward autonomy and independence. One of the most important tasks for the family is to provide the child with opportunities for exploration and to allow attempts at mastery of the environment. This must be tempered with a realistic appraisal of the child's still undeveloped judgment and lack of experience, as accidents account for a major portion of the morbidity and mortality in this age group. Except under the most extreme conditions of deprivation or pathological parent–child relationships, it should always be assumed that developmental abnormalities during this period have a biological, rather than a psychosocial, origin. It is difficult to stand in the way of normal development.

The DDST remains an excellent tool for the initial screening of developmental progress up to 4–5 years of age. Referral for more detailed testing is important if there are any suspicions concerning developmental progress, as the number of items at any given age is limited. Reference to the DDST form will provide an overview of the major landmarks expected to be achieved in the preschool years.

SCHOOL-AGE CHILDREN

The basic tools for complex motor, language, and cognitive function are present by the time the child enters school. The child should feel comfortable about mastering the environment and be able to separate from the family and face the new academic demands. Major developmental problems are generally recognized prior to this time, but careful monitoring during the first few years in school is most important. The child will now be exposed to higher-level cognitive demands, and the developmental acquisitions of the preschool years, with the possible exception of those relating to language, are poor predictors of success in attaining these higher-order skills. Learning disabilities can only be defined when there is an inability to meet academic demands.

Whether or not the physician should administer tests of language and visual–motor skills in the office to children who are not doing well in school is a matter of personal preference. The school system is clearly responsible for evaluating any child who is not meeting academic expectations appropriate to his age. The school system must also develop remedial plans and provide periodic reevaluation. The physician, however, has an obligation to refer any child with developmental abnormalities to the school system in those states in which early-childhood programs exist. It is also important to make the school aware of any suspicion of developmental problems occurring in older children. Parents often approach the physician first, as the only professional with whom most families have had a consistent long-term relationship.

Some physicians, because of their specific interests, provide screening in major areas of development for all children or for those having problems in school. Table 7-2 lists a number of useful tests, the abilities tested, and the ages for which they are appropriate. The specific tests listed were chosen because they are easy to administer, well standardized, and easy to score. In most cases,

TABLE 7-2
Screening Tests, School-Age Child

Wide Range Achievement Test
Reading, spelling, arithmetic
Preschool to early college
Beery–Buktenica Test of Visual Motor Integration (VMI)
Visual motor abilities
2 years 10 months to 15 years 11 months
Bender Gestalt Test
Visual motor abilities
3 years to adult
Peabody Picture Vocabulary Test
Receptive language
2 years 3 months to 18 years 5 months

they can be administered by office personnel. Table 7-3 provides a somewhat more informal approach. The most important screening tests, which *must* be provided for all school-age children, are those which assess vision and hearing.

SCREENING TESTS

The DDST is a screening test, not a standardized diagnostic instrument. Screening tests all share certain important characteristics, which must be kept in mind to prevent their misuse. First, they must be given in standardized fashion and scored according to the instructions provided. Validity is lost if these guidelines are not followed. Second, screening tests cannot be used for setting a developmental level, but merely indicate whether a child has or has not passed the required number of items at that level. Finally, it is inappropriate to use repeated administrations of a screening test to document developmental progress or response to therapy. It is important to emphasize that these tests can only raise the suspicion that the child has a developmental problem and needs further evaluation. If the test failure can be confirmed, the child should be referred for standardized developmental testing by a qualified professional.

PATTERNS OF DEVELOPMENTAL ABNORMALITIES

Although the use and limitations of screening tests must always be kept in mind, the pattern of delays will often provide a clue as to the most efficient direction for further evaluation. The following are some of the more common patterns.

Global Delay

A diagnosis of mental retardation is suggested if the child fails to achieve age-appropriate scores in all areas. Severe impairment of the motor system (e.g.,

TABLE 7-3
Cognitive Screening

First grade (6 years)

Spelling words		Reading words	
go		cat	work
cat		see	book
and		red	eat
will		to	was
		big	him

Arithmetic
  Counts objects
  Reads two-digit numbers
General knowledge
  Knows five pennies in a nickel
  Knows where sugar is bought

Second grade (7 years)

Spelling words		Reading words	
make	cook	then	even
him	light	open	spell
say	must	letter	awake
cut		jar	block

Arithmetic
  Adds single-digit numbers
  Subtracts single-digit numbers
General knowledge
  Knows 7 days in a week
  Knows who discovered America

Third grade (8 years)

Spelling words		Reading words	
chess		weather	felt
reach		should	start
order		lip	cliff
watch		finger	lame
enter		tray	struck

Arithmetic
  Adds two-digit numbers
  Subtracts two-digit numbers
  Multiplies two-digit by one-digit numbers
General knowledge
  Knows 12 objects in a dozen
  Knows seasons of the year

Fourth grade (9 years)

Spelling words		Reading words	
correct	nature	approve	sour
grown	explain	plot	apply
circle		huge	urge

Arithmetic
  Divides one-digit number into three-digit number
  Adds simple fractions
General knowledge
  Knows color of rubies
  Knows where sun sets

(continued)

TABLE 7-3
(Continued)

Fifth grade (10 years)			
Spelling words		Reading words	
edge	surprise	bulk	exhaust
kitchen	result	collapse	abuse
educate		glutton	clarify
Arithmetic			
Multiplies two-digit by three-digit numbers			
Subtracts simple fractions			
Reduces fractions			
General knowledge			
Knows what stomach does			
Knows why oil floats on water			

cerebral palsy, infantile spinal muscular atrophy) may mimic a global delay, because the examination of the young child relies heavily on the testing of motor skills. In most instances, however, language and personal–social development will progress normally.

Gross Motor Delay

If the delay is restricted to gross motor skills, this is indicative of neuromuscular disease. One confounding feature, however, is that major involvement of upper-extremity function also delays fine motor–adaptive function as well as many aspects of personal–social development.

Fine Motor–Adaptive Delay

The child who is clumsy or apraxic will have difficulties in this area and, if it continues, will have problems with writing and related skills in school. This may or may not be associated with an overall learning disability. In the young child, predominant delay in this area may be an early sign of mental retardation, although an associated language delay is also usually present.

Personal–Social Delay

Specific delays in this area are unusual and suggest major behavioral or psychiatric abnormalities involving the child or the family. Autistic children are severely impaired in this area, but also invariably have abnormalities of language. If the child is both autistic and mentally retarded, there will, of course, be global delays.

Language Delay

Isolated delays in language are among the most sensitive indicators of abnormalities of cognitive development. A large number of factors may cause problems. The basic differential diagnosis includes hearing handicaps, mental retardation, autism, developmental language disorders, and major psychosocial problems in the home. If language abnormalities persist, and only a developmental language disorder is found, the child is at high risk for having a learning disability when school age is reached.

One footnote is important. The term "delay" has been used in this chapter, although it should always be used with great caution. The implication, for both the parents and the professional, is that given enough time, the child will "catch up" and function normally. The prognostic tools are not precise enough to allow this prediction in many cases, however. If a developmental function is clearly disordered, the term "delay" should be avoided, and the abnormality confronted directly.

REFERENCES

1. Knobloch, H., and Pasamanick, B., 1974, *Developmental Diagnosis,* 3rd ed., Harper and Row, Hagerstown, MD.
2. Knobloch, H., Stevens, F., and Malone, A. F., 1980, *Manual of Developmental Diagnosis,* Harper & Row, Philadelphia.
3. Frankenburg, W. K., Dodds, J. B., Fandal, A. W., Kazuk, E., and Cohrs, M., 1975, *Denver Developmental Screening Test: Reference Manual,* University of Colorado Medical Center, Denver.
4. Elkind, D., 1973, Infant intelligence, *Am. J. Dis. Child.,* **126:**143–144.

8

Neurodiagnostic Techniques

This chapter will present a brief discussion of the major neurodiagnostic techniques as they relate to children. It is not meant to be a complete atlas of laboratory diagnosis, but to provide an overview of the use and abuse of special studies in pediatrics and the range of normal values expected in this age group. More detailed discussion of many procedures may be found in chapters relating to specific disease processes.

The last 10 years have seen a proliferation of new, highly sophisticated, and rather expensive procedures. Some have been truly revolutionary, others remain techniques in search of an indication.

NEURORADIOLOGY

Skull x rays, long the mainstay of neuroradiology, are now of rather limited usefulness. They are the preferred diagnostic procedure only when searching for abnormalities of the bony skull, cranial sutures, sinuses, or mastoids. Many traditional applications of skull x rays, such as the demonstration of intracranial calcification, have been supplanted by computerized-tomography (CT) scans. Although more expensive, CT scans provide higher sensitivity, clearer definition, and greater localizing ability, all without any increase in radiation dose.

The skull x ray of the young child differs from that of older individuals in the proportion of the size of the cranial vault to the face. The cranial vault of the newborn infant appears to encompass approximately three times the area of the face on a lateral view; in the mature individual, its area is twice that of the face. Suture lines and synchondroses, radiolucent cartilaginous plates separating bones at the base of the skull, are seen in x-ray studies of the infant and child and are easily confused with fractures.

Skull x rays are indicated if it is important to demonstrate any of the following:

- Congenital anomalies of the bone
- Fractures

- Suture synostosis or separation
- Enlargement of foramina
- Pituitary fossa expansion or destruction
- Lytic lesions of skull bones
- Bone diseases involving skull bones
- Abnormalities of sinuses or mastoids

Congenital anomalies of the skull best visualized with skull x rays are those producing a defect in bone, such as a cranial encephalocele. Structure of the facial bones is also abnormal in conditions such as Crouzon and Apert syndromes.

Linear skull fractures lie over the convexity and tend to be delimited by suture lines. Unlike vascular markings, they often become wider as they move distally from the base of the skull. The sutures found in the young child are a major source of confusion and should be carefully differentiated from fractures. Depressed fractures are best seen with a view taken tangential to the depression. Fractures of the base of the skull are rarely visualized with clinical x-ray studies; if it is necessary to confirm the diagnosis, tomography can be used, but the yield is still low.

Cranial synostosis, in its early stages, begins with sclerosis on either side of the suture line. As the condition progresses, the suture becomes obliterated. Other features on x ray include characteristic abnormalities of head shape and, in the case of Crouzon or Apert syndrome, changes in facial bones.

Enlargement of the optic or auditory canals is an early sign of tumors of the second and eighth cranial nerves, respectively. Optic gliomas are well visualized by CT scan. Acoustic neuromas, while they remain within the bony canal, require specialized diagnostic techniques such as cisternography.

Lesions involving the pituitary region cause expansion of the pituitary fossa, destruction of the floor of the sella, and erosion of the anterior clinoids and dorsum sellae. Calcification is often seen, especially in the case of craniopharyngioma.

Lytic lesions of the bone are most commonly present in histiocytosis and metastatic neuroblastoma; other common childhood tumors rarely metastasize to the skull. Leukemia and anemias associated with an increased rate of erythrocyte turnover expand the marrow-containing diploic spaces and give a "hair-on-end" appearance to the bones of the cranial vault.

Primary diseases of bone are rare in children, but characteristic findings are seen in osteopetrosis. The bones of the base of the skull are dense and sclerotic, and there is impingement on the foramina. In osteogenesis imperfecta, there is an increased number of wermian bones, islands of bone occurring within suture lines. These are also present in hypothyroidism and cleidocranial dysostosis.

Radiological criteria of sinusitis include opacification of the sinus, thickening of the lining membranes, and the presence of an air–fluid level. Knowledge of the normal development of the sinuses is needed before the criterion of opacification can be applied. Although mastoiditis is now relatively uncommon, it still occurs. Opacification of the mastoids and bone destruction are seen. It is unwise to make a diagnosis of either mastoiditis or sinusitis on the basis of minimal x-ray changes in the absence of clinical signs and symptoms.

The interpretation of *spine x rays* is also dependent on knowing the normal anatomy in the young child. The major area of potential confusion is the presence of synchondroses and multiple centers of ossification, which may appear to be fractures in the vertebral bodies and posterior arches. This study is useful in the evaluation of

- Congenital anomalies
- Intraspinal tumors
- Infections of the vertebral body or disc
- Trauma
- Metabolic disorders

The major congenital anomalies of the spine are spina bifida and scoliosis. Spina bifida occulta is a frequent finding and, if isolated, is not accompanied by neurological disease. Scoliosis in the preadolescent patient is almost always associated with abnormalities of the bony spine or neuromuscular disorder. X-ray studies may reveal the presence of an anomaly such as a hemivertebra and will also allow the progression of the scoliosis to be followed. Abnormal vertebrae in the cervical region are often associated with anomalities of the base of the skull. Diastematomyelia can be suspected if the calcified spicule is seen, but myelography or a CT scan is required to make a definitive diagnosis.

The typical changes found with intraspinal tumors are widening of the interpedicular distance, erosion of the pedicles and vertebral bodies, and widening of the neural foramina. If there is a strong clinical suspicion of intraspinal pathology, myelography, CT scan of the spine, or magnetic resonance imaging (MRI) of the spine is required, even in the absence of bony changes.

Infections of the vertebral bodies are rare in children. The changes are the same as seen in adults, with areas of lucency and sclerosis and eventual collapse of the involved vertebrae. Infection, as opposed to tumor, is usually associated with destruction of the intervertebral disc. Low-grade disc infections (discitis) can present with back pain for many months before any narrowing of the disc space is seen.

Accurate diagnosis of traumatic lesions of the bony spine also depends on understanding normal developmental anatomy. Vascular grooves in the vertebral bodies and lack of fusion of the epiphyses at the margin of the body are often mistaken for fractures. Delayed fusion of portions of the arches also can lead to a similar misdiagnosis.

Certain metabolic disorders produce characteristic changes in the vertebral bodies. The most important are the mucopolysaccharidoses and generalized gangliosidosis. This is obviously not the primary diagnostic tool, but can point out the need for specific metabolic studies.

CT scan has revolutionized diagnostic radiology by greatly reducing the need for more invasive procedures, such as pneumoencephalography and ventriculography, that are difficult to perform on children. It also allows definition of intracranial structures and pathological lesions well beyond that previously possible. The level of radiation exposure is less than that of many of the older techniques, and the volume of contrast material required is also greatly reduced.

The procedure is not completely without hazard, however. As each section takes several seconds and the child must lie absolutely still, anesthesia is often required, introducing an element of risk. The child must be carefully positioned in the apparatus to prevent respiratory obstruction. The use of contrast medium adds the possibility of allergic reactions. Finally, there is no portable apparatus available, and so it is frequently necessary to move a critically ill child with all of the associated tubes and life-support equipment to the radiology suite. For these reasons, and because of the considerable expense, a firm indication should be required before a CT scan is ordered. It is not a neurological screening procedure and does not replace a careful history and neurological examination.

The value of a CT scan can now be enhanced by the computer-assisted reconstruction of sections in the coronal and sagittal planes, a capability of later-generation scanners. If abnormalities involving the parenchyma of the brain or vascular structures are being sought, an unenhanced and an enhanced scan (following the intravenous injection of contrast medium) should be obtained. This is also important if an extracerebral hematoma is suspected, as it may be iso-dense with the brain and not be easily visualized. In selected cases, such as the diagnosis of a small cerebellopontine angle tumor or as part of a CT scan of the spine, the procedure is performed following the subarachnoid instillation of a contrast agent such as metrizamide.

A listing of some of the major conditions in which CT scans are useful is presented in Table 8-1. The majority of these conditions are discussed in the relevant chapters.

Arteriography remains the only procedure that will give detailed definition of vascular structures. The usual approach in children is retrograde catheterization of the femoral artery; this allows small injections of contrast medium to be made selectively into the appropriate vessels. Complications include vascular injury and thrombosis, infarction of cerebral tissue, seizures, and a hypersensitivity reaction to the contrast agent. The amount of agent used in young children must be carefully limited because of its high osmolarity.

The major indications for angiography are

- Intrinsic vascular disease
- Aneurysm
- Vascular malformation
- Definition of vessels supplying a tumor

On occasion, arteriography must be used to determine whether a lesion is vascular or avascular, if this distinction cannot be made on an enhanced CT scan. This can be important in differentiating a neoplasm from an abscess or area of infarction.

Intravenous digital subtraction angiography reduces the volume of contrast medium needed and eliminates the requirement for arterial puncture. Follow-

TABLE 8-1
Conditions Diagnosed by Computerized-Tomography Scan

Intracerebral pathology	Orbit
Congenital anomalies	Optic atrophy
Calcifications	Optic nerve tumor
Tumors	Orbital tumor
Hematomas	Intraocular tumor
Vascular malformations	Orbital infection
Intraventricular hemorrhage	Proptosis
Cerebral edema	Spine
Atrophy	Congenital anomalies
Encephalomalacia	Intraspinal tumor
Demyelination	Spinal vascular malformation
Ventricular enlargement	Hematoma
Extracerebral intracranial pathology	Disc protrusion
Hematomas	
Subarachnoid hemorrhage	
Meningitis	
Cysts	
Tumors	

ing intravenous administration of the contrast agent, a series of x rays is taken. The images are digitized, and the computer program subtracts the overlying nonvascular structures, giving a clear picture of the blood vessels. The technique is promising, although there is still little experience with it in pediatric neuroradiology.

Air encephalography (ventriculography and pneumoencephalography) has been replaced almost entirely by the CT scan. This has eliminated the morbidity associated with these procedures. Virtually all children suffer headache, obtundation, irritability, fever, and meningismus, especially following pneumoencephalography. Ventriculography requires inserting a needle or catheter through brain tissue and produces focal damage. Porencephalic cysts developing along the needle tract have been reported. Although the mortality rate associated with these studies is low, herniation and brain stem compression is a risk if increased intracranial pressure is present.

Myelography is not commonly performed in children, but is useful in the following conditions:

- Congenital anomalies
- Intraspinal tumors
- Intraspinal hematomas
- Intraspinal vascular malformations
- Intraspinal abscesses
- Syringomyelia
- Vertebral infections
- Impingement on the spinal canal following trauma
- Disc protrusion

Use of the water-soluble contrast agent metrizamide allows excellent definition of intraspinal structures, and it does not have to be removed following the procedure. Removal was necessary with the iodinated oils that were previously in use, to reduce the risk of arachnoiditis. There is now also little need to perform air myelography. The major hazard associated with the use of metrizamide is the precipitation of seizures. A loading dose of an anticonvulsant is generally administered before the procedure is carried out.

SPECIAL IMAGING PROCEDURES

Radionuclide brain scans have also largely been replaced by CT scans. They can be used to give an approximation of cerebral blood flow dynamics in cases where angiography may not be indicated or is difficult to obtain. This would be useful in the demonstration of

- Hemispheric blood flow asymmetry
- Cerebral death

Vascular disease in children is uncommon, but major asymmetries in blood flow can be demonstrated if vascular disease is present. This is obviously no substitute for quantitative studies if they are required.

The absence of any intracranial flow demonstrated by the radionuclide scan is a confirmatory sign of cerebral death. Some centers rely on angiography, but this requires transporting the patient to the neuroradiology suite.

MRI is now available in many clinical centers. As with CT scan, this procedure gives excellent definition of brain as well as intracerebral and extracerebral intracranial lesions. The spinal cord may also be clearly visualized. The few studies available support predictions of levels of resolution much better than those obtainable with the latest generation of CT scanners. Low-grade glial brain tumors, such as pontine gliomas, are clearly visualized. This technique appears to be extremely valuable for demonstrating areas of demyelination, as are found in multiple sclerosis.

Another new technique, *positron emission tomography,* is less likely to come into clinical use in the near future. It relies on the use of radioisotopes, many of which have short half-lives and must be produced locally. The advantage of this procedure is that the anatomical location and metabolism of specific substances can be defined under a variety of functional conditions.

ULTRASONOGRAPHY

Real-time ultrasonography is an important procedure for the diagnosis of intracranial pathology in the infant. The fontanelle provides an acoustic window through which the study can be performed. Images of the cerebral hemispheres and cerebellum can be made in planes which are roughly coronal, sagittal, and parasagittal. The portability of the instrument allows it to be brought to the special-care nursery, and the procedure can be carried out without sedation of the infant, restraint, or the use of contrast agents. The major limitation is in identifying pathological lesions that lie peripherally, such as subdural hematomas. There are no recognized complications at this time.

Important uses of ultrasonography in the infant are in the diagnosis of

- Intraventricular/subependymal hemorrhage (IVH/SEH)
- Intracerebral hemorrhage
- Infarction
- Vascular malformations
- Ventricular dilatation
- Congenital anomalies

Ultrasonography has become the preferred tool in the diagnosis and follow-up of IVH/SEH and hydrocephalus, especially in the premature or critically ill infant. Studies have shown excellent correlation with CT scans.[1] Infarction may actually be visualized before it appears on CT scan.

ELECTROENCEPHALOGRAPHY

The *electroencephalogram* (EEG) undergoes major changes between the time of birth and adulthood. These developmental patterns are closely correlated with the patient's age. There is also evolution of specific findings related to sleep. Finally, there are a number of age-specific abnormal features that are restricted to childhood.

The EEG is a useful tool in the evaluation of

- Seizures
- Pseudoseizures
- Sleep disorders
- Focal neurological disease
- Metabolic encephalopathy
- Coma
- Brain death

Seizure disorders, and the role of the EEG in diagnosis and management, are discussed in detail in Chapter 16. An important method of differentiating seizures from pseudoseizures is recording the EEG during an attack while simultaneously videotaping the patient's activity and behavior. Ambulatory EEG monitors are now available and can also be useful, although the information is limited because only a few channels can be recorded.

Sleep studies are becoming an important tool in the understanding of sudden infant death syndrome (SIDS), near-miss SIDS, and sleep apnea. Documentation of nocturnal seizures is also possible. Sleep is an excellent tool for activating epileptogenic foci in some patients, even if their seizures occur only when they are awake.

EEG can provide ancillary assistance in an attempt to define the nature of a focal lesion. There are few absolutely specific patterns, although the extreme slowing in the region of a cerebral abscess and the presence of spikes near an area of focal slowing in brain tumor are examples of features with some degree of predictive value.

Metabolic disorders that produce a change in the level of consciousness should invariably be associated with changes in the EEG. Clinical recovery usually precedes improvement in the EEG by several days. A normal EEG is incompatible with the diagnosis of coma and suggests a conversion reaction or the locked-in syndrome.

Whether or not an EEG is always required in the diagnosis of brain death is a source of controversy, some workers stating that findings on neurological examination are fully adequate. A diagnosis of an isoelectric EEG should not be made unless it is possible to document that the patient is not significantly hypothermic and that there is not a toxic serum level of barbiturates.

Sensory evoked potentials are recorded from scalp electrodes in response to auditory, visual, or somatosensory stimuli. There is a consistent pattern of developmental changes. This is a new technique, and its value is still being determined. The major areas in which diagnostic assistance can be obtained are

- Testing hearing and vision
- Screening for brain stem pathology
  - Trauma
  - Demyelination
  - Tumor
- Testing spinal cord integrity
  - Trauma
  - Demyelination
  - Tumor
- Prediction of recovery from coma
- Peripheral neuropathy

The use of evoked potentials to test vision and hearing does not depend on the patient's cooperation or understanding, and it can provide an "objective" measure of these sensory functions. Studies have shown a high degree of diagnostic accuracy in most cases. There are children, however, who have normal evoked responses but no behavioral evidence of functional vision or hearing. The significance of this is not understood.

The accuracy of this procedure in assessing the integrity of the brain stem and spinal cord and in suggesting the presence of demyelination of portions of the neuraxis has also not been tested in large series of children. It appears as if those patients who have absent evoked responses are unlikely to recover from coma and will die or be left with serious residua.[2]

Electroretinography is a technique in which electrical potentials are recorded

from the retina in response to flashes of light. This is performed with the eye
both light adapted and dark adapted. An early diagnosis of retinal degeneration,
either hereditary or associated with neuronal storage diseases, can be assisted
by this procedure.

CEREBROSPINAL FLUID EXAMINATION

Valuable information can be obtained from examination of the cerebrospinal fluid (CSF). There is little risk to the patient, except in the face of increased
pressure. If pressure is elevated, and especially if a unilateral temporal lobe
swelling or mass is present, there is a risk of herniation and brain stem compression. It should be obvious that a lumbar puncture should not be performed
through an infected area. It is also probably best to always use a needle with a
stylet, even in very small infants. This avoids the possibility of implanting small
pieces of skin in the spinal canal, which can lead to the formation of epidermoid
tumors.

The normal values of cell and protein content of CSF vary with the patient's
age (Table 8-2). Although 25% of children have two or three leukocytes/mm^3,
only 5% have three or more polymorphonuclear leukocytes.[3] Infants less than 6
weeks of age may have slightly higher counts.

The major indications for CSF examination include evaluation of

- Infection
- Subarachnoid hemorrhage
- Leukemia and tumor
- CSF protein
- CSF pressure

The signs of infection and subarachnoid hemorrhage are discussed in the
appropriate chapters. Two points require emphasis, however. First, it is most
important to document the presence or absence of xanthochromia if the CSF
appears bloody. This is the only certain way of determining whether blood has
been in the subarachnoid space for a period of time or was introduced at the
time of the lumbar puncture. Obviously, if the CSF clears entirely, it can be

TABLE 8-2
Normal Cerebrospinal Fluid
Values

Cell count	0–5 per ml^3
Glucose	45–80 mg/dl
Total protein	
Premature	50–200 mg/dl
Newborn	40–120 mg/dl
Older	15–45 mg/dl[a]

[a]In children beyond the first year of life, values of total protein above 30 mg/dl should
be viewed with suspicion.

assumed that the procedure was traumatic. The more usual situation is one of partial clearing, and in that case, it cannot be assumed that the blood was produced by the procedure. To properly evaluate xanthochromia, a sample of CSF is centrifuged and the supernatant examined. A test tube should be used, as the column of fluid in a microhematocrit tube is not wide enough to permit the observation of any but the most dense discoloration.

The second issue is that of crenated erythrocytes in the CSF. It has been clearly shown that this does not differentiate recent hemorrhage from old. Crenation of cells can occur quite rapidly and is a function of osmotic differences between the cell's interior and the CSF, and membrane changes resulting from the lack of lipids in the cerebrospinal fluid.

Elevated CSF protein is seen in any disorder that alters the integrity of the blood–brain barrier. These include infections, tumors, anoxia, trauma, and a host of other conditions. Electrophoretic determination of different classes of globulin and a search for specific antibodies is useful in some diseases, such as subacute sclerosing panencephalitis (SSPE). Monoclonal antibodies can be found in demyelinating diseases, especially sclerosis.

Evaluation of the levels of various enzymes in the CSF in different pathological conditions has been studied, but these techniques are not in general clinical use. Lactic dehydrogenase (LDH) is increased in partially treated bacterial meningitis but remains normal in viral meningitis, aiding the differential diagnosis. This technique is less important now that rapid methods for detecting bacterial antigens are easily available. Creatine phosphokinase-BB isoenzyme (CPK-BB) is elevated in cases of perinatal asphyxia.

ELECTRODIAGNOSIS

Electrodiagnosis refers to procedures that are used primarily for diagnosis of disorders of the motor unit. They rely on electrical stimulation of nerves and recording of electrical potentials from nerve and muscle. The results of these tests allow localization of motor and sensory disorders to the

- Anterior horn cell
- Peripheral nerve
- Myoneural junction
- Muscle

The *nerve conduction velocity* is determined by stimulating a peripheral nerve and recording the time required for the onset of contraction of an associated muscle. This is repeated with the stimulus applied at a more distal site on the same nerve. By calculating the difference in time between the onset of the contraction evoked by each of two stimuli, and knowing the distance between the two points, the rate of conduction of the stimulus along the nerve can be calculated. As is the case with all physiological phenomena, norms are age specific.[4] In preterm infants, they correlate with gestational age.[5] The conduction velocity is slowed most markedly in any condition associated with demyelination of the nerve.

Electromyograhy requires the insertion of a coaxial needle into the muscle. Recording of electrical potentials is made during insertion, with the muscle at rest, and during voluntary contraction of the muscle. The last portion of the test obviously is of limited usefulness in young children. Fasciculations are the result of spontaneous firing of single motor neurons. The group of muscle fibers innervated by that neuron contract and a complex potential is recorded. Fibrillations are seen when a muscle has lost its innervation, because of either death of the anterior horn cell or disruption of the nerve. Abnormal insertion activity and polyphasic potentials are seen in many myopathic conditions; in myotonic dystrophy, characteristic features are present.

Diagnosis of disorders of the myoneural junction is aided by measuring the muscle response to rapidly repeated stimuli applied to the nerve. In myasthenia gravis, there is a decremental muscle response with the application of supramaximal stimuli. The Eaton–Lambert syndrome is rare in children. This presents like myasthenia gravis clinically, but electrodiagnostic studies show an incremental response to nerve stimulation.

The picture of botulism is complicated. In severe cases, there is a decremental response to low rate of stimulation. This is not found in mildly affected patients, but they have an incremental response to high rates of stimulation.

REFERENCES

1. Silverboard, G., Horder, M. H., Ahmann, P. A., Lazzara, A., and Schwartz, J. F., 1980, Reliability of ultrasound in diagnosis of intracerebral hemorrhage and posthemorrhagic hydrocephalus: Comparison with computed tomography, *Pediatrics* **66:**507–514.
2. Frank, L. M., Furgiuele, T. L., and Etheridge, J. E., Prediction of chronic vegetative state in children using evoked potentials, *Neurology* **35:**931–934.
3. Portnory, J. M., and Olson, L. C., 1985, Normal cerebrospinal fluid values in children: Another look, *Pediatrics* **75:**484–487.
4. Moosa, A., and Dubowitz, V., 1971, Postnatal maturation of peripheral nerves in preterm and full-term infants, *J. Pediatr.* **79:**915–922.
5. Schulte, F. J., Michaelis, R., Linke, I., and Nolte, R., 1968, Motor nerve conduction velocity in term, preterm, and small-for-dates newborn infants, *Pediatrics* **42:**17–27.

ADDITIONAL READING

Garson, L. P., and Singleton, E. B., 1979, Computerized tomography in the pediatric patient, *Curr. Probl. Pediatr.* **9:**1–32.
Mizrahi, E. M., and Dorfman, L. J., 1980, Sensory evoked potentials: Clinical applications in pediatrics, *J. Pediatr.* **97:**1–10.
Wallach, J., 1983, *Interpretation of Pediatric Tests*, Little Brown and Co, Boston.

II

Major Disease Categories

9

Static Encephalopathies

Many of the neurological problems of childhood are manifestations of static abnormalities of the central nervous system. These can be genetically determined or result from any insult to the developing brain occurring from the time of fertilization of the ovum to the end of postnatal development. The clinical manifestations may change with time; this is a function of the interaction between normal developmental processes, attempts at functional reorganization, and the specific nature of the cerebral abnormality. It is not necessarily an indication of progressive disease.

Abnormalities in specific functional areas are traditionally given different labels for ease in clinical classification. A global deficit in cognitive ability, for instance, is called mental retardation, impairment of the motor system is labeled cerebral palsy, and loss of function of the occipital cortex produces cortical blindness. These can all result from the same underlying central nervous system abnormality, however. Rather than being separate conditions, they represent varying perspectives taken when evaluating the same patient. Despite this somewhat artificial construct, diagnostic terms with broad acceptance are needed to simplify communications between professionals and for administrative purposes when seeking services for the child and family.

MENTAL RETARDATION

It has always been recognized that human beings differ in abilities in all areas. The concept that there could be quantitation of the abilities that make up intellectual functioning was introduced in 1890 by Cattell as "mental tests." Binet and Simon in 1906 developed additional tests that were meant to be used to predict school abilities. This was the forerunner of modern intelligence testing. There has always been a great deal of argument about what is actually being tested, the role of past life experiences, the impact of genetic, environmental, and socioeconomic factors, and the biases introduced by the tester. These are important issues, but largely beyond the scope of this book. It should be noted, however, that despite these many problems, intelligence tests are still a reasonably reliable predictor of school achievement.

A useful operational definition of mental retardation is that developed by the American Association on Mental Retardation.[1] This has three components:

1. There is significantly subaverage intellectual functioning. This is defined as scores on age-appropriate IQ tests that are below 70–75.
2. There is impairment in adaptive behavior. This is demonstrated by limitations in meeting expected standards of maturation, learning, personal independence, and/or social responsibility.
3. The problem is manifested during the developmental period.

Tests of adaptive function measure the individual's abilities in the areas of independent functioning, physical skills, communications, and social interactions. In older individuals, such factors as occupation, economic activities, and self-direction are evaluated. A number of standardized scales, such as the Vineland Social Maturity Scale and the AAMD Scales of Adaptive Behavior, are available and provide quantitative data.

The diagnosis of mental retardation requires that *both* intellectual and adaptive function be impaired. An individual who is functioning with independence in daily life and is economically self-sufficient is not classified as being mentally retarded regardless of the score on an IQ test.

This dependence on a two-part definition accounts for variations in the prevalence of mental retardation defined at different ages. In the preschool years adaptive demands are fairly simple, and only the most obviously impaired children are brought for diagnostic evaluation. The prevalence before age 5 years is approximately 1%. During the school years adaptive tasks increase and become more complex. These include the ability to perform adequately in school and in the community and to progress toward autonomy. Approximately 3% of the population fail these demands and are found, when evaluated, to be mentally retarded. In adulthood, many mildly retarded individuals disappear into the general population and carry out the activities of daily living at a simple level; only 1% of adults are defined as being mentally retarded.

IQ level, functional level, and expectations for school performance can be correlated, as shown in Table 9-1. The table also indicates the percentage of individuals with mental retardation at each level.

The term educable implies that, with special education, the child will learn the basics of reading, writing, and arithmetic and will be able to develop the abilities needed for unskilled or semiskilled employment. Many of these people will, as adults, be able to live independently but lack the ability to manage all but the most simple financial affairs.

The trainable level implies that no functional academic skills will be developed, but that the individual can be trained to be independent in self-help areas and can carry out simple routinized tasks under supervision. Adults and children whose IQ falls in the severe range of mental retardation will only be indepen-

TABLE 9-1
Levels of Mental Retardation[a]

IQ	Adaptive deficit	School function	Percent of MR population
50–55 to approx. 70	Mild	Educable	89.0
35–40 to 50–55	Moderate	Trainable	6.0
20–25 to 35–50	Severe	—	3.5
Below 20–25	Profound	—	1.5

[a]Modified from Grossman.[1]

dent for the simplest self-help activities and will need lifelong supervision. Profound mental retardation implies almost complete dependence on others for all aspects of care.

Approach to the Patient

The approach to the diagnosis of the underlying cause of mental retardation is based on history, physical and neurological examinations, and the selective use of laboratory tests and special studies. A specific etiological diagnosis is important, as the information is needed for genetic counseling, determining the prognosis, and, in some cases, treatment. The first task is to decide whether the condition is of prenatal, perinatal, postnatal, or indeterminate onset. Table 9-2 lists many of the major conditions in each category. Specific entities that are common or illustrate important points will be discussed.

Prenatal factors are involved in 40–50% of all cases. The history should focus on abnormalities related to the pregnancy, such as the level of fetal activity, gestational problems, excessive or insufficient weight gain, and the duration of the pregnancy. A three-generation pedigree should always be constructed with the age, educational and vocational history, and evidence of neurological disease indicated for each individual. The IQ of each of the parents should be estimated. They should also be examined for stigmatizing features, and their head circumferences should be measured.

TABLE 9-2
Factors Associated with Mental Retardation

Prenatal	Perinatal	Postnatal
Intrauterine infection	Fetal distress from any cause	Infection
Medication	Birth trauma	Trauma
Drugs of abuse, including alcohol	Perinatal asphyxia	Toxins
Eclampsia		Anoxia
Chromosomal disorder		Metabolic disease
Congenital malformations		Hyperbilirubinemia
Maternal PKU		

Examination of the child is directed toward finding dysmorphic features. These may be typical enough to allow the diagnosis of a specific syndrome or may only be nonspecific major or minor congenital anomalies. If more than three anomalies are present, it is highly significant and further evaluation is needed. A number of atlases of mental retardation syndromes are available and are useful in correlating dysmorphic features with specific diagnoses.

Computerized tomography and magnetic resonance imaging are the most valuable neuroradiological techniques for defining major defects in brain development. Chromosome studies, with the use of banding techniques, are indicated if a specific syndrome associated with chromosomal abnormalities is suspected, if there are multiple congenital anomalies, or if there was poor intrauterine growth. In the neonatal period, antibody studies for toxoplasmosis, rubella, cytomegalovirus, herpes, and syphilis (TORCH titers) must be obtained. Metabolic screening tests are rarely indicated if major dysmorphic features are present.

Specific etiological factors are discussed in detail in the appropriate chapters.

Fragile X chromosome syndrome presents as mental retardation with an X-linked pattern of inheritance.[2] There is great variation in associated dysmorphic features, but the early reports include pale blue irides, large ears, and macrorchidism. These are inconstant, however, and studies for this syndrome should be carried out on any mentally retarded male with affected brothers or male cousins, or if no other etiology can be determined. The female carriers also may be mentally retarded. Special laboratory techniques are required for diagnosis.

Intrauterine infections include toxoplasmosis, cytomegalovirus, rubella, herpes, and syphilis. Features raising suspicion of these infections include low birth weight for gestational age, chorioretinitis, hepatosplenomegaly, and intracranial calcifications. These are best visualized with computerized tomography. Acquired immune deficiency syndrome can be transmitted transplacentally. The children fail to thrive in early life.[3]

Perinatal insult to the brain accounts for 3% of cases of mental retardation. In almost all cases, this is associated with cerebral palsy. Many problems can occur in the perinatal period, are well known, and need little elaboration. One caution is that children with prenatal abnormalities may have difficulty initiating respirations at birth, and perinatal factors are often incorrectly implicated. Few special studies are indicated if there is unequivocal evidence for major perinatal problems.

Postnatal damage is involved in 4–5% of cases of mental retardation. The etiology is usually obvious (e.g., head trauma, meningitis).

In approximately 40% of cases, no etiological factors can be found to explain the mental retardation. Sociocultural causes are often postulated, but this brings with it serious controversy. There is overrepresentation of mental retardation in lower socioeconomic groups. One hypothesis is that these children suffer from intrauterine problems resulting from poor prenatal care and have themselves had poor medical care and inadequate nutrition. Another speculation is that they have not been exposed to adequate learning experiences during critical phases of their development. Discussion of a possible genetic component has produced the most acrimonious debate. All of these factors seem to make some contribution, but do not explain the major part of the variance in large studies.

Management of mental retardation involves the physician, especially at the state of initial diagnosis and treatment. The physician is the only professional with whom most children will have contact in the preschool years and is in the best position to find early evidence of delayed development and to respond to the parents' concerns in this area. After the diagnosis has been made and specific treatment, if any, instituted, other issues arise.

All families are concerned about the genetic implications of the child's disability, whether or not a hereditary condition is present. Specialized consultation is often useful, as an empirical risk figure can be set for many conditions that are not inherited by simple genetic mechanisms.

Management of the family may be taken on by the physician, or referral made to professionals in social work or mental health. All families are devastated by a diagnosis of mental retardation. Many of them will go through a stereotyped series of responses, which include shock, denial, anger, and then some accommodation to the disability. Full acceptance is rarely achieved. These are similar to the stages associated with a diagnosis of terminal illness. In this case, however, there is no termination of the problem, and many of the feelings can never be satisfactorily resolved. This is important to understand, so that the parents' feelings and actions are not misinterpreted.

The physician is responsible for the ongoing medical needs of the child, many of which are no different than those of any other patient. Special needs may include problems with nutrition due to chewing and swallowing difficulties, repeated respiratory tract infections, and decubitus ulcers, especially in the nonambulatory patient. Many severely retarded children develop joint contractures and scoliosis. Seizures are also a common concomitant.

Early-intervention programs have become an integral part of the management of most children with delayed development. Although these have not been rigorously studied, the parents can be taught many useful skills, have an opportunity to interact with other parents and concerned professionals, and take an active part in the child's care. An intervention program without a major component of parental involvement will have little impact on the ultimate outcome.

Public-school systems are now required to provide services to all mentally retarded children, regardless of the severity of the retardation and associated problems. The child is entitled to an appropriate, free, public education under the mandate of the Education for All Handicapped Children Act (PL 94-142). In addition to the educational component, the child must receive necessary related services, including physical therapy, occupational therapy, speech therapy, transportation, and counseling. In many states eligibility begins at age 3 years. This has helped parents maintain handicapped children at home without the need for seeking residential placement during the school years.

Many families, especially if the child is severely retarded, reach a point where they can no longer manage the child at home. This may be related to the degree of handicap, physical size, behavior, parental health, or any of a large number of other factors. There has been considerable movement toward alternatives to placement in large residential state developmental centers. These include group living facilities, halfway houses, and small, decentralized residential units. Unfortunately, these have been difficult to organize and operate in many areas and are not appropriate for all mentally retarded individuals.

Mental Retardation Syndromes

Many syndromes that are associated with mental retardation are discussed in other chapters. Some are not easily classified, however, and are presented here as selected examples of the broad range of abnormalities associated with mental retardation. These syndromes appear to have their origins in abnormal morphogenesis.

Specific diagnosis is important, as this allows the physician to provide the parents with information concerning the expected intellectual level, associated disabilities, and life-span. It also allows ascertainment of genetic risk for the family.

Cornelia de Lange syndrome is characterized by severe mental retardation, bushy eyebrows which meet over the nasal bridge (synophrys), anteverted nostrils, thin lips, and micrognathia. There is also hirsutism and abnormalities of the extremities. These range from shortening of the distal portion of the arms with small hands to phocomelia. The condition is sporadic. Reports of chromosomal abnormalities have been inconsistent.

Rubinstein–Taybi syndrome is moderate to severe mental retardation associated with broad thumbs and toes. This broadening is quite pronounced and is characteristic. A beaklike nose, minor facial anomalies, and cryptorchidism are also found. The condition is sporadic in almost all reported cases.

Seckel syndrome (bird-headed dwarfism) is distinguished by microcephaly, hypoplastic facial bones, and a prominent, beaklike nose. Mental retardation is mild to moderate. There is intrauterine growth failure, and the children achieve a final height of no greater than 100–110 cm. Life-span is not compromised. Genetic transmission is as an autosomal recessive trait.

Laurence–Moon–Biedl syndrome consists of pigmentary degeneration of the retina, polydactyly, obesity, and mental retardation which ranges from minimal to severe. There is genital hypoplasia and cryptorchidism. Visual loss is progressive, but life-span is normal. An autosomal recessive gene is involved.

Another condition associated with obesity is the *Prader–Willi syndrome*. The children are severely hypotonic at birth, and feeding is difficult. Except for hypogonadism, dysmorphic features are not pronounced. Obesity develops in infancy or the preschool years and is most pronounced in the lower trunk, buttocks, and thighs. There is an abnormal glucose tolerance test, although frank diabetes does not always occur. The condition is sporadic.

Cerebrohepatorenal syndrome also presents with hypotonia at birth. There is a characteristic facial appearance with a high forehead, hypertelorism, flat facies, high arched palate, and abnormal auricular helices. Hepatomegaly with cirrhosis is present, and the children may be jaundiced. There are cystic changes in the kidneys and proteinuria. The patients die in the first few months of life, so the degree of mental retardation cannot be assessed. This is an autosomal recessive condition.

Smith–Lemli–Opitz syndrome is associated with moderate to severe mental retardation. The children are small for gestational age and hypotonic, and they grow poorly. Physical stigmata are microcephaly, epicanthal folds, ptosis, low-set ears, a nose with a broad tip and anteverted nostrils, and micrognathia. Abnormalities of the fingers and toes, cryptorchidism, and a simian crease are common. The hereditary pattern is not clear, but there is some evidence that it is autosomal recessive.

Hypercalcemia, present only in infancy, is associated with moderate to severe mental retardation, supravalvular aortic stenosis, and dysmorphic facial features. This "elfin facies" consists of hypertelorism, epicanthal folds, large mouth, and prominent ears. The condition is sporadic.

Cerebral gigantism (Sotos syndrome) is characterized by increased size for gestational age at birth and rapid growth during the first years of life. The head, hands, and feet are large. Bone age is advanced and is consistent with the height age. The rapid rate of growth slows after the first few years, although the children are always well above average height. Typical facial features are dolicocephaly, hypertelorism, an antimongoloid slant to the palpebral fissures, and prognathism. Intelligence is in the borderline-to-mild range of mental retardation. No hereditary pattern has been defined.

Incontinentia pigmenti (Bloch–Sulzberger disease) is easily identified by the characteristic skin lesions. Shortly after birth, erythematous linear streaks of vesicles appears, especially on the limbs. These then become verrucous and remain in this state until age 6 months. Finally, areas of hyperpigmentation develop. These appear as streaks, whorls, and reticulated areas. Approximately 20% of these children have skeletal anomalies, and 30% are mentally retarded or have seizures.

CEREBRAL PALSY

Cerebral palsy can be operationally defined by three features:

1. There is an abnormality of motor function. This can involve strength, tone, posture, or coordination. A dyskinesia may also be present.
2. The underlying cerebral pathology is static.
3. The pathological changes occur during the developmental period.

The overall incidence of cerebral palsy is approximately 2.5/1000 live births.[4] The relative risk for males is 1.3; that for multiple births, 3.2. There is also a strong association with low birth weight. The relative risk for infants weighing less than 2000 g is 26.0; for infants weighing 2000–2499 g, it is 9.2.

It should be apparent from the discussion of mental retardation that the developing brain can be damaged by a large number of factors. The insults caus-ing mental retardation and those leading to cerebral palsy are the same, and the diagnostic approach is identical.

There are three factors to analyze when clinically evaluating patients with cerebral palsy. These are the exact nature of the motor abnormality, the topog-raphy of the limb involvement, and the suspected etiology. When this is done, it will become apparent that certain clusters are found. The syndromes defined are constant enough that the presence of associated problems such as mental retardation and seizures can be predicted with reasonable certainty.[5]

The early diagnosis of cerebral palsy is difficult. During the first 4–6 months of life the child is usually hypotonic and presents as a floppy infant with feeding difficulties. Muscle tone then begins to increase in those children who will become spastic. An important early sign of spasticity is hyperextension of the spine, especially if the child is crying or agitated. Children who will become ath-etoid or ataxic generally remain hypotonic. It is not until 6–12 months of age that the exact type of cerebral palsy and the extent of involvement begin to become clear.

Another problem for the clinician is that the signs characteristic of cerebral palsy may be found in the infant and then disappear. A group of 229 1-year-old children with a diagnosis of cerebral palsy were reexamined at age 7 years. No motor handicap could be detected in 118 (52%) of the children.[6] Resolution was most common if the symptoms were mild and the clinical manifestations were monoparesis, ataxia, dyskinesia, or diplegia. Many of these patients were not entirely normal on follow-up evaluation, however. Mental retardation was pres-ent in 13% of white children and 25% of black children. Other common prob-lems were seizures, behavior disorders, poor articulation, and abnormalities of extraocular movements.

Spastic diplegia refers to the condition in which there is spasticity involving the lower extremities almost exclusively. There are increased tone, hyperre-flexia, and Babinski signs. Lifting the child rapidly in vertical suspension causes marked hyperextension and adduction of the legs with scissoring.

The feet are held in an equinovarus position, and shortening of the Achilles tendon occurs, as do flexion contractures at the hips and knees. The upper extremities are relatively spared.

Severe mental retardation is present in only 6% of children with spastic diplegia, although an additional 33% have some intellectual impairment. Sei-zures are uncommon. Strabismus is frequently found.

This type of cerebral palsy is most commonly associated with prematurity; 80% of premature infants with motor abnormalities have spastic diplegia. Pre-mature infants with and without diplegia do not differ significantly on analysis of most perinatal and neonatal factors.[7] The affected children did have a lower birth weight, smaller head circumference at birth, and a high incidence of Apgar scores below 3 at 1 min. They also were more likely to have intracranial hem-orrhage, neonatal seizures, and transient neurological depression on examina-tion. Eighty-three percent of the babies with spastic diplegia were thought to be neurologically normal on nursery discharge, however.

The underlying pathological change is periventricular leukomalacia, which is usually the result of subepenhdymal/intraventricular hemorrhage. The motor system is organized so that the descending fibers from the portion of the motor cortex representing the legs are periventricular in location and bear the brunt of the damage. Diffuse cortical injury is not present, accounting for the low incidence of seizures and mental retardation.

Spastic quadriplegia occurs following a severe hypoxic or ischemic insult. The clinical features are spasticity of all limbs and pseudobulbar palsy, which produces swallowing difficulty. Mental retardation is associated in 93% of patients, and seizures, often difficult to control, are present in 50% of the children. Many of the children are also blind and deaf.

These patients are generally extremely hypotonic in early infancy and may remain so, with little or no evidence of spasticity. This condition, *atonic diplegia,* is associated with profound mental retardation.

Spastic hemiplegia involves the limbs on one side of the body. The earliest sign is usually the premature development of hand preference. This should be considered to be abnormal prior to 18 months of age. Fine skilled movements of the hand are affected. The gait is characteristic with flexion at the hip and knee, an equinovarus position of the foot, and circumduction of the leg when walking. The arm is pronated and flexed at the elbow and wrist. Right hemiplegia is present 65% of the time.

If there are associated deficits in cortical sensory functions, such as stereognosis and graphesthesia, the arm is disabled out of proportion to the degree of spasticity and weakness. There also will be growth failure of the affected side. Seizures are present in 33% of these children, and mild or moderate mental retardation in 31%.

A number of different etiological factors can be involved. Some children have apparently suffered an intrauterine vascular accident with replacement of the injured brain by a porencephalic cyst. Birth trauma, postnatal head trauma, and acute infantile hemiplegia all produce the same outcome.

Athetoid cerebral palsy usually presents with a mixture of athetosis, chorea, and dystonia. The most severe involvement is of the limbs and neck, which show varying muscle tone and involuntary movements associated with contraction of both agonist and antagonist muscles. This dyskinesia occurs at rest and also interferes with voluntary movement. The voice is frequently involved, and speech intelligibility may be extremely poor.

The classical form of athetoid cerebral palsy is the result of bilirubin encephalopathy and kernicterus. There is almost pure athetosis; deafness and absent upward gaze are frequently associated, and seizures and mental retardation are uncommon. This syndrome is now rare, as strict attention is paid to bilirubin levels in neonates and treatment instituted before significant hyperbilirubinemia can occur. Most athetoid cerebral palsy, at this time, is also associated with evidence of spasticity. There frequently are mental retardation and seizures in addition. The usual etiology is diffuse hypoxia, with or without accompanying hyperbilirubinemia.

Ataxic cerebral palsy is the least common form, accounting for only 10% of all cases. The children present with a major delay in the development of gross motor skills and are obviously ataxic when they begin to stand and walk. Intelligence is usually not impaired, and seizures are unusual. No specific etiological factors have been associated. Because ataxic cerebral palsy is rare, full evaluation should always be carried out so that a more serious neurological condition is not overlooked.

Management of cerebral palsy requires the skills of many professionals including pediatricians, neurologists, physiatrists, orthopedists, ophthalmologists, physical and occupational therapists, speech pathologists, and orthotists. It should be obvious that such a large team can only work effectively if there is assignment of a single case manager who will coordinate the efforts of the others.

There have been few controlled studies documenting the efficacy of physical therapy. It appears that children with the highest intellectual function make the most gains during treatment.[8] Older children also fare better, but this may be due to the fact that the younger patients are more severely and globally involved.

A number of neurophysiologically based techniques, such as chronic cerebellar stimulation, have been tried, particularly in an attempt to reduce spasticity. Their usefulness has not been documented in placebo-controlled studies.[9]

It is difficult to define the prognosis of patients with cerebral palsy because of the great variability in clinical manifestations and severity of the deficit. The level of independence required before assigning a patient to the "good-outcome" group also varies greatly with each investigation.

The most important negative prognostic indicators for children with hemiplegic cerebral palsy are abnormalities on the EEG and computerized-tomography scan.[10] These correlate highly with mental retardation and the development of seizures. The worst outcome is found if the abnormalities involve commissural pathways, association pathways, or cerebral cortex.

The ultimate prognosis for ambulation and independent function depends as much on the child's intellectual abilities and associated medical problems as on the degree of motor disability. The level of physical handicap is, however, a crucial factor in work and social adjustment.[11] Speech handicap is less important. Life expectancy correlates inversely with the degree of mental retardation.[5]

REFERENCES

1. Grossman, H. J. (ed.), 1983, *Classification in Mental Retardation,* American Association on Mental Deficiency, Washington DC, 1983.
2. de la Cruz, F., 1985, Fragile X syndrome, *Am. J. Ment. Def.* **90:**119–123.
3. Epstein, L. G., Sharer, L. R., and Joshi, V. V., 1985, Progressive encephalopathy in children with acquired immune deficiency syndrome, *Ann. Neurol.* **17:**488–496.
4. Kudrjavcev, T., Schoenberg, B. S., Kurland, L. T., and Groover, R. V., 1983, Cerebral palsy: Trends in incidence and changes in concurrent neonatal mortality (Rochester, MN, 1950–1976), *Neurology* **33:**1433–1438.
5. Kudrjavcev, T., Schoenberg, B. S., Kurland, L. T., and Groover, R. V., 1985, Cerebral palsy: Survival rates, associated handicaps, and distribution by subtype (Rochester, MN, 1950–1976), *Neurology* **35:**900–903.

6. Nelson, K. B., and Ellenberg, J. H., 1982, Children who "outgrew" cerebral palsy, *Pediatrics* **69:**529–536.
7. Bennett, F. C., Chandler, L. S., Robinson, N. M., and Sells, C. J., 1981, Spastic diplegia in premature infants, *Am. J. Dis. Child.* **135:**732–737.
8. Scherzer, A. L., Mike, V., and Ilson, J., 1976, Physical therapy as a determinant of change in the cerebral palsied infant, *Pediatrics* **58:**47–52.
9. Gahm, N. H., Russman, B. S., Cerciello, R. L., Fiorentino, M. R., and McGrath, D. M., 1981, Chronic cerebellar stimulation for cerebral palsy: A double-blind study, *Neurology* **21:**87–90.
10. Cohen, M. E., and Duffner, P. K., 1981, Prognostic indicators in hemiparetic cerebral palsy, *Ann. Neurol.* **9:**353–357.
11. Andrew, G., Platt, L. J., Quinn, P. T., and Neilson, P. D., 1977, An assessment of the status of adults with cerebral palsy, *Dev. Med. Child. Neurol.* **19:**803–810.

ADDITIONAL READING

Goodman, R. M., and Gorlin, R. J., 1983, *The Malformed Infant and Child,* Oxford University Press, New York.
Holmes, L. B., Moser, H. W., Halldorsson, S., Mack, C., Pant, S., and Matzilevich, B., 1972, *Mental Retardation. An Atlas of Diseases with Associated Physical Abnormalities,* Macmillan, New York.
Smith, D. W., 1982, *Recognizable Patterns of Human Malformations,* 3rd ed., W. B. Saunders, Philadelphia.

10

Congenital Malformations of the Central Nervous System

Malformations of the central nervous system (CNS) are among the most common of the major congenital anomalies and are an important source of chronic disability in childhood. Exact incidence figures are difficult to determine, as they vary with geographical location, the population group under study, and the epidemiological techniques used. In addition, there are unexplained changes in incidence over long periods of time. It now appears, for instance, that the frequency of occurrence of spina bifida has been decreasing.[1]

Neural tube defects, encompassing spina bifida, encephalocele, and anencephaly, occur in approximately 2/1000 live births. Other anomalies are less common. Another method of ascertaining the impact of these lesions is to determine death rates. The combined death rate for all of the major congenital malformations ranges from 6.8/100,000 population in Ireland to 0.6/100,000 population in Japan. The rate for the United States is 3.1/100,000 population in Caucasians and 2.1/100,000 population in non-Caucasians. The overwhelming majority of these deaths occur in the first year of life.[2] Major malformations of the CNS are also found in 4% of all first-trimester spontaneous abortions.[3]

The mechanisms producing these anomalies are still largely speculative and appear to be quite complex. Classical mendelian inheritance is occasionally found. More frequently, the pattern of occurrence is consistent with polygenic mechanisms, exposure to environmental substances, or a combination of the two. The teratogenic influence disrupts the complex series of interrelated steps outlined in Chapter 1. Interference with normal development at any point will adversely influence all subsequent developmental programs, so, as a general rule, the earlier in embryonic development the insult, the more extensive and severe the malformation. Even a clearly defined, time-limited event will not usually produce a simple anomaly, but will adversely affect the entire subsequent chain of developmental progress.

The underlying mechanisms of teratogenesis have been set into a number of conceptual frameworks, such as that proposed by Zwilling[4]:

1. Abnormal initial stimulus (absent, deficient, or excessive)
2. Abnormal response of reacting tissues (absent, deficient, or excessive)
3. Abnormality of both stimulus and response
4. Abnormal differentiation
5. Abnormal growth of structures
6. Degenerative processes (abnormal, absent, or excessive)
7. Abnormal functional activity

Another method of analysis is to search for the initiating factor.[5] This is a more fundamental approach, as it allows definition of the etiology of the malformation. Among the most important such factors are

1. Mutation
2. Chromosomal abnormality
3. Mitotic interference
4. Altered nucleic acid synthesis or function
5. Lack of precursors, substrates, or coenzymes
6. Altered energy sources
7. Enzyme inhibition
8. Osmolar imbalance
9. Changed membrane characteristics

Evidence is now becoming available that supplementation of the mother's diet with folic acid may reduce the incidence of neural tube defects.[6] If this can be documented, it will provide a simple but powerful tool for prevention and also allow the generation of hypotheses concerning the causation of these lesions.

APPROACH TO THE PATIENT

When faced with a patient with a developmental malformation of the CNS, a series of interrelated questions must be answered. These are:

1. What are the anatomical abnormalities?
2. What are the functional abnormalities?
3. Are there associated malformations?
4. What is the etiology?
       Are there genetic factors?
       Are there environmental factors?

Many malformations, such as myelomeningocele and anencephaly, are immediately apparent at birth. Others, such as hydrocephalus, may not make their presence known for several months. More subtle anomalies can remain undetected during the individual's entire life and produce no functional deficit. Now that CT scans are frequently performed for conditions such as headaches and seizures, unsuspected and unrelated anatomical abnormalities are often discovered.

The computerized-tomography (CT) scan is currently the major diagnostic tool for clinical investigation of CNS malformations. If possible, a high-resolution scan using a late-generation scanner is desirable. As magnetic resonance imaging (nuclear magnetic resonance) scanning becomes increasingly available, more detailed information will be obtainable. It is now possible to visualize a great deal of anatomical detail, especially that of the ventricular system, with real-time ultrasonography in the infant. This is also a useful tool for following ventricular size if progressive hydrocephalus is suspected. Angiography is an important adjunct for the understanding of complex malformations. This procedure can help document a vascular etiology for lesions associated with destruction of brain tissue. It also provides the neurosurgeon with valuable information prior to surgery if this should be required.

The evaluation of the functional deficit comes from a detailed history, neurological examination, and developmental examination. These must be repeated on a regular basis, as the impact of the anatomical abnormality on development and neurological function often is not fully apparent initially. This makes firm prognostic statements impossible, except in the case of the most severe malformations.

Congenital anomalies involving the CNS can occur as isolated lesions or be associated with additional major or minor malformations. If other abnormalities are present, careful evaluation directed toward defining a specific syndrome is important. This is more than just an exercise in classification, but will clarify the possible etiology of the condition and expectations for the child's future progress. Syndrome identification requires meticulous cataloging of all congenital anomalies. There are standards for measuring and classifying physical features, and these, rather than clinical impressions, should be used. The search is assisted by any one of a number of atlases (see Additional Reading, Chapter 9).

The remaining task is to attempt to determine the etiology of the condition. The question of a genetic basis for the problem concerns all families, whether or not hereditary factors are actually involved. Evaluation should always include a complete three-generation pedigree and examination of as many family members as possible. Partial forms of specific syndromes are frequently found. The need for special studies, such as karyotyping, depends on the results of the initial evaluation.

There is a growing tendency to attempt to blame environmental agents for serious developmental anomalies. Cause and effect have only been proven with a limited number of agents, and attempts to prove such relationships are fraught with many hazards. The physician who goes beyond the evidence often diverts the family from coming to an accommodation with the situation and may precipitate unwarranted litigation.

NEURAL TUBE DEFECTS

Neural tube defects result from failure of the normal processes that form the neural tube in the embryo. There is also failure of induction of the proper development of overlying mesodermal structures as bone and muscle. These are complicated lesions and clearly represent more than simply incomplete closure of the neural tube at one end or the other.

Anencephaly is the most severe of the neural tube defects. The abnormality, obvious at birth, consists of major defects in the cranial vault exposing a mass of abnormal tissue made up of blood vessels, ependyma, and a membrane which represents portions of the meninges. The cerebral hemispheres are absent. Brain stem and cerebellum, though present, are abnormal, as is the spinal cord. The eyes appear normal, although there is no optic nerve. In most cases, no other major extracranial malformations are present.

There may be sufficient intact brain stem function to allow crying, swallowing, and a response to sound. The majority of children die in 1 or 2 days.

Prenatal diagnosis of anencephaly is easily made with ultrasonography. Elevation of α-fetoprotein in the amniotic fluid is found in this condition, as well as in the other neural tube defects. This is a glycoprotein that is synthesized by the fetal liver and yolk sac and is excreted in the fetal urine. Detectable levels are found at 6 weeks of gestation, and peak levels at 12–14 weeks. Concentrations are increased in the face of open neural tube defects. Elevated levels of acetylcholinesterase are confirmatory. If the lesions are skin covered, which occurs in 10–15% of cases, a false negative determination is possible. False positive elevations are found in a number of conditions, including fetal distress, fetal death, erythroblastosis, atresia of the upper gastrointestinal tract, omphalocele, congenital nephrosis, and maternal liver disease.

Acetylcholinesterase, another enzyme present in amniotic fluid, is also elevated if the fetus has an open neural tube defect. An elevation of both α-fetoprotein and acetylcholinesterase reduces the rate of false positive examinations and increases diagnostic accuracy.

If there is a clinical reason to suspect a neural tube defect, ultrasonography and amniocentesis should be used as complementary procedures. High-risk patients include mothers who have previously given birth to a child with a neural tube defect and women with relatives who have borne such children. A screening assay using maternal serum is now available. Positive findings should always be confirmed with ultrasonography and amniocentesis.

No specific etiological factors have been found. There is an increased incidence among individuals of English and Irish descent and a relatively low incidence among American blacks. Studies suggest a polygenic mode of inheritance, and an empirical recurrence risk of 5% applies to most families with an affected child.

Spina bifida is a generic term referring to a series of congenital malformations that have in common incomplete formation of the posterior arches of the bony spine. This is often associated with abnormalities of the spinal cord and defects of the overlying skin.

Spina bifida occulta is a common abnormality found fortuitously on x-ray studies of the lumbar spine. Neurological abnormalities are not present. If neurological function is in any way impaired, the lesion must be more extensive.

Meningocele presents as a soft mass, most commonly over the lumbar spine. Examination shows it to be a skin-covered, fluid-filled sac. The underlying spinal cord is intact. Several nerve roots often course along the wall of the sac, but their function is not seriously impaired. Examination is usually normal or may show isolated weakness of individual muscle groups or bladder dysfunction.

Myelomeningocele is accompanied by neurological deficits, as associated abnormalities of the spinal cord and nerve roots are always present (Figure 10-1). The sac may be covered by intact skin, but more commonly consists of only meninges. On occasion, no sac is present, and an abnormal mass of neural tissue is exposed. Neurological examination reveals severe motor and sensory abnormalities below the level of the lesion. There may be complete paraplegia and anesthesia or a spotty, irregular distribution of signs. Bowel and bladder function are almost invariably impaired. Muscle atrophy in the affected limbs is apparent, and bony deformities, most frequently talipes equinovarus, are common. Scoliosis usually accompanies thoracic lesions.

Hydrocephalus is frequently associated with myelomeningocele. The overall concordance is 75%, but the exact risk varies with the level of the spinal lesion. It is almost always present in conjunction with high cervical or thoracic lesions and is much less frequently associated with small sacral defects. The underlying

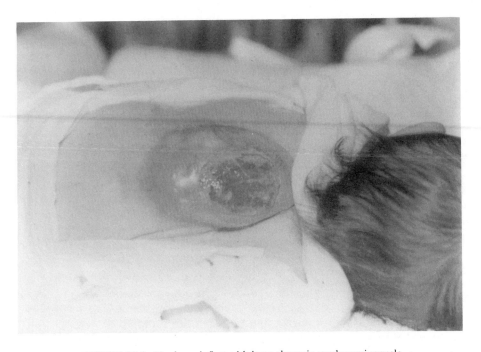

FIGURE 10-1. Newborn infant with large thoracic myelomeningocele.

pathology causing the hydrocephalus is the Arnold–Chiari malformation. There are several variations, all involving abnormalities in the structure and position of the brain stem and cerebellum. The variant associated with myelomeningocele is type 2; the medulla and cerebellum are elongated and enter the cervical canal, overlapping the cervical spinal cord. Aqueductal stenosis is also frequently present, contributing to the hydrocephalus.

Seizures occur in approximately 25% of children. Risk factors appear to be shunt infection, the number of shunt revisions, and the presence of additional brain malformations. Developmental delay appears to be more common among the children with seizures.[7]

Treatment is complex and requires the close coordination of a number of medical and surgical specialists. The first task is closure of the defect and covering of the area with skin. Surgery has generally been recommended in the first 24 hr of life to reduce the risk of meningitis. There is also some evidence that early closure will prevent further loss of neurological function. This has been questioned, however, and a delay in surgery has the advantage of allowing more time for making treatment decisions.[8] It has been stated that stopping the leak of cerebrospinal fluid (CSF) causes the hydrocephalus to become more rapidly progressive, but the evidence for this is not strong.

Attempts to develop triage criteria to withhold active treatment from infants who are predicted to have a poor outcome have been made in Great Britain. The trend in this country is to offer treatment to all children, regardless of the severity of the functional deficit or presence of associated medical and surgical problems.

The severely affected child enters life with a complex series of handicaps. The most obvious is paralysis of the lower extremities. Functional ambulation is difficult without braces, as the hip extensors (L_5–S_1 roots) are involved even in relatively low lesions. Mobility of children with paraplegia is greatly improved by the use of a wheelchair, either manual or electric.

Orthopedic surgery to correct deformities of the lower extremities should be carried out only if there are clear-cut functional goals. These can be either improved mobility or facilitation of nursing care and personal hygiene.

Severe kyphoscoliosis often results from vertebral abnormalities. New procedures utilizing the implantation of flexible rods will partially correct this and prevent progression, even in the presence of anomalies as severe as hemivertebrae. Plastic surgery is often required to revise the repair of the back as the child grows and may be needed if decubitus ulcers become a problem. Before extensive surgical procedures are planned, it is important to assess the goals and determine whether they are functional or cosmetic.

Hydrocephalus accompanies myelomeningocele in approximately 75% of cases. The therapeutic approach is the same as that for hydrocephalus of any cause. Intellectual function in these children is not substantially altered by the presence of hydrocephalus, but is clearly reduced if ventriculitis occurs. A group of children who did not require a shunt had a mean IQ of 102. Children with a shunt but no history of ventriculitis had a mean IQ of 95; it was 72 in the group with a shunt and ventriculitis.[9]

Urinary tract dysfunction and chronic infection are major causes of disability and death in children with myelomeningocele. It is extremely important that regular bladder emptying be accomplished. The Credé maneuver often suffices early on, but the majority of children need a more reliable approach. Intermittent clean catheterization of the urinary bladder can be taught to the child's caretakers, and eventually to the child. Results of this approach are superior to those obtained by urinary diversion procedures such as ileal conduits or indwelling catheters.[10,11] The possibility of infection must be investigated with the slightest clinical suspicion and, if found, treated vigorously. Prophylactic treatment should be considered if the child has had repeated infections.

Fecal incontinence can be ameliorated by rigorous bowel-training regimens, but a significant percentage of children will not obtain reliable continence.

The causes of myelomeningocele have not been determined. The highest incidence is among families from England and Ireland, and girls are affected more frequently than boys. Advanced maternal age has some effect. The empirical risk figure for recurrence is 5%, but increases with each affected child. The only teratogen regularly associated with this lesion in the human is valproate.[12]

Recent evidence appears to implicate a deficiency of folic acid as a possible etiological factor. Supplementation with folic acid has been reported to reduce the number of children with myelomeningocele born to mothers who previously had an affected infant.[13]

Prenatal diagnosis can be made by ultrasonography in many cases, and by finding increased levels of α-fetoprotein in amniotic fluid. As with anencephaly, screening of maternal serum appears to be a useful screening technique.

Analogous lesions involving the skull include *cranial meningocele,* in which there are no abnormalities of neural tissue, and *encephalocele,* in which the sac contains malformed brain tissue. These are most commonly present in the midline, in either the occipital or nasal regions. Functional deficits depend on the amount of neural tissue in the sac, and with extensive lesions there are major neurological abnormalities. Hydrocephalus is also commonly associated with encephalocele. Even in the case of the most severely involved children, surgical removal of the sac and treatment of the hydrocephalus is important for cosmetic purposes and to allow the provision of optimal nursing care. Maternal hyperthermia early in pregnancy has been implicated as a causative factor.[14]

Diastematomyelia refers to a bifid spinal cord, either complete or partial. The halves of the cord are separated by a septum of fibrous tissue, cartilage, or bone which is attached to the vertebral bodies and often to the posterior elements. The clinical presentation is one of lower motor neuron weakness and sensory loss involving the legs and feet. Bladder disturbances are common. A useful diagnostic clue is the presence of any one of a number of cutaneous abnormalities in the midline of the back. These include hemangiomas, nevi, tufts of hair, and lipomas.

X-ray studies often show spina bifida and scoliosis. A calcified spicule is diagnostic, but not frequently seen. Myelography, generally supplemented by a CT scan, allows definition of the lesion and provides the neurosurgeon with important information. The standard operative approach is to remove the septum and free up the spinal cord. This will usually, but not always, prevent progression of the neurological deficit.

Lumbosacral lipomas are frequently associated with diastematomyelia or myelomeningocele, but can occur as isolated lesions. There often is an intradural extension of the tumor, which can produce bladder dysfunction or weakness in the legs. On rare occasions the signs are progressive and surgical intervention is required.

Syringomyelia rarely produces symptoms in childhood. There is a cavity in the central region of the spinal cord, most commonly in the cervical or lumbar levels, but sometimes involving the entire extent of the cord. This progressively enlarges and is associated with gliosis. No etiological mechanism has been agreed upon.

The initial complaint is weakness and sensory loss in the hands. Atrophy and areflexia are present, and dystrophic changes in the skin are prominent. The sensory abnormalities involve pain and temperature sensation, while leaving light touch intact. This phenomenon, dissociation of sensation, results from the location of the syrinx, which spares the dorsally located uncrossed fibers mediating light touch.

Syringomyelia is often associated with the Arnold–Chiari malformation. These children present with hydrocephalus.

CT scan assists in diagnosis, although the syrinx can collapse and the typical widening of the cord not be visualized. Air myelography is sometimes required. Surgical treatment to decompress the cavity does not always halt progressive loss of function.

HYDROCEPHALUS

CSF is formed predominantly in the choroid plexuses of the lateral, third, and fourth ventricles. It is not a passive transudate of plasma but is produced by active, energy-dependent mechanisms. Movement of the fluid is from the lateral ventricles through the foramina of Monro to the third ventricle, and then to the fourth ventricle by way of the aqueduct of Sylvius. Exit from the fourth ventricle is via the midline foramen of Magendie and the lateral foramina of Luschka into the basal cisterns. The CSF then circulates around the spinal cord and over the convexity of the hemispheres in the subarachnoid space. It enters the superior sagittal sinus through the arachnoid villi. This appears to be a relatively passive, pressure-dependent process, although there is now evidence that resorption may be more complex.

Progressive ventricular enlargement is most frequently due to an imbalance between CSF production and absorption.[15] Possible mechanisms include increased production, block of the normal pathways of flow, and impaired absorption (Table 10-1). The first mechanism, increased production, rarely occurs, although it may possibly be seen with choroid plexus papillomas. There is reserve absorptive capacity amounting to approximately four times the normal

TABLE 10-1
Causes of Hydrocephalus[a]

Site of pathology	Mechanism
Arachnoid villi	Failure of development
	Obstruction
	Infection
	Hemorrhage
Subarachnoid spaces	Meningitis
	Subarachnoid hemorrhage
	Subependymal–intraventricular hemorrhage
Fourth ventricle outlet	Meningitis
	Arnold–Chiari malformation
	Dandy–Walker malformation
	Neoplasm
Fourth ventricle	Neoplasm
Aqueduct of Sylvius	Empendymitis
	X-linked trait
	Arteriovenous malformation of the vein of Galen
	Tumor
	Mesencephalon
	Pineal
	Gliosis following shunt
Third ventricle	Tumor
Foramina of Monro	Tumor
	Ventriculitis
Lateral ventricles	Tumor
	Subependymal hemorrhage

[a]From Lemire et al.[15]

rate of production, and unless this were exceeded, hydrocephalus would not result.

A block at the level of the foramina of Monro is most frequently associated with tumors. These can arise in the basal ganglia, hypothalamus, third ventricle, or suprasellar area. Lesions associated with tuberous sclerosis are commonly present in this region.

Aqueductal stenosis results from a number of problems. Brain stem tumors, intraventricular hemorrhage, and infections all can produce this lesion. The origin of the congenital form, which is associated with forking of the aqueduct, is not clear. An X-linked hereditary variant has been reported. Symptoms can occur at almost any age, depending on the specific etiology.

The *Dandy–Walker syndrome* consists of abnormalities of the cerebellar vermis, cystic dilatation of the fourth ventricle, failure of formation of the outlet foramina, and hydrocephalus. It represents a complex malformation and is not just a result of occlusion of the foramina. A protuberant occiput provides a diagnostic clue, and this area will often transilluminate if a strong light is used.

Inflammatory changes in the arachnoid secondary to infection or hemorrhage also interfere with the flow of CSF and produce hydrocephalus. The block can also be at the level of the arachnoid villi. This is referred to as communicating hydrocephalus, as there is no obstruction to the egress to CSF from the ventricular system.

No specific etiology can be determined for many cases of congenital hydrocephalus. Retinoic acid, an analog of vitamin A used to treat severe acne, has been reported to produce several types of hydrocephalus.[16]

The symptoms of hydrocephalus depend more on the age of onset than on the specific underlying cause. In early infancy, the most prominent finding is excessively rapid growth of the head. The most sensitive clinical tool is regular measurements of the head circumference; these should always be plotted on an appropriate head growth chart. Early symptoms include irritability, poor feeding, vomiting, and incessant crying. Physical signs, other than the rapidly enlarging head circumference, may not be present or may be quite prominent. These include frontal bossing, tense fontanelle, spreading of sutures, dilated scalp veins, and involuntary conjugate downward deviation of the eyes so that the sclera is visible above the iris. This is referred to as the "setting-sun sign." Papilledema is quite uncommon in infants.

The onset of hydrocephalus in older patients is marked by headache, vomiting, and lethargy. This may be chronic or acute, with rapid progression to coma, decerebrate posturing, and tentorial herniation. Head circumference may be abnormally large with a chronic presentation, but this is a slow process in the child older than 5 years. Papilledema is commonly present, and paresis of lateral gaze results from compression of the sixth nerve.

Medical approaches to treatment are rarely successful. These include the administration of acetazolamide and isosorbide. The majority of children, if the hydrocephalus is progressive, will require surgery. The most widely used approach, independent of the etiology or level of block, is a ventriculoperitoneal shunt. A catheter is inserted into the lateral ventricle through a burr hole, a connecting valve sets the ventricular pressure and allows flow in only one direction, and a second tube is run subcutaneously to the abdomen where it enters the peritoneal cavity. The CSF is then resorbed into the circulation.

Although this approach is simple, the apparatus frequently becomes occluded and requires revision. In addition, several revisions will be required as the child grows. An unusual, but serious, complication is perforation of the bowel and ventriculitis caused by enteric organisms.

Ventriculoatrial shunts are still performed on occasion, but have a number of additional serious complications. These include bacteremia, perforation of the myocardium, nephritis, which may be due to an immune reaction, and pulmonary vascular disease from multiple pulmonary emboli.

It is difficult to determine prognosis in any specific case, as it depends on etiology and the success of treatment. The children who do well are those who have hydrocephalus that is not the result of infection or intracranial hemorrhage, have a shunt placed in early life, do not need multiple shunt revisions, and do not have ventriculitis.[17] Normal intelligence and academic performance are quite possible under optimal conditions.

OTHER STRUCTURAL MALFORMATIONS

Structural malformations of the brain are extremely complex, and although there are a number of systems of classification, each patient shows unique features.[15] This section will present the most common of these lesions, focusing on those with specific clinical features. Many important abnormalities, such as lissencephaly and polymicrogyria, are pathological, rather than clinical, diagnoses and will not be specifically discussed.

Microcephaly refers to a small brain, usually defined by a head circumference two or more standard deviations below the mean for the child's age. This should be viewed as an absolute figure, independent of other anthropometric measures. Using this defining criterion alone, 86.5–92.5% of microcephalic children will have subnormal intelligence.[18]

Microcephaly can be caused by any insult that interferes with brain growth or causes destruction of cerebral tissue. The physical finding itself is not a specific diagnosis, but is merely a clue to the need for further investigation.

An autosomal recessive form of microcephaly has been described. There is an extremely small brain and obvious lack of growth of the cranial vault. This is especially noted in the frontal region, where there is little expansion above the supraorbital ridges. Mental retardation is always present.

Ionizing radiation appears to be an environmental teratogen. Studies on children exposed *in utero* to the Hiroshima atomic bomb show a strong correlation between microcephaly, maternal exposure within 1500 m of the blast, and gestational age less than 15 weeks.[19] Experimental evidence using laboratory animals suggests that small doses of ionizing radiation can have profound effects on the development of the CNS. The human data support this hypothesis, although time–dose relationships have not been clearly defined.[20]

Hydranencephaly has a clinical presentation similar to that of hydrocephalus. Studies reveal that the cerebral hemispheres are absent, although islands of cortex sometimes remain (Figure 10-2). The head is filled with a sac made up of leptomeninges and remnants of what had been the cerebral cortex. Abnormal thalamus, brain stem, and cerebellum are present at the base of the skull. It had been originally postulated that this state represented the end stage of severe intrauterine hydrocephalus. More recent evidence suggests a vascular etiology.

Despite the severity of the defect, the neurological examination at birth is often nearly normal. Clinical features that then develop are an abnormally increasing head circumference, progressive irritability, and spasticity. Visual tracking fails to develop. The diagnosis can be made by transillumination of the head, and it is confirmed by a CT scan. Only the most primitive developmental progress occurs.

Megalencephaly is a poorly understood condition. It is diagnosed when the head circumference is three or more standard deviations above the mean for the child's age and there is no evidence of a space-occupying intracranial lesion or hydrocephalus. Both familial and sporadic forms are found. Intelligence is normal or borderline in most affected children, although all levels of mental retardation can be found.

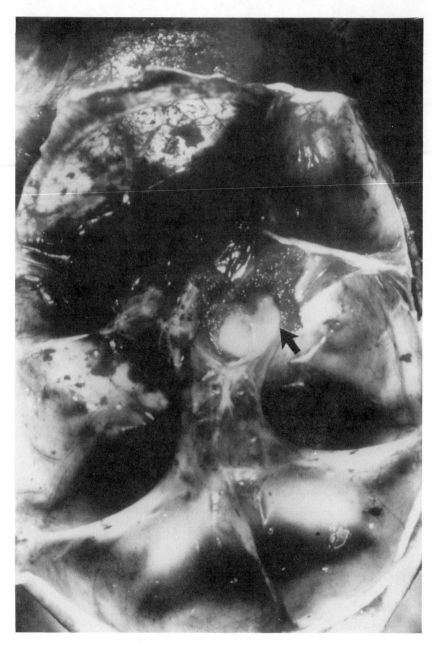

FIGURE 10-2. Base of skull of a hydranencephalic infant. The arrow indicates the only remaining neural tissue.

Agenesis of the corpus callosum, either partial or complete, is probably more frequent than had been thought. With a large number of CT scans being performed on children for various reasons, this lesion is often an unexpected finding. Minor congenital anomalies, particularly hypertelorism, are associated in some cases. There is no consistent cognitive deficit, although detailed neuropsychological testing has shown problems with skilled bimanual tasks.

CHROMOSOMAL DISORDERS

Chromosomal abnormalities are a factor in over 50% of human spontaneous abortions.[21] These are especially prevalent in the case of early fetal deaths, being found in 70% of abortions of less than 6 weeks of gestation.

Many of the disorders of chromosome number or structure are associated with multiple congenital anomalies, and the central nervous system is often involved. For this reason, it is essential that a karyotype, preferably with chromosomal-banding studies, be obtained whenever neurological dysfunction occurs in the presence of one or more major or minor anomalies.

Clinical features suggesting the need for chromosomal studies include[21]:

1. Congenital anomalies of multiple organ systems
2. Moderate to severe mental retardation
3. Intrauterine or postnatal growth retardation
4. Endocrine abnormalities
5. Unusual dysmorphic features

Trisomy 21 (Down syndrome) was the first chromosomal abnormality to be described in humans. This condition is the most frequently occurring cause of mental retardation that can be specifically diagnosed; the incidence is approximately 1/600 to 1/1000 live births. The rate of occurrence increases as maternal age passes 35 years, and still more dramatically after age 40. In women older than 45 years of age, the risk is 1/20 live births.

Prenatal diagnosis can be made by karyotyping cells obtained by amniocentesis. This fact should be brought to the attention of all pregnant women age 35 years or older. Failure to inform them of this option has resulted in a number of malpractice suits.

The diagnosis can be made in most children at the time of birth. There is striking hypotonia and a constellation of typical physical features, which include a flat face with slanted palpebral fissures and epicanthal folds, a brachycephalic head with flattened occiput, and small ears. Other features include incurved fifth fingers with a hypoplastic or absent middle phalynx, and a single transverse palmar crease (simian line).

Developmental progress is slow, and the rate appears to fall off in the middle of the preschool years; this is due to a disproportionate delay in the acquisition of expressive language. The range of IQ scores is great, and children with Down syndrome can be mildly retarded, profoundly involved, or at any level in between. Social skills are often good, and this can cause overestimation of the expected level of academic skills. Early prognostication is a hazardous venture.

A large number of medical and neurological complications can occur. Duodenal atresia presents in the neonatal period and requires surgical correction. One-half of children with Down syndrome have congenital heart disease; the most common lesion is an atrioventricular canal. An increased incidence of acute myelogenous leukemia has been reported, although cases in infancy that appear to resolve spontaneously have also been documented. Seizures are infrequent, but there is an association with infantile spasms.

There has been recent interest in the finding of atlantoaxial instability, which is present in 15–20% of children with Down syndrome. Spinal cord compression has been reported, but appears to be rare, despite this finding on x-ray studies. Adults with Down syndrome are at risk for the early development of Alzheimer's disease (presenile dementia). The reason for this is not known.

The majority of patients with Down syndrome (90–95%) have trisomy 21 on chromosome karyotyping. The remainder have a translocation which, in many cases, is carried by one of the parents. This substantially increases the risk of having another affected child; the magnitude of this risk varies with the specific translocation. If either parent is the carrier of a 21:21 translocation, the risk is 100%. Genetic counseling should not be attempted until all of the appropriate biological information is obtained.

Trisomy 13 (trisomy D, Patau syndrome) occurs much less frequently than trisomy 21, with an incidence of 1/10,000 to 1/20,000 live births. There are multiple congenital anomalies, the most characteristic of which are midline cleft lip and palate, microphthalmos, abnormal ears, congenital heart disease, renal abnormalities, polydactyly, and rocker-bottom feet. The infants are small for gestational age and grow poorly. Seizures and apneic spells are common. Death usually occurs in the first year of life.

The most common abnormality of brain structure is holoprosencephaly, a state in which the two cerebral hemispheres have not separated and there is a single midline ventricle. This is usually associated with arhinencephaly, absence of the olfactory bulbs and tracts. The majority of children have trisomy 13, rather than translocations.

Trisomy 18 (trisomy E, Edwards syndrome) is characterized by a dolicocephalic head; abnormal ears, hands, and feet; micrognathia; and renal and cardiac malformations. Seizures are common. Although death usually occurs in the first year, a few long-term survivors have been reported. Karyotypes generally show a trisomy. A broad range of structural and histological defects of the central nervous system has been reported.

The *cri du chat* syndrome is associated with a partial deletion of the short arm of chromosome 5. The condition, which is rare, is named for the kittenlike cry produced by the infants. This is due to laryngeal abnormalities and disappears as the child grows. There are characteristic facial features, which include an antimongoloid slant of the eyes, strabismus, and micrognathia. The children are small for gestational age and grow poorly. Prolonged survival is possible, although mental retardation is severe.

Abnormalities of *sex chromosomes* should be suspected in any child with excessive or inadequate growth and abnormalities of sexual maturation. Turner syndrome (45, XO) is not associated with mental retardation, but these children have problems with visuopractic skills and frequently have learning disabilities. Individuals with an excessive number of X chromosomes (polysomy X) have been reported. As a general rule, the greater the number of X chromosomes, the greater the degree of mental retardation.

Boys with Klinefelter syndrome (47, XXY) have mild degrees of mental retardation in 20–30% of cases, with disproportionate problems in language skills. There is controversy concerning the relationship of the 47, XYY syndrome to mental retardation and antisocial behavior.

The *fragile* X syndrome has recently gained prominence in the literature.[22] It has been known for many years that boys are overrepresented among populations of mentally retarded individuals, both in institutions and in the community. This suggests X-linked inheritance, and this pattern has been documented in many families. It was found that some of these boys have an abnormal X chromosome, which shows a constriction near the end of the long arm when cells are grown in a special medium. The initial descriptions of the patients included mental retardation and a characteristic phenotype consisting of large ears, light blue irides, and macrorchidism. It is now evident that this phenotype is not always present and that macrorchidism is often not seen until puberty. Mild mental retardation has been reported in some of the female carriers of the abnormal chromosome.

CRANIOSYNOSTOSIS

Premature closure of one or more cranial sutures is referred to as craniosynostosis. This condition occurs in 0.6/1000 live births.[23] This always produces abnormalities of head shape which can be predicted by using Virchow's law: growth of a skull bone is perpendicular to the suture line. A consistent and early physical finding is palpable ridging of bone over the suture. Diagnosis is made on x-ray study of the skull. The first radiological sign is increased density on either side of the suture. The suture then becomes obliterated. It is important to differentiate this from closely approximated cranial bones or narrow suture lines associated with failure of growth of the cranial vault in microcephaly.

Premature closure of the sagittal suture produces a long, narrow head, which is referred to as scaphocephaly or dolicocephaly (Figure 10-3). This is rarely associated with any neurological deficit.[24] Treatment, strip craniectomy and wrapping the edges of the bone with polyethylene film, is often recommended for cosmetic purposes, although the necessity of this procedure and its success are a continual source of controversy.

A short, broad head, brachycephaly, results from closure of the coronal suture. Increased intracranial pressure and optic atrophy have been associated but are rare. Treatment is warranted to prevent these complications if they occur. A markedly asymmetrical head, plagiocephaly, results from premature closure of a single lambdoid or coronal suture.

Closure of multiple cranial sutures and abnormalities of facial bones are

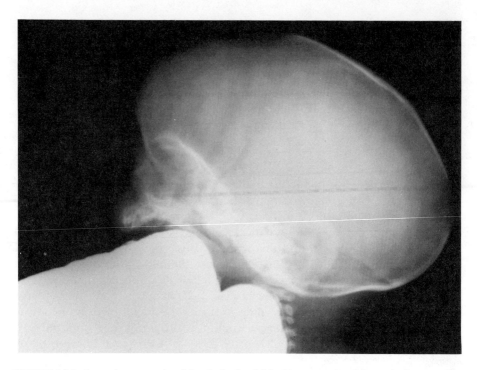

FIGURE 10-3. Lateral x-ray study of the skull of a child with synostosis of the sagittal suture. The dolicocephalic shape of the head is obvious.

present in Crouzon disease. A similar condition, associated with syndactyly, is called Apert syndrome. Extensive surgery is necessary to open the sutures, and a radical approach to correction of the facial deformities has been developed. Hydrocephalus and mental retardation are more likely to occur in conditions associated with premature synostosis of multiple sutures.[24]

TERATOGENIC AGENTS

A large number of chemical and physical agents produce major malformations of the CNS in experimental animals. The situation in the human is not as clear, although certain relationships appear to be valid.[25] Known human teratogens are listed in Table 10-2. Exposure of the fetus to sufficient quantities of *ionizing radiation* in the first or second trimester of gestation is a well-documented cause of microcephaly.

The *fetal alcohol syndrome* was initially described as affecting children of women who had heavy consumption of alcohol during pregnancy. It now appears that less intense exposure can affect the fetus, and it is not certain whether there is any threshold level that is safe. The features of this condition are poor prenatal and postnatal growth, delayed development, behavioral

TABLE 10-2
Human Teratogenic Agents[a]

Drugs and experimental chemicals	Maternal disease
Androgenic hormones	Iodine deficiency goiter
Aminopterin	Diabetes
Cyclophosphamide	Phenylketonuria
Busulfan	Alcohol ingestion
Thalidomide	Phencyclidine ingestion
Organic mercury	Virilizing tumors
PCBs	Infections
Diethylstilbestrol	Rubella
Coumarin	Cytomegalovirus
Phenytoin	Toxoplasmosis
Phenobarbital	Syphilis
Primidone	Physical agents
Trimethadione	Radiation
Valproate	Hyperthermia
Retinoic acid	

[a]Modified from Shepard.[25]

abnormalities, and a number of characteristic physical features. These include short palpebral fissures; short, upturned nose; thin upper lip; and hypoplastic philtrum. Some patients have abnormal palmar creases and hypoplasia of the fingernails.

The teratogenic effects of *anticonvulsant drugs* are a subject of some controversy, as it has been shown that women with epilepsy have twice the expected rate of stillbirths and infants with congenital anomalies. This increase is independent of drug ingestion during pregnancy. Phenytoin has been most frequently implicated. Consistent features are prenatal and postnatal growth deficiency, mental retardation, microcephaly, and hypoplastic nails. The risk of fetal malformation is 10%. Attempts to radically change the mother's drug regimen should only be carried out if medically indicated, however, so that the lives of the mother and fetus are not put at risk from loss of seizure control or status epilepticus.

Phenobarbital and primidone have been reported to produce a similar syndrome, but the data are less convincing. Valproate has been clearly associated with the development of neural tube defects. Trimethadione produces multiple severe anomalies and is contraindicated if pregnancy is planned.

Maternal diabetes mellitus is associated with a two- to fourfold increase in congenital anomalies of the fetus. The caudal regression syndrome is one of the most characteristic. Lumbar, sacral, and coccygeal vertebrae are abnormal or missing, and the associated segments of the spinal cord also fail to develop or are severely dysmorphic. Abnormalities of the legs, gastrointestinal tract, kidneys, and genitalia are present. Retinoic acid is a potent teratogen with a relative risk for major malformations of 25.6.[16] Hydrocephalus is the most common anomaly of the CNS. Others include abnormalities of cell migration and major malformations of the brain stem and cerebellum. There are also abnormalities of the face, ears, heart, thymus, and retina or optic nerve.

REFERENCES

1. Windham, G. C., and Edmonds, L. D., 1982, Current trends in the incidence of neural tube defects, *Pediatrics* **70:**333–337.
2. Kurtzke, J. F., and Goldberg, I. D., 1973, The distribution of deaths from congenital malformations of the nervous system, *Neurology* **23:**483–496.
3. Bell, J. E., 1979, Central nervous system defects in early human abortuses, *Dev. Med. Child. Neurol.* **21:**321–332.
4. Zwilling, E., 1955, Teratogenesis, in: *Analysis of Development* (B. H. Willier, P. A. Weiss, and V. Hamburger, eds.), WB Saunders, Philadelphia, pp. 699–719.
5. Wilson, J. G., 1973, Mechanisms of teratogenesis, *Am. J. Anat.* **136:**129–131.
6. Smithells, R. W., 1982, Neural tube defects: Prevention by vitamin supplements, *Pediatrics* **69:**498–499.
7. Bertoshesky, L. E., Haller, J., Scott, R. M., and Wojick, C., 1985, Seizures in children with meningomyelocele, *Am. J. Dis. Child.* **139:**400–402.
8. Charney, E. B., Weller, S. C., Sutton, L. N., Bruce, D. A., and Schut, L. B., 1985, Management of the newborn with myelomeningocele: Time for a decision-making process, *Pediatrics* **75:**58–64.
9. McLone, D.G., Czyzewski, D., Raimondi, A. J., and Sommers, R. C., 1982, Central nervous system infections as a limiting factor in the intelligence of children with myelomeningocele, *Pediatrics* **70:**338–342.
10. Ehrlich, O., and Brem, A. S., 1982, A prospective comparison of urinary tract infections in patients treated with either clean intermittent catheterization or urinary diversion, *Pediatrics* **70:**665–669.
11. Uehling, D. T., Smith, J., Meyer, J., and Bruskewitz, R., 1985, Impact of an intermittent catheterization program on children with myelomeningocele, *Pediatrics* **76:**892–895.
12. Bjerkedal, T., Czeizel, A., Goujard, J., Kallen, B., Mastroiacova, P., Nevin, N., Oakley, G., and Robert, E., 1982, Valproic acid and spina bifida, *Lancet* **2:**1096.
13. Smithells, R. W., 1982, Neural tube defects: Prevention by vitamin supplements, *Pediatrics* **69:**498–499.
14. Fisher, N. L., and Smith, D. W., 1981, Occipital encephalocele and early gestational hyperthermia, *Pediatrics* **68:**480–483.
15. Lemire, R. J., Loeser, J. D., Leach, R. W., and Alvord, E. C., 1975, *Normal and Abnormal Development of the Human Nervous System*, Harper and Row, Hagerstown, MD.
16. Lammer, E. J., Chen, D. T., Hoar, R. M., Agnish, N. D., Benke, P. J., Braun, J. T., Curry, C. J., Fernhoff, P. M., Grix, A. W., Lott, I. T., Richard, J. M., and Sun, S. C., 1985, Retinoic acid embryopathy, *N. Engl. J. Med.* **313:**837–841.
17. Shurtleff, D. B., Foltz, E., and Loeser, J. D., 1973, Hydrocephalus: A definition of its progression and relationship to intellectual function, diagnosis, and complications, *Am. J. Dis. Child.* **125:**688–693.
18. Martin, H. P., 1970, Microcephaly and mental retardation, *Am. J. Dis. Child.* **119:**128–131.
19. Wood, J. W., Johnson, K. G., and Omori, Y., 1967, *In utero* exposure to the Hiroshima atomic bomb, *Pediatrics* **39:**385–392.
20. Yamazaki, J. N., 1966, A review of the literature on the radiation dosage required to cause manifest central nervous system disturbances from *in utero* and postnatal exposure, *Pediatrics* **37**(Suppl.):877–903.
21. Lemieux, B. G., 1982, Chromosomal aberrations, in: *The Practice of Pediatric Neurology* (K. S. Swaiman and F. S. Wright, eds.), C.V. Mosby, St. Louis, pp. 344–402.
22. de la Cruz, F., 1985, Fragile X syndrome, *Am. J. Ment. Def.* **90:**119–123.

23. Shuper, A., Merlob, P., Grunebaum, M., and Reisner, S. H., 1985, The incidence of isolated craniosynostosis in the newborn infant, *Am. J. Dis. Child.* **139:**85–86.
24. Noetzel, M. J., Marsh, J. L., Palkes, H., and Gado, M., 1985, Hydrocephalus and mental retardation in craniosynostosis, *J. Pediatr.* **107:**885–892.
25. Shepard, T. H., 1982, Detection of human teratogenic agents, *J. Pediatr.* **101:**810–815.

ADDITIONAL READING

Gorlin, R. J., Pindborg, J. J., and Cohen, M. M., 1976, *Syndromes of the Head and Neck,* 2nd ed., McGraw-Hill, New York.

11

Neurocutaneous Disorders

A number of heterogeneous conditions characterized by abnormalities of the skin and central nervous system are traditionally classified as the neurocutaneous disorders, or phakomatoses. These are distinct entities, however, with no genetic overlap. The occurrence of two of these conditions in the same individual or family probably represents the workings of chance.

The central nervous system and skin are both products of the ectodermal layer of the embryo. Abnormal development that involves both of these systems is, therefore, easy to conceptualize. Unfortunately, the problem is not quite as simple as it first appears. Many of these disorders also have associated abnormalities of blood vessels and other tissues of mesodermal origin. This illustrates the complex interrelationships of developmental insults that occur early in morphogenesis.

The decision as to which disorders fall into this broad category is somewhat arbitrary. Those presented in this chapter were chosen because they are relatively common or because of the severity of involvement of the central nervous system.

Tuberous sclerosis is characterized by the triad of mental retardation, seizures, and adenoma sebaceum. The disorder typically becomes clinically apparent in infancy with the onset of infantile spasms or other types of seizures. Depigmented nevi are frequently present, even in the neonatal period (Figure 11-1), and a computerized-tomography (CT) scan will show typical subependymal intracranial calcifications (Figure 11-2).

Older children typically present for evaluation of delayed development or with a seizure disorder. In addition to the depigmented nevi, physical examination often shows a shagreen patch, which is an area of raised, roughened skin over the lumbar spine. Subungual and periungual fibromas may be present on the hands and feet (Figure 11-3). The characteristic adenoma sebaceum are rarely prominent before age 5 years. These are actually angiofibromas and have the appearance of acne, but without comedones. Small tumors of the retina, phakomas, can sometimes be visualized. CT scan is diagnostic, demonstrating one or more discrete subependymal calcifications.

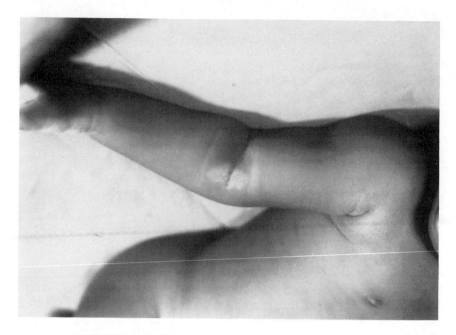

FIGURE 11-1. Depigmented areas in a child with tuberous sclerosis.

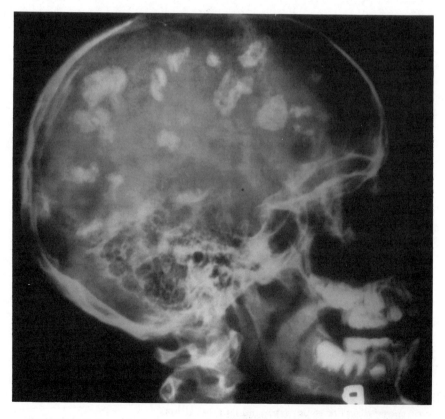

FIGURE 11-2. Extensive intracranial calcifications in a patient with tuberous sclerosis.

The disorder is transmitted by an autosomal dominant gene. The literature suggests that 80% of cases represent new mutations, but with the use of the CT scan, it has now become clear that the parents are frequently affected but have neither seizures nor mental retardation. Genetic evaluation should include a complete physical examination of both parents and all of the child's siblings, as well as CT scans and EEGs of all available family members. Prenatal diagnosis is not possible, and the family needs complete information in order to rationally evaluate reproductive options.

Pathological findings in the brain consist of subependymal nodules and multiple firm lesions (tubers) within the cerebral hemispheres. The nodules consist of whorls of glial fibers; the tubers contain bizarre glial cells and neurons. Both types of lesions frequently calcify. Malignant changes can occur.

Many other organs are involved, including the bones, kidneys, lungs, and gastrointestinal tract. Rhabdomyoma of the heart often presents with cardiac arrhythmias and can be the cause of death.

Management consists mainly of treatment of the seizure disorder, which may be most difficult to control, and the provision of special-education services for the mental retardation. Many of these children develop serious behavior disorders which require intervention. The child must be followed carefully for the development of a brain tumor or hydrocephalus produced by blockage of a foramen of Monro by a subependymal nodule. Tumors of other organs occasionally become symptomatic.

Neurofibromatosis is diagnosed clinically by the presence of multiple café-au-lait spots on the skin. Smaller fibromas along the course of peripheral nerves and large swellings due to plexiform neuromas are present in many cases.

The major neurological problem for the patient with neurofibromatosis is development of neoplasms. The most common are neurofibromas, which may involve any peripheral nerve. These do not often produce paralysis, but can become quite sensitive to pressure. These tumors also occur on spinal nerve roots and frequently have an intraspinal component which produces spinal cord compression. This causes a progressive myelopathy.

Optic glioma typically presents with monocular loss of vision. Extension into the orbit produces proptosis, although this sign is also seen with congenital absence of the sphenoid wing, a commonly associated malformation. Funduscopic examination reveals optic atrophy. Hypothalamic involvement is associated with growth failure, precocious puberty, or hydrocephalus.

The best known intracranial tumor associated with neurofibromatosis is an acoustic neuroma. The most common presentation is progressive loss of hearing. This is insidious, and the child rarely has any complaints. Suspicion is typically raised by the parents or schoolteacher. Tinnitus and vertigo occur, but are less common. Findings on audiometric evaluation are a sensorineural hearing loss with poor speech discrimination, and marked impairment of vestibular function. If diagnosis is delayed, the tumor grows into the posterior fossa and produces signs and symptoms referable to dysfunction of the brain stem and cerebellum.

Routine x-ray studies of the skull are often normal. Special views or tomo-

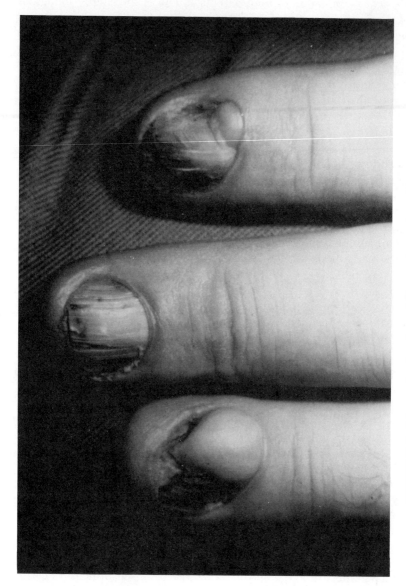

FIGURE 11-3. Subungual and periungual fibromas in a patient with tuberous sclerosis.

grams of the internal auditory canal show expansion and erosion of the walls of this structure. Some patients with neurofibromatosis have abnormally expanded canals without tumors, however. Early diagnosis requires cisternography. Metrizamide is introduced into the lumbar subarachnoid space, and the patient positioned so that it flows into the posterior fossa. This fills the internal auditory canals and permits visualization of small tumors. CT scan is a useful adjunct to metrizamide cisternography when the tumor has grown beyond the confines of the canals.

The operating microscope has greatly improved the results of surgical treatment. The facial nerve can be preserved, unless there is extensive involvement by the tumor. It is sometimes possible to save the auditory division of the eighth nerve, as the tumor typically begins on the vestibular division.

If acoustic neuromas are bilateral, it is virtually diagnostic of neurofibromatosis. Tumors of the cerebral hemispheres are less common, but do occur.

In addition to periodic reevaluation to detect early signs of tumors, patients with this condition should be screened for hypertension, which can be due to renal artery stenosis or pheochromocytoma. Scoliosis is also common and, if progressive, requires surgical intervention.

Neurofibromatosis is transmitted as an autosomal dominant condition. Penetrance is high, but there is great variability of expressivity.

There is now genetic evidence to support the concept that there are discrete peripheral and central forms of neurofibromatosis.[1] The central type is manifested by mild skin changes and bilateral acoustic neuromas. Symptoms begin at approximately 20 years of age. The peripheral type is the familiar classical form of the disorder.

Sturge–Weber syndrome is the association of a port-wine nevus of the face and a superficial vascular malformation involving the surface of the ipsilateral cerebral hemisphere. The facial nevus always involves part of the territory of the first division of the trigeminal nerve, although it has a different embryological origin.[2] Common clinical manifestations include contralateral hemiparesis, seizures which are typically focal, mental retardation, and glaucoma of the eye on the involved side.

CT scan (Figure 11-4) or x-ray studies (Figure 11-5) of the skull reveal the classic superficial intracranial calcifications, which have a "railroad track" configuration. The hemicranium is often smaller on the involved side than on the other, and the hemisphere is atrophic.

The condition appears to be sporadic, and no specific teratogenic agents have been described. Treatment of the seizures is difficult but should be pursued aggressively. Physical therapy will help maintain optimal function of the hemiparetic limbs. There is some evidence that early hemispherectomy in the child with uncontrolled seizures and a dense hemiparesis will improve the eventual outcome.

Studies of cerebral blood flow indicate reduced perfusion in the affected areas. This may be associated with progressive loss of cerebral tissue. If this finding can be replicated, criteria for early radical surgical intervention might be developed.

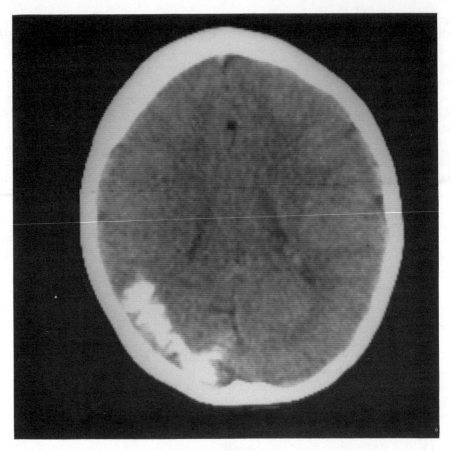

FIGURE 11-4. Computerized-tomography scan of the head showing a large area of calcification in the parietooccipital region of the brain of a patient with Sturge–Weber syndrome.

Ataxia–telangiectasia is generally included among the neurocutaneous disorders. This autosomal recessive condition presents in the first few years of life with progressive ataxia and choreoathetosis. Prominent telangiectasiae develop on the bulbar conjuctivae in the preschool years and also can be found on other areas of the face and the limbs. Ocular movements are abnormal, with impaired ability to smoothly follow a moving object or to shift gaze rapidly from one object to another. This pattern is referred to as oculomotor apraxia.

An associated abnormality involves the immune system. The thymus is absent, and cellular immunity is impaired. In addition, there are decreased levels of IgA and IgE, which result in repeated sinopulmonary infections. As with many of the immunodeficiency states of childhood, these patients have an increased incidence of lymphoreticular malignancies.

Hereditary hemorrhagic telangiectasia (Osler–Weber–Rendu syndrome) is associated with several types of vascular anomalies within the central nervous system, including telangiectasiae and arteriovenous malformations. Among the neurological complications are seizures, cerebrovascular accidents, and sub-arachnoid hemorrhage. The diagnosis can be suspected by demonstrating the characteristic telangiectasiae of the skin and mucous membranes. This is an autosomal dominant disorder.

There are other conditions which have prominent vascular malformations involving the skin and the central nervous system. *Cutaneous spinal angiomatosis* (Cobb syndrome) occurs sporadically. A hemangioma over the back is associated with a hemangioma of the spinal cord at the same segment. The *Wyburn–Mason syndrome,* also occurring sporadically, has vascular malformations involving the retina and brain. A facial angioma is sometimes present, in addition.

Neurocutaneous melanosis can be suspected at the time of birth. The child has a giant pigmented nevus or large multiple nevi. Melanotic cells in the lep-tomeninges most commonly produce hydrocephalus but can also cause spinal cord compression. There is no evidence that the condition is hereditary.

Incontinentia pigmenti (Bloch–Sulzberger syndrome) presents initially with skin lesions which begin as vesicular or bullous pigmented areas and then resolve to form characteristic pigmented whorls. CT reveals low-density areas, repre-senting edema, shortly after birth. Cerebral atrophy is found in older children.[3] Approximately one-third of patients are mentally retarded. Seizures are fre-quently a complicating factor. A number of ocular abnormalities are associated

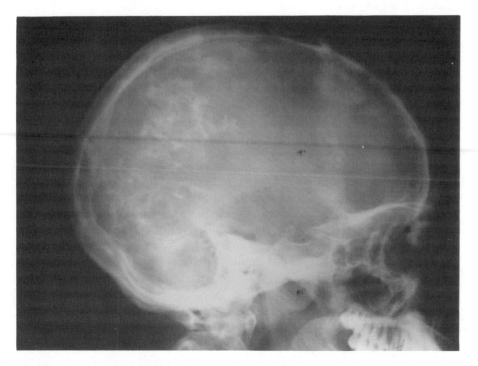

FIGURE 11-5. Lateral x-ray study of the skull showing extensive calcifications in the parietooccipital region in a patient with Sturge–Weber syndrome.

and include retinal pigmentation, optic atrophy, and corneal or lenticular opacification. The condition is transmitted by a dominant gene. It is not clear whether this is autosomal or X-linked with lethality for the affected males.

Incontinentia pigmenti achromians (hypomelanosis of Ito) differs in that there are no preceding vesicular or bullous lesions. Characteristic areas of hypopigmented skin are present. Mental retardation and seizures are common. No clear hereditary pattern has been established.

Linear nevus sebaceous predominantly affects the midline of the face, although other areas may also be involved. The nevus is hyperkeratotic and does not assume the bizarre shapes of those seen with the incontinentia pigmenti syndromes. There is a strong association with seizures and mental retardation. This appears to be a sporadic condition.

REFERENCES

1. Kanter, W. R., Eldridge, R., Fabricant, R., Allen, J. C., and Koerber, T., 1981, Central neurofibromatosis with bilateral acoustic neuroma: Genetic, clinical and biochemical distinctions from peripheral neurofibromatosis, *Neurology* **30:**851–859.
2. Enjolras, O., Riche, M. C., and Merland, J. J., 1985, Facial port-wine stains and Sturge–Weber syndrome, *Pediatrics* **76:**48–51.
3. Avrahami, E., Harel, S., Jurgenson, U., and Cohn, D., 1985, Computed tomographic demonstration of brain changes in incontinentia pigmenti, *Am. J. Dis. Child.* **139:**372–374.

ADDITIONAL READING

Berg, B. O., 1982, Neurocutaneous syndromes, in: *The Practice of Pediatric Neurology* (K. S. Swaiman and F. S. Wright, eds.), C.V. Mosby, St. Louis, pp. 914–934.
Rapin, I., and Chalhub, E. G., 1982, Phakomatoses and other neurocutaneous syndromes, in: *Pediatrics,* 17th ed. (A. M. Rudolph and J. I. E. Hoffman, eds.), Appleton-Century-Crofts, Norwalk, CT, pp. 1762–1766.

12

Infections of the Central Nervous System

Infections of the CNS are relatively common in children and many are potentially life threatening. Early diagnosis and treatment are essential to limit damage from the infection itself and from complications such as seizures, increased intracranial pressure, and infectious vasculitis.

Children appear to be at increased risk, as compared to adults, for a number of reasons. The major one is lack of immunity to many of the organisms involved. Most adults are immune to these pathogens, previously having had infections that did not involve the CNS. In addition, children have a higher incidence of specific illnesses, such as acute otitis media, which often precede CNS infections.

Invasion of the nervous system is generally through hematogenous spread and follows bactermia or viremia. Penetrating head wounds, sinusitis, mastoiditis, and osteomyelitis can introduce bacteria directly into the subarachnoid space or brain. Retrograde thrombophlebitis can follow infections of the scalp, face, sinuses, or mastoids. Migration along nerves to the central nervous system is a rare mechanism, but is involved in the pathogenesis of rabies.

Localization of the infection depends on both the mechanism of entry and the biological characteristics of the agent. Herpesvirus, for example, has a tendency to localize in the temporal lobes in older children and adults.

APPROACH TO THE PATIENT

An infection of the CNS should be suspected when a child has fever and any sign or symptom suggesting CNS involvement. These can be as subtle as lethargy and irritability or as obvious as seizures or coma. Only by constantly remembering to include infection in the differential diagnosis will diagnostic errors be minimized.

115

The threshold of suspicion should be further lowered in certain clinical situations. The neonate often manifests subtle behavioral changes, such as poor feeding or brief apneic spells, and frequently will not have fever. Hypothermia, in fact, is equally common. Infection should also be considered if behavioral or neurological abnormalities appear in any child who has a disorder associated with impairment of immune mechanisms or is being treated with drugs that suppress immunity.

Knowledge of illnesses prevalent in the community is important, as aseptic meningitis often occurs in epidemics. Every child still deserves a thoughtful and thorough diagnostic approach, but this knowledge may assist decision making and prevent unnecessary hospitalization and treatment.

Signs on examination that suggest the presence of a CNS infection are lethargy, irritability, confusion, and nuchal rigidity. It is often difficult to demonstrate a stiff neck in infants and young children, as they will actively resist any movement of their head. If a child is placed supine with his head hanging over the edge of the bed, he will allow the examiner to support and lift it, and the nuchal rigidity can often be elicited. The Brudzinski sign is involuntary flexion of the legs when the neck is flexed; the Kernig sign is pain and limitation of motion demonstrated by flexing the hip and knee and then attempting to straighten the leg at the knee. The tripod sign is seen when the child is placed in a sitting position and leans back on the outstretched arms. These are all nonspecific indicators of meningeal irritation.

If increased intracranial pressure is present, sixth-nerve palsies or signs of uncal herniation, such as a third-nerve palsy or hemiparesis, can be found. The presence of focal neurological signs suggests either localized infection or vascular occlusion as a complication of the infection.

Diagnosis ultimately depends on examination of the CSF and, whenever possible, isolation and identification of the offending organism. Many other routine and specialized laboratory tests can help document the presence of an infection, but *lumbar puncture* is required to document involvement of the nervous system.

A common clinical situation is the presence of signs suggesting both infection and increased intracranial pressure. Although lumbar puncture is potentially dangerous in the face of elevated CSF pressure, in this situation the procedure should still generally be performed. Intravenous mannitol can be administered to rapidly lower the pressure before the lumbar puncture is done. The minimum amount of fluid necessary for important studies should be taken. If focal neurological signs and increased intracranial pressure are both present in a patient suspected of having a CNS infection, a computerized-tomography (CT) scan and emergency neurosurgical consultation should be obtained.

Pleocytosis in the CSF is the major laboratory finding in the patient with nervous system infection. In bacterial infections there are mainly polymorphonuclear leukocytes and total counts of several hundred to thousands of cells. Viral infections are associated with a lymphocytic pleocytosis and cell counts no greater than several hundred. Early in the course of a viral illness, a preponderance of polymorphonuclear leukocytes is occasionally found, although cell counts are not extremely high.

The CSF glucose level is depressed in bacterial infections. Normal levels are greater than 40% of the corresponding serum glucose level. A level in the CSF less than 40 mg/dl is strong presumptive evidence for a bacterial infection; a normal level does not rule one out. Viral infections rarely cause a significant decrease in the glucose level, although this may occasionally be seen with mumps meningoencephalitis.

A marked increase in CSF protein content is strongly suggestive of a bacterial infection. Viral infections are accompanied by only a modest rise.

A Gram stain should always be performed on the fluid, and the yield will be increased if the specimen is first centrifuged. This is now being supplemented, in many centers, by a number of techniques that can rapidly give an exact bacteriological diagnosis. These depend on the detection of bacterial antigen in the CSF or other body fluids. Culture of the fluid is still mandatory, however, not only to allow an exact etiological diagnosis but also to determine the pattern of antibiotic susceptibility and resistance of the organism.

The child who has signs and symptoms suggestive of meningitis, but who has been receiving antibiotic therapy, presents a special diagnostic problem. In some cases, the CSF findings are ambiguous and are more consistent with a viral than a bacterial infection. Cultures and Gram stain are often negative. Antigen detection techniques are of value in such cases, but if the issue cannot be resolved, therapy appropriate for meningitis should be instituted empirically. The possibility of tuberculous or fungal meningitis should always be considered if CSF abnormalities are not typical of a bacterial infection.

BACTERIAL MENINGITIS

The most common organism producing bacterial meningitis in children beyond the neonatal period is *Hemophilus influenzae type b*. This accounts for over 60% of cases, although the incidence decreases rapidly after 4 years of age. The onset of the illness may be insidious, and early diagnosis difficult. There is some evidence that a delay in initiating treatment is associated with more severe sequelae, and so there should always be a vigorous attempt to rapidly obtain a diagnosis in all cases.

The standard treatment has been ampicillin, 200–400 mg/kg per day in divided doses. The emergence of ampicillin-resistant strains now mandates the simultaneous administration of chloramphenicol, 100 mg/kg per day. When the organism has been cultured and antibiotic sensitivity determined, one or the other drug can be discontinued. Moxalactam appears to be an adequate drug for initial therapy.[1]

Complications of *H. influenzae* meningitis include mental retardation, sensorineural deafness and other cranial nerve palsies, hydrocephalus, and static motor deficits. In some cases there is occlusion of arteries over the convexity of the hemispheres, with multifocal brain destruction. One common complication is subdural effusion. This presents with prolonged fever and evidence of increased intracranial pressure. Diagnosis by CT scan has virtually replaced diagnostic subdural taps. In most cases, the collections resolve on their own, and no treatment is necessary. If increased intracranial pressure becomes severe, or there is progressive excessive head growth, therapeutic taps may become necessary.

Following appropriate and effective treatment, the child may still carry the organism in the nasopharynx and represent a risk to household contacts, especially other children under 4 years of age. Treatment of the patient with rifampin, 20 mg/kg per day (maximum dose 600 mg), once daily for 4 days, will eliminate the carrier state. Although it is somewhat controversial, some investigators recommend that all household, day-care, and nursery-school contacts under 4 years of age should also be treated.

Streptococcus pneumoniae (pneumococcus) is the second most common organism causing bacterial meningitis in childhood. The preceding infection is usually otitis media, pneumonia, or sepsis. Children who have had a splenectomy for any reason, or have decreased splenic function such as in sickle cell disease, are at increased risk, as are children with nephrotic syndrome.

Pneumococcal meningitis is the most common bacterial complication of basilar skull fractures. If a child has repeated episodes of infection with this organism, a fracture or a congenital anomaly such as a dermal sinus which connects the subarachnoid space with the external environment should be suspected. Thin-section CT scans can help delineate defects in the sinuses.[2]

The onset of the illness is usually acute, and the course is fulminant if untreated. Initial therapy with ampicillin is adequate, but when the organism is isolated, this should be changed to penicillin G. Pneumococci resistant to penicillin have been identified, but this is not yet a common problem in this country. The mortality rate in children is under 20%, but is higher if there is an underlying illness. Basilar meningitis with deafness, cranial nerve palsies, and hydrocephalus are the most common complications.

Meningitis caused by *Neisseria meningitidis* (meningococcus) occurs at any age, but is more common in older children. The illness most often follows meningococcal sepsis and has an acute onset. Multiple petechiae and purpuric lesions are present in over one-half of cases, and there may be other evidence of disseminated disease such as arthritis and pericarditis. Vascular collapse, often with evidence of adrenal hemorrhage (Waterhouse–Friderichsen syndrome), and disseminated intravascular coagulation are sometimes present and associated with an extremely high mortality rate.

Initial treatment with ampicillin is effective in meningococcal meningitis also, although this should be changed to penicillin G when a specific diagnosis is made. If the patient survives, serious sequelae are rare. Rifampin is given orally at the end of treatment to eliminate the carrier state and should be used to treat contacts prophylactically. Initial studies on the use of a vaccine are quite promising.

It should be apparent from the preceding discussion that initial therapy with ampicillin and chloramphenicol provides adequate empirical therapy for the most common organisms associated with meningitis in childhood. The therapeutic protocol can then be modified based on the organism isolated and the specific pattern of antibiotic sensitivity and resistance. Treatment is continued for 2 weeks.

General management, preferably in an intensive-care unit, is also most important. Cerebral edema with herniation is the most common feature associated with death in meningitis. Careful attention to fluid therapy, with limitation of fluid replacement to the minimum needed, and supplementary use of osmotic diuretics such as mannitol are usually effective. Seizures should be treated promptly and vigorously.

NEONATAL MENINGITIS

The neonate is at high risk for the development of sepsis and meningitis. This is at least partially due to the failure of placental transfer of IgM and IgA antibodies. Other pathogenetic factors include prolonged rupture of the membranes with chorioamnionitis, maternal sepsis, and infections of the umbilical stump. The signs of meningitis in the neonate may be subtle and include poor feeding and either elevated temperature or hypothermia. The infant then becomes acutely ill with seizures, apneic spells, and a bulging fontanelle. Systemic signs of sepsis are usually present, and death may quickly ensue. Sepsis and meningitis must be strongly suspected in any infant not doing well in the nursery.

The most common organisms are Gram-negative bacilli and group B *streptococcus*. The latter presents either with symptoms in the neonatal period or in the first few months of life. Because of the broad range of bacteria potentially involved, penicillin and an aminoglycoside antibiotic are used in combination. Although aminoglycosides do not readily cross the blood–brain barrier, studies of intraventricular and intrathecal administration of these agents have shown no additional benefit.

Prognosis depends on the specific organism involved. Gram-negative bacilli are associated with a mortality rate of over 50% and a high incidence of serious sequelae among the survivors. Group B streptococcal meningitis has a more favorable outcome. The mortality rate is closer to 15%, and few survivors have major disabilities.

TUBERCULOUS MENINGITIS

Tuberculous meningitis has become a difficult diagnostic problem as its incidence has decreased in this country and patients are seldom encountered. It is still a common condition in less developed nations and is seen among recent immigrants from these countries. Meningitis most often occurs as part of miliary tuberculosis, and usually within 1 year of the primary infection. The majority of children are under 2 years of age.

Onset is typically insidious, with fever, lethargy, irritability, headache, and vomiting. Progression is marked by further obtundation, signs and symptoms of increased intracranial pressure, meningeal signs, and, finally, coma. Death occurs within 3–5 weeks. The mortality rate is high, ranging between 20 and

50%, and serious residua are common. These include deafness, mental retardation, cerebral palsy, and hydrocephalus.

Initial diagnosis is often complicated by the finding of only a few hundred leukocytes in the CSF, with a lymphocytic pleocytosis. CSF glucose also may be normal initially, but then rapidly falls to very low levels. Protein becomes markedly elevated. Acid-fast bacilli may be seen in a centrifuged specimen of CSF, but diagnosis ultimately depends on the results of culture. Tuberculous meningitis should be considered in any child with a preponderance of lymphocytes in the cerebrospinal fluid.

Treatment must be rapidly instituted and carried out for as long as 18–24 months. The current recommendation is isoniazid, 20 mg/kg per day, and rifampin, 20 mg/kg per day (up to a maximum dose of 600 mg daily). Streptomycin, 40 mg/kg per day, is also administered for the first 4 weeks. It is then discontinued to prevent damage to the vestibular and cochlear apparatus. Pyridoxine supplements are not necessary for children treated with isoniazid. There is some evidence that prednisone, 1 mg/kg per day, given for 30 days reduces mortality.

BRAIN ABSCESS

A brain abscess can present either as an acute CNS infection or as an expanding mass lesion. If the child is symptomatic during the first stage, cerebritis, there will be fever, lethargy, headache, and meningeal signs. Seizures and focal findings on neurological examination are common. Lumbar puncture is dangerous in this situation, and if an abscess is suspected, an emergency CT scan should be the initial diagnostic procedure. The characteristic finding is an area of lucency surrounded by an enhancing ring. EEG almost always shows an extremely slow focus over the affected region.

Clinical presentation often does not include signs of infection. There are, instead, increased intracranial pressure and progressive focal neurological signs. Lumbar puncture, if performed, shows a low cell count with lymphocytic preponderance, normal glucose, and an elevated protein concentration. CT scan is similar to that outlined for cerebritis, and these findings are characteristic.

Abscesses can develop from contiguous spread of infection in the mastoids or paranasal sinuses, by the hematogenous route, or from a penetrating head wound. Predisposing conditions include cyanotic congenital heart disease, bronchiectasis, and intravenous drug use. Any child with a right-to-left intracardiac shunt who is over 2 years of age and presents with focal neurological signs should be considered to have a brain abscess until proven otherwise. Under age 2 years, children presenting with this clinical constellation are more likely to have venous thromboses.

Treatment relies on antibiotics and surgery. Organisms most frequently involved include *Streptococcus,* pneumococcus, *Staphylococcus,* and anaerobes, so broad-spectrum coverage is required. Infection with multiple organisms is not rare. Initial therapy usually includes large doses of penicillin, methicillin, and gentamycin. This regimen will sometimes lead to resolution of cerebritis without formation of a frank abscess, and surgery will not be required. Surgical removal of fully formed abscesses is strongly recommended, although there is disagreement as to how early this procedure should be carried out. If abscesses are multiple, surgery may be impossible.

Life-threatening complications of abscess include transtentorial herniation and the tendency to track through the white matter and rupture into the ventricular system. Even after prompt and effective treatment, there is a high risk of residual neurological signs and seizures.

SUBDURAL EMPYEMA

Subdural empyema most frequently occurs as a complication of frontal or ethmoid sinusitis or mastoiditis and spreads to the subdural space by direct extension or as thrombophlebitis. The onset of symptoms is acute and progression is rapid. The major signs are infection, increased intracranial pressure, and focal neurological disease. The localizing findings result from thrombophlebitis with infarction or from the abscess acting as a mass lesion.

Diagnostic evaluation is approached as an emergency if empyema is suspected. CT scan identifies the lesion in most cases. X-ray studies of the sinuses and mastoids demonstrate the source of the infection. Treatment is centered around the use of large doses of antibiotics and an aggressive attempt to control intracranial pressure. Initial antimicrobial therapy must provide coverage for staphylcocci, anaerobic streptococci, and Gram-negative organisms. This should then be modified when culture and sensitivity determinations are available. Surgical drainage is required if there is a significant mass effect.

Penetrating head wounds also can be the forerunner of subdural empyema. In those patients, surgical debridement is necessary to allow removal of any foreign material.

In infants subdural empyema is most frequently a complication of meningitis. Diagnosis can be made by CT scan and confirmed by subdural taps. This also provides material for culture.

VIRAL MENINGOENCEPHALITIS

The brain, spinal cord, and meninges can be infected by several groups of viruses. There is an acute illness, which, if the brain is involved, is characterized by impairment of consciousness, fever, and headache. Focal neurological signs are also frequently present. If the infection is restricted to the meninges, the signs and symptoms are indistinguishable from those of acute bacterial meningitis, although the patient is generally not as seriously ill.

The usual clinical picture of encephalitis begins with a prodromal illness, which is followed, within 1 week, by the acute onset of neurological symptoms and signs. Changes in mental status range from lethargy and confusion to coma. Seizures are common. The patient also will have fever, headache, and meningeal signs. Neurological examination documents involvement of cerebral cortex, subcortical structures, brain stem, or spinal cord, in any combination.

Severity of the illness and outcome depend on the specific virus involved. Among the *arboviruses,* eastern equine encephalitis can have a mortality rate as high as 35%. The mortality rate is 5% for St. Louis encephalitis and somewhat less for western equine and California encephalitis. Death is rare in Venezualan encephalitis. *Enteroviruses* (echovirus and coxsackievirus) also have mortality rates of less than 5%. Residua can result from damage to any portion of the CNS and are most common with the arbovirus infections.

The most important diagnostic tool is a lumbar puncture, and examination of the CSF is required to eliminate the possibility of a bacterial infection. The typical findings are 50–500 white blood cells/mm^3, normal glucose content, and slightly elevated protein levels. Although there may be a preponderance of polymorphonuclear leukocytes present initially, they soon are replaced by mononuclear cells. A useful technique for determining the exact etiological agent is demonstration of a rise in serum antibody titers against a specific virus. Enteroviruses can sometimes be isolated from the CSF, but this is much less common for arboviruses. If the child should die, pathological examination shows inflammation of the brain and meninges, and necrosis of neurons.

Specific treatment is not available. Important aspects of management include attempts to reduce intracranial pressure, treatment of seizures, and the types of general medical and nursing care that are appropriate for any seriously ill patient. As soon as the child's condition is stable, a vigorous rehabilitation program should be begun.

Herpesvirus hominis (HSV) produces three distinct types of CNS infection, depending on the patient's age and the type of herpesvirus. Neonatal encephalitis is associated with HSV-2 (genital) in 75% of cases and HSV-1 (nongenital) in the remainder. Infection is by contact with herpetic lesions of the genital tract in the mother; these may be asymptomatic and unrecognized. The illness presents as an acute, severe encephalitis with coma, seizures, and abnormal neurological signs. Skin lesions or disseminated herpes are present in one-half of cases. The mortality rate is approximately 60%, and at least one-half of survivors have serious residua. It is now recommended that if the woman has active genital herpes, the baby be delivered by cesarean section. If membranes have been ruptured for several hours, operative delivery is probably not useful. The child should be isolated and observed, and meticulous isolation techniques used in nursing care.

The older individual infected with HSV-2 generally will only have aseptic meningitis. Recovery is rapid and the prognosis is excellent.

HSV-1 causes severe encephalitis. Typical signs include a change in the state of consciousness, fever, and headache. Seizures and focal neurological signs are common. There is often localization of the infection to one or both temporal lobes (Figure 12-1), and the clinical presentation may resemble that of an acute bacterial cerebritis.

Lumbar puncture is associated with some risk in the face of temporal lobe swelling and increased intracranial pressure and should probably not be performed if CT scan is rapidly available. This shows swelling and decreased density

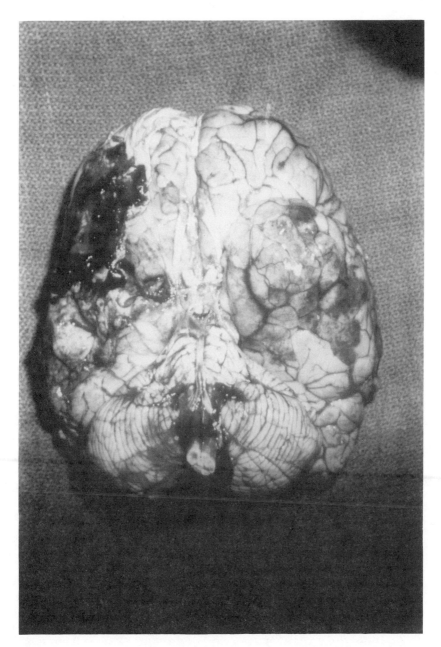

FIGURE 12-1. Base of the brain of a patient dying from herpesvirus encephalitis. There is extensive hemorrhagic necrosis of the temporal lobes, especially the right.

in the affected temporal lobe. If CSF is obtained, it reveals, in addition to the typical findings of encephalitis, red blood cells. Definitive diagnosis is made by temporal lobe biopsy with demonstration of typical intranuclear inclusions in infected neurons and isolation of the virus in tissue culture.

Therapy with adenine arabinoside can reduce mortality and, to some extent, morbidity. The best results are obtained if treatment is begun early in the course of illness, before the patient becomes comatose. Whether or not biopsy should always be performed before beginning therapy is controversial. Needle biopsy can be carried out with relative safety and is routinely done in many centers. General aspects of management, as with any encephalitic illness, are also most important.

Rabies, endemic in many wild animals, is likely to become an increasingly important pediatric problem. Children often attempt to play with a wild animal, such as a raccoon, that approaches them, not realizing that this is abnormal behavior and indicates that the animal may be ill. The incubation period following a bite varies according to the distance from the CNS, as the virus appears to travel retrograde along nerves. The usual delay before the onset of symptoms is 3–8 weeks. There is a flulike prodromal illness followed by pain at the site of the bite. The patient next develops severe anxiety, salivation and perspiration, and changes in mental status. There is then progressive paralysis, seizures, coma, and death. Approximately one-half of patients have severe spasm of pharyngeal muscles when attempting to swallow (hydrophobia).

Diagnosis is difficult if the history of exposure to a sick animal is not available. CSF may be normal or show typical findings of encephalitis. Antibody studies on serum or blood are helpful, but it is difficult to isolate the virus, except from cerebral tissue.

No specific treatment is available, and the mortality rate is nearly 100%. For this reason, prevention is extremely important. The first step in this process is to educate children (and adults) to avoid any wild animal that does not flee from human contact. Laws concerning vaccination of domestic pets also must be enforced. If the child is bitten, the use of immune globulin and passive immunization with human diploid cell vaccine should be considered. Current recommendations are outlined in Table 12-1.

TABLE 12-1
Postexposure Rabies Treatment[a]

Wild animals
    Regard as rabid unless laboratory tests are negative
    Rabies immune globulin and human diploid cell vaccine
Domestic dog or cat
    Healthy: no treatment
    Unknown: consult local health official for level of risk
    Rabid or suspected rabid: treat with immune globulin and vaccine
Livestock, rodents, lagomorphs
    Rarely affected

[a]Modified from Klein *et al.*[9]

Poliovirus infections are rare because of the high immunization rate in this country. The problem remains potentially serious, however, because of the continuous immigration of unimmunized children from less developed countries. There is, classically, a biphasic course. The prodrome consists of a flulike illness associated with myalgias. The patient appears to improve, but there is then a secondary rise in fever and onset of paralysis. This is typically asymmetrical and spotty in distribution and can involve both bulbar and spinal musculature. Respiratory paralysis may occur when the brain stem is affected.

Although the mortality rate is low, many children are left with severe residua. In addition to paralysis and atrophy of muscles in the extremities, scoliosis is common. Some patients are left with respiratory insufficiency and remain partially or fully dependent on ventilatory assistance. Specific treatment is not available. An intensive rehabilitation program should be begun as soon as the acute illness is over. Immunization is highly effective, and polio should remain a rarity, although an identical disease can be produced by other enteroviruses.

Progressive loss of anterior horn cells with increasing weakness has been reported in patients with residua of poliomyelitis. This appears as long as 20–30 years after the acute infection. It is not clear whether these patients will have periods of stability, or if loss of strength will be relentless.

Encephalitis can be caused by the *Epstein–Barr virus* (EBV), the agent producing infectious mononucleosis. This may be very mild or severe and life threatening. The diagnosis is confirmed by serological studies. EBV also has been associated with meningitis, myelitis, and the Guillain–Barré syndrome.

Approximately 30% of patients with *acquired immune deficiency syndrome* (AIDS) have involvement of the nervous system. The usual clinical manifestation is a subacute encephalopathy with progressive dementia. Myelopathy, chronic meningitis, and peripheral neuropathy have also been reported. Human immunodeficiency virus (HIV) can be isolated from brain tissue and CSF, and specific antibodies can also be found in the CSF.

Children with AIDS also have a progressive encephalopathy.[3,4] Common features include loss of cognitive function, developmental milestones, and motor skills; spasticity and ataxia; secondary microcephaly; and seizures. Cortical atrophy can be demonstrated on CT scans.

Opportunistic infections of the CNS are common in patients with AIDS, which can cause problems in diagnosis. Cytomegalovirus encephalitis in a child with AIDS has been reported.[4]

CONGENITAL INFECTIONS

A number of infectious agents can cross the placenta and infect the infant. Those most frequently affecting the brain have been referred to as the TORCH organisms. The acronym refers to toxoplasmosis, rubella, cytomegalovirus, and herpes. Syphilis should be included in this group of organisms, but there has been disagreement as to what the new acronym should be. Herpesvirus infections have already been discussed.

Toxoplasma gondii is an obligate intracellular protozoan. Congenital toxo-plasmosis presents with chorioretinitis, intracranial calcifications, mental retar-dation, and seizures. The children may have either hydrocephalus or micro-cephaly. X-ray and CT studies show a pattern of fine scattered intracranial calcifications. Elevated levels of IgM in the infant's serum provide presumptive evidence for an intrauterine infection. Specific serological diagnostic techniques are available. Treatment with sulfadiazine and pyrimethamine has been recom-mended, but there is no strong evidence that this is effective in congenital toxoplasmosis.

Congenital *rubella* has a wide range of manifestations. The classic triad is mental retardation, deafness, and cataracts. Common additional findings are microphthalmia, chorioretinitis, and seizures. Involvement of other organ sys-tems is seen and includes patent ductus arteriosus, peripheral pulmonary artery stenosis, abnormal teeth, and osteitis. Infective virus can be isolated from throat washings and urine, so it is important that unimmunized women in the child-bearing age group avoid contact with the infant or take appropriate precautions. Congenital rubella cannot be treated, but can be effectively prevented by assur-ing the immunization of all girls as they approach adolescence and adulthood. It is important that the vaccine, a live-virus preparation, not be administered during pregnancy or several months before a pregnancy is planned.

Cytomegalovirus (CMV) infections also vary in severity. The most severely affected children have spastic cerebral palsy, mental retardation, and choriore-tinitis. CT scan reveals microcephaly with enlarged ventricles, indicating severe cerebral atrophy. The ventricles are lined by a thin rim of calcium. Recent stud-ies have shown that most cases of CMV infections are probably less severe, the major residua being sensorineural deafness and school problems. The virus is excreted by the patient for a prolonged period, and appropriate precautions must be taken. Pregnant hospital personnel must be especially careful.

Congenital *syphilis* is becoming more common as a result of the general increase in the incidence of sexually transmitted diseases. Involvement of the CNS in the neonatal period is restricted to meningitis. Other important prob-lems include keratitis and sensorineural deafness. Treatment is important to prevent tertiary luetic neurological problems.

SLOW VIRUS INFECTIONS

Viral infections are generally considered to be acute monophasic illnesses that may or may not leave residua and are followed by a high degree of immunity to the offending organism. Research carried out over the last 30 years has proven that certain viruses can infect the individual, have a prolonged incuba-tion period, and then produce a slowly progressive, degenerative disease. The only one of these disorders that is common in children is *subacute sclerosing pan-encephalitis* (SSPE). This is due to rubeola virus, which appears to have a specific defective protein.

The average age of onset is currently 12–16 years, although it was under

12 years of age prior to 1976. Boys are affected twice as frequently as girls; the disease is rare among blacks. Children who live in rural areas are at highest risk. Over 80% of patients have a history of a documented rubeola infection, often at an early age.

The clinical course of SSPE can be divided into four stages. In the first, the child presents with the sudden onset of learning and behavior problems. A psychiatric diagnosis is commonly made. The most typical feature of stage 2 is seizures, especially myoclonic or atonic. A characteristic EEG is found with regularly occurring periodic bursts of epileptogenic activity, each burst having a stereotyped morphology. Spasticity and athetosis occur.

The third stage is associated with progressive dementia, paralysis, and adventitious movements. The child may become comatose. A chronic vegetative state marks stage 4, and the majority of patients die within 5 years of pneumonia, sepsis, or hypothalamic dysfunction with impaired temperature regulation, respiratory arrest, or cardiac abnormalities.

Variations in this stereotyped pattern have recently been described. Patients may have an acute, chronic, or stuttering course.

Diagnosis can be made by the demonstration of high levels of rubeola antibodies in the CSF and very high levels in the serum. Treatment has become somewhat controversial, and analysis is complicated by the observation that the disorder has a variable rate of progression, may become static in some patients, and has been reported to partially remit in others.[5] The majority of patients, however, do not survive, regardless of treatment.

A similar disorder, caused by the *rubella* virus, has been reported.[6] It is characterized by dementia and progressive abnormalities on neurological examination. The diagnosis is made by demonstrating rubella antibodies in the CSF.

Progressive multifocal leukoencephalopathy affects patients with chronic illnesses, malignancies, and immunosuppressed states. The causative organism is a papovavirus. The clinical course is one of seizures, progressive spasticity, and dementia. Death usually occurs within a year.

A number of other persistent viral infections occur in patients with compromised immunity. Patients with X-linked hypogammaglobulinemia appear to have increased susceptibility to enteroviruses, especially poliomyelitis. Chronic ECHO type 5 virus has been reported in children with this disorder.[7]

UNUSUAL INFECTIONS

The life-cycle of a number of parasites includes a phase during which the organisms enter the circulation and are carried to parts of the body distant from the gastrointestinal tract. They can then infest various organs, including the brain and spinal cord, and produce neurological signs and symptoms by causing inflammation or by acting as a mass lesion. *Visceral larva migrans,* due to the dog or cat ascarid *(Toxocara),* is the most common tissue parasite affecting children in this country. Preschool children are usually involved. The patient typically presents with attacks resembling asthma. The diagnosis should be suspected when hepatosplenomegaly, marked eosinophilia, and increased serum IgG levels are present. Involvement of the brain produces meningoencephalitis and seizures. The organism frequently enters the eye and may be mistaken for retinoblastoma. Mild cases are self-limited. Treatment with thiabendazole or diethylcarbamazine may shorten the course.

Cysticercosis, caused by the pork tapeworm *(Taenia solium),* is rare in this country but is seen in children coming from Latin America or India. The usual presentation is as a mass lesion. CT scan often shows multiple areas of lucency, which subsequently calcify. Other patients have signs of a meningeal reaction and can develop arachnoiditis and hydrocephalus. There is no effective medical treatment, and surgery is quite dangerous, as rupturing a cyst will cause widespread dissemination of the contents. Conservative therapy is usually followed by resolution of the symptoms.

Echinococcus (dog tapeworm) infestations are also rare in this country. When they occur, the clinical picture is that of a mass lesion. *Trichinosis* occasionally presents as a diffuse meningoencephalitis. The most common presentation is with myalgia, weakness, and marked eosinophilia.

Amebic meningoencephalitis has been reported from the middle Atlantic states in this country. The causative organism, *Naegleria fowleri,* enters the CNS through the cribriform plate. A severe meningitis and hemorrhagic necrosis of brain occur. The course is relentlessly progressive, and the great majority of patients die. A diagnostic clue is CSF findings of meningitis and a large number of red blood cells in the fluid.

Rocky mountain spotted fever is the most common rickettsial disease in this country and is being reported from an increasing number of geographical areas. The organism, *Rickettsia rickettsii,* is transmitted by either the wood tick or the dog tick. The initial symptoms are fever and headache, and 1–5 days later a characteristic rash appears. This begins on the ankles and wrists and spreads to involve the entire body, including the palms and soles. The rash then becomes petechial. Muscle pain and weakness, disturbances of consciousness and cognition, and multiple neurological signs can occur. Despite the seriousness of the illness, the mortality rate is low and major residua are infrequent. Treatment with tetracycline or chloramphenicol will shorten the course, and reduce the severity of the disease.

A large number of *fungi* can invade the CNS. These are extremely rare in children unless there is compromise of the immune system due to a specific disease or secondary to the administration of immunosuppressive drugs.

Mycoplasma appear to be involved in a number of acute infections of the CNS, such as meningitis and encephalitis. These can potentially be treated with erythromycin or tetracyclines. *Mycoplasma* have also been implicated in postinfectious diseases such as the Guillain–Barré syndrome and transverse myelitis.

Lyme disease is a spirochetal infection characterized by three stages. Initially, the patient presents with a characteristic rash (erythema chronicum migrans), malaise, fatigue, fever, headache, stiff neck, myalgias, or arthralgias. Weeks to months later, many patients develop arthritis.

During the initial phase, meningoencephalitis, cranial neuritis, or radiculoneuritis may be found.[8] Ataxia, chorea, and myelitis have also been reported. A lymphocytic pleocytosis is present in the cerebrospinal fluid. A rise in serum antibody titers confirms the diagnosis. Symptoms persist for several months, although resolution is more rapid following administration of penicillin.

REFERENCES

1. Kaplan, S. L., Mason, E. O., Mason, S. K., Catlin, F. I., Lee, R. T., Murphy, M., and Feigin, R. D., 1984, Prospective comparative trial of moxalactam versus ampicillin or chloramphenicol for treatment of *Haemophilus influenzae* type b meningitis in children, *J. Pediatr.* **104:**447–453.
2. Steele, R. W., McConnell, J. R., Jacobs, R. F., and Mawk, J. R., 1985, Recurrent bacterial meningitis: Coronal thin-section cranial computed tomography to delineate anatomical defects, *Pediatrics* **76:**950–953.
3. Epstein, L. G., Sharer, L. R., Joshi, V. V., Fojas, M. M., Koenigsberger, M. R., and Oleske, J., 1985, Progressive encephalopathy in children with acquired immune deficiency syndrome, *Ann. Neurol.* **17:**488–496.
4. Belman, A. L., Ultmann, M. H., Horoupian, D., Novick, B., Spiro, A. J., Rubinstein, A., Kurtzberg, D., and Cone-Wesson, B., 1985, Neurological complications in infants and children with acquired immune deficiency syndrome, *Ann. Neurol.* **18:**560–566.
5. DuRant, R. H., Dyken, P. R., and Swift, A. V., 1982, The influence of inosiplex treatment on the neurological disability of patients with subacute sclerosing panencephalitis, *J. Pediatr.* **101:**288–293.
6. Jan, J. E., Tingle, A. J., Donald, G., Kettyls, M., Buckler, W. St. J., and Dolman, C., 1979, Rubella panencephalitis: Clinical course and response to isoprinosine, *Dev. Med. Child. Neurol.,* **21:**648–652.
7. Bodensteiner, J. B., Morris, H. H., Howell, J. T., and Schochet, S. S., 1979, Chronic ECHO type 5 virus meningoencephalitis in X-linked hypogammaglobulinemia: Treatment with immune plasma, *Neurology* **29:**815–819.
8. Pachner, A. R., and Steere, A. C., 1985, The triad of neurologic manifestations of Lyme disease: Meningitis, cranial neuritis, and radiculoneuritis, *Neurology* **35:**47–53.

ADDITIONAL READING

Bell, W. E., and McCormick, W. F., 1975, *Neurologic Infections in Children,* W. B. Saunders, Philadelphia.
Klein, J. O., Brunell, P. A., Cherry, J. D., and Fulginiti, V. A., 1982, *Report of the Committee on Infectious Diseases,* 19th ed., American Academy of Pediatrics, Evanston, IL.

13

Postinfectious and Immunological Disorders

A number of acute neurological disorders of childhood are regularly associated with a preceding illness, either one of the classic exanthematous diseases or a "nonspecific" upper respiratory tract infection. Although other family members may share the same prodromal symptoms, they rarely go on to manifest involvement of the CNS.

The conditions arbitrarily included in this chapter are postinfectious (parainfectious) encephalitis and myelitis, Guillain–Barré syndrome, Reye syndrome, and postimmunization encephalopathy, although the underlying pathophysiology is probably quite different for each disorder. Some cases of acute cerebellar ataxia (Chapter 25) may be postinfectious in origin, rather than due to viral invasion of the cerebellum.

Consistent pathological changes in postinfectious encephalitis and myelitis include diffuse perivenous demyelination associated with infiltration of mononuclear cells and macrophages. The majority of the changes are in the white matter, and affected areas also show reactive gliosis.

Understanding of these disorders has been enhanced by an animal model, experimental allergic encephalomyelitis. This is a monophasic demyelinating disease produced by injecting myelin and Freund's adjuvant into the animal. After a delay of several days, there is progressive neurological disability; pathological changes are similar to those of the human condition. Fractionation of myelin has shown that the major encephalitogenic component is in myelin basic protein and, even more specifically, is a polypeptide of eight amino acid residues. It is reasonable to speculate that the disease in children also results from an immunological mechanism. This could be due to a subclinical attack of the virus on myelin, a shared antigen in the virus, or an antigen that causes production of an antibody that cross-reacts with myelin.

131

Acute allergic polyneuritis is produced in animals by using peripheral nerve rather than brain tissue. This disorder has many analogies to Gullain–Barré syndrome and, like the latter, is a monophasic illness.

The pathology of Reye syndrome is quite different. The major feature of CNS involvement is cerebral edema, without inflammation, vasculitis, cellular necrosis, or infarction. The liver shows massive intracellular accumulation of neutral fat in microvesicular droplets. Other organs, including the kidneys and heart, also have fatty infiltration. Electron microscopy of brain and liver shows swelling of mitochondria with disruption of the cristae. As the patient recovers, these changes revert to normal.[1] Experimental models have largely relied on the administration of toxins, such as octanoate, to animals. Relevance to the human disorder is still speculative.

APPROACH TO THE PATIENT

The differential diagnosis applied to any patient with acute onset of dysfunction involving any portion of the nervous system includes

- Trauma
- Infection
- Vascular disease
- Toxicity
- Metabolic disorders
- Seizures
- Demyelinating disease
- Postinfectious disorders

Historical data are most important. The signs and symptoms of postinfectious disorders typically occur within 1 week following an antecedent illness. There is no history of trauma or ingestion of a toxin, although the latter must always be considered with children in the preschool-age group. The neurological examination will help rule out trauma or a structural lesion. Metabolic coma (Chapter 27) is often associated with characteristic signs on examination, but diagnosis is largely dependent on laboratory evaluation.

The major task for the physician at this point is to differentiate infectious from postinfectious disorders. Bacterial meningitis can easily be eliminated as a diagnostic consideration, but it is more difficult to rule out viral encephalitis with certainty. Knowledge of the exact nature of the prodromal illness, season of the year, and types of viral infections prevalent in the community are all useful bits of information. As will be discussed, the approach to treatment is generally the same, and an exact etiological diagnosis will make little practical difference. There are exceptions with conditions such as herpesvirus encephalitis, however, in which specific therapy is available.

POSTINFECTIOUS ENCEPHALITIS

Postinfectious encephalitis following *rubeola* has dramatically decreased in incidence in the United States since the introduction of effective measles immunization. The incidence of encephalitis following infection with wild-strain measles is approximately 1/1000 cases. The majority of patients are under 8 years of age, and boys are affected slightly more frequently than girls. The typical presentation, within the first week after the onset of the infection, is with seizures, irritability, and depressed consciousness.

Examination of the CSF generally reveals cell counts up to 500/ml, with lymphocytic preponderance. Glucose content is normal. Protein content is elevated on admission in one-half of patients and rises over the next week in most of the remainder. The γ-globulin component of the CSF protein is increased. EEG is markedly abnormal, with high-voltage slow waves.

Treatment is supportive. This includes strict attention to the patient's cardiorespiratory status, control of intracranial pressure, prompt treatment of seizures, and maintenance of nutrition. There is no proven benefit to the use of corticosteroids. Reported mortality rates have ranged from 10 to 33%. Major sequelae are found in one-third of the survivors, the most frequent including mental retardation, cerebral palsy, seizures, and blindness. Serious behavior disturbances are common.

Identical disorders occur following the other exanthematous diseases of childhood, although they differ in certain specific details. *Mumps* may present as a benign viral meningitis, or as a postinfectious demyelinating encephalitis. It is a fairly mild illness; the only major complication is deafness in a small percentage of cases. *Varicella* and *rubella* encephalitis are both uncommon, but are associated with significant mortality and morbidity. Acute cerebellar ataxia following varicella is the exception; death is most unusual in this syndrome, and the majority of patients make a complete recovery.

A similar disorder also follows respiratory infections in which the specific viral agent is not defined. The term *acute toxic encephalopathy* has been used to refer to children who present with the sudden onset of seizures, coma, and increased intracranial pressure. Pathological examination shows severe cerebral edema, without perivenous demyelination. The majority of reports are from the period prior to the definition of Reye syndrome, so the relationship to that condition is not clear. It should be noted, however, that seizures do not occur in the majority of cases of Reye syndrome.

ACUTE TRANSVERSE MYELITIS

Acute transverse myelitis presents with the sudden onset and rapid progression of signs and symptoms of spinal cord dysfunction. It is grouped with the postinfectious disorders, as it sometimes is preceded by one of the exanthematous diseases and can also be associated with postinfectious encephalitis. A prodromal illness is not always present, however.

Children of any age can be affected, although the incidence is higher in adolescence. There is no predominance by sex. The initial presentation includes weakness, sensory loss, back pain, or radicular pain. The symptoms progress, and maximum paralysis is present within the first 24 hr in one-half of patients. Motor disability is severe in two-thirds of patients, and sensory examination defines a level in all cases. The lesion is most commonly thoracic, but a cervical level is found in 20% of patients.

Lumbar puncture should be approached with great caution. If the patient has an unsuspected mass lesion in the spinal canal, this can precipitate acute paraplegia. Arrangements should be made in advance so that metrizamide can be introduced and myelography carried out. Computerized-tomography (CT) scan of the spine following the introduction of metrizamide also will help in obtaining clear definition of the lesion. The usual finding is swelling of the spinal cord, either localized to one area or rather diffuse. The study is sometimes normal, however.

Findings on examination of the CSF are quite variable. The fluid may be acellular, or there may be several thousand cells present. Either lymphocytes or polymorphonuclear leukocytes can predominate. CSF protein levels are elevated in one-half of patients. The variability in findings suggests that more than one pathophysiological mechanism is involved in this condition.

Death is unusual if the patient is provided with skilled medical and nursing care. No specific treatment appears to provide any benefit. Prognosis for complete recovery is not good, however. Approximately one-third of patients make little or no recovery, one-third a fair recovery, and one-third a good recovery.

GUILLAIN–BARRÉ SYNDROME

The acute onset of polyneuropathy is frequently preceded by a viral infection. A similar condition has been reported following influenza immunization, although the majority of these cases were associated with the use of swine flu vaccine in adults in 1977. The relationship to other strains of influenza vaccine and other types of immunization is less certain. Guillain–Barré syndrome may also follow *Mycoplasma* infections.

Diagnostic criteria were formalized by an ad hoc committee of the National Institutes of Health.[2] Table 13-1 is a summary of this report.

In a typical case the child appears to be recovering uneventfully from an upper respiratory infection. Weakness of the legs is noted when the child begins to stumble and has difficulty walking. There are often some complaints of paresthesiae. The weakness progresses, appearing to ascend the lower extremities and then involve the arms. This is often followed by involvement of the sixth and seventh cranial nerves. Examination reveals weakness and areflexia. Findings on sensory examination are not prominent, although many patients will have slight hypesthesia distally. Unusual associated features include hypertension or hypotension, hyponatremia, and vasomotor symptoms.

The major threat to the patient is ventilatory insufficiency due to weakness of the respiratory muscles. Frequent measurements of vital capacity will allow

TABLE 13-1
Criteria for Diagnosis of Guillain–Barré Syndrome[a]

I. Features required for diagnosis
   A. Progressive motor weakness of more than one limb
   B. Areflexia
II. Features strongly supportive of the diagnosis
   A. Clinical features
      1. Progression
      2. Relative symmetry
      3. Mild sensory signs or symptoms
      4. Cranial nerve involvement
      5. Recovery
      6. Autonomic dysfunction
      7. Absence of fever
   B. CSF features supporting diagnosis
      1. Elevated protein
      2. Few or no cells
   C. Electrodiagnostic features
      1. Nerve conduction slowing or block
III. Features casting doubt on diagnosis
   A. Marked persistent asymmetry
   B. Persistent bowel or bladder dysfunction
   C. Bladder or bowel dysfunction at onset
   D. More than 50 cells/ml in CSF
   E. Presence of PMN in CSF
   F. Sharp sensory level
IV. Features that rule out the diagnosis
   A. Current history of hexacarbon abuse
   B. Abnormal porphyrin metabolism
   C. Recent diphtheritic infection
   D. Evidence of lead intoxication
   E. Occurrence of a purely sensory syndrome
   F. Definite diagnosis of another condition

[a]Modified from Asbury *et al.*[2]

ventilatory support to be instituted before an emergency situation arises. As a general rule, if bulbar musculature becomes involved, or marked weakness of the deltoids is present, intubation and assisted respiration will probably become necessary.

Examination of CSF early in the course of the illness may be normal. The characteristic finding of an elevated protein concentration in an acellular fluid is found almost invariably by the end of the first week.

Supportive treatment in an intensive-care setting is the most important part of management. Although corticosteroids are often administered, controlled studies do not confirm the usefulness of these agents.[3]

There is now evidence in adults that plasmapheresis can shorten the course of the illness and improve the outcome.[4] Maximum benefit is seen if treatment is begun within 7 days of the onset of symptoms, and it is most effective in the severely involved group, that needing mechanical ventilation.

Meticulous attention must be paid to the patient's respiratory status. Excellent skin care to prevent decubitus ulcers, maintenance of optimal nutrition, and physical therapy to prevent contractures are also important. Three-quarters of children will make a complete recovery. The major factor predicting an adverse outcome is the length of time between maximum weakness and the start of recovery. If this is longer than 18 days, there will probably be significant residua.[5]

An unusual variant of the Guillain–Barré syndrome is the *Fisher syndrome*. These children present with ataxia, ophthalmoplegia including ptosis, and areflexia. There is no muscle weakness, and the sensory examination remains normal. CSF examination, like that in the Guillain–Barré syndrome, reveals an elevated protein concentration and few cells. The prognosis for complete recovery is good.

REYE SYNDROME

Reye syndrome is an acute encephalopathy with a stereotyped clinical presentation. The child has a viral infection, frequently varicella or influenza type b. Within a few days following the onset of the illness, the child suddenly begins to vomit and becomes disoriented and irritable. The condition may remain mild or progress rapidly with impairment of consciousness, coma, and irreversible loss of CNS function. The clinical signs are accompanied by a marked increase in intracranial pressure. Seizures and focal neurological signs are uncommon. A system of staging (Table 13-2) has been of value in investigating treatment methods and predicting outcome.[6]

There are a number of laboratory and pathological concomitants of the condition.[7] Serum ammonia is elevated, especially early in the course. The SGOT and SGPT levels are markedly increased, and there often is mild prolongation of the prothrombin time. Bilirubin levels are normal, and there is no other evidence of hepatic dysfunction. Hypoglycemia is occasionally a severe problem, especially in young patients.

TABLE 13-2
Stages of Reye Syndrome[a]

0	Neurologically normal	4	Coma
	Elevated serum transaminases		Decerebrate posturing
1	Lethargy		Pupillary reactions sluggish
	Vomiting		Discs blurred
2	Slurred speech	5	Flaccid and unresponsive
	Alternating agitation and lethargy		Fixed dilated pupils
3	Coma less than 3 hr		Respiratory arrest
	Seizures		
	Babinski signs present		

[a]Modified from Brunner *et al.*[6]

The most characteristic pathological finding is massive accumulation of microvesicular droplets of neutral fat in hepatocytes. There is no evidence of inflammation, necrosis, or cirrhosis. This can easily be seen on liver biopsy. Neuropathological changes are restricted to cerebral edema and its complications, such as uncal herniation.

The etiology of the condition is not clear. Its association with varicella and influenza suggests specific biological effects of those viral agents, but the majority of cases follow common respiratory infections. A pathogenetic role for salicylates has been suggested on the basis of epidemiological studies.[8] These compounds produce mitochondrial injury *in vitro,* similar to that seen in Reye syndrome. A similar disorder occurs with inherited metabolic defects, such as carnitine deficiency, and as a toxic response to certain drugs, such as valproic acid.

The most important aspect of management is effective treatment of increased intracranial pressure. If the child is seriously ill, intracranial pressure monitoring is a vital adjunct. The details of therapy are outlined in Chapter 24. Hypoglycemia should be treated promptly and aggressively. This may require administration of large volumes of a concentrated glucose solution. There appears to be no place at this time for techniques such as exchange transfusion and peritoneal dialysis. It is most probable that Reye syndrome is a generalized metabolic disorder with hepatic and CNS involvement as coprimary effects, and that the neurological symptoms do not represent hepatic encephalopathy.

Mortality and morbidity rates vary considerably over time, even in the same center. Data are also difficult to analyze because of constant changes in treatment protocols. One consistent finding is that the mortality rate varies directly with the stage of illness on admission. The outcome for those patients who survive appears quite good, although cognitive deficits and attention deficit disorder have been reported as sequelae in the patients who were youngest at the time of the illness.[9]

POSTIMMUNIZATION COMPLICATIONS

A major area of controversy is the role of pertussis immunization in producing an encephalopathy and infantile spasms. A demyelinating encephalopathy appears to occur in 1/300,000 children receiving DTP immunization. There is no evidence for an association with myoclonic seizures. The current recommendation is that there be no change in immunization schedules for most children. Pertussis remains a serious disease and can itself be associated with a severe encephalopathy, chronic pulmonary disease, and death. Subsequent doses of pertussis vaccine should not be administered if the child has a convulsion, frank encephalopathy, fever greater than 40.5°C, or a period of several hours of inconsolable crying following the injection. There is no contraindication to immunizing most children with static neurological deficits.

Tetanus antitoxin has been reported to produce a painful brachial neuritis. Paralysis of the arm is severe, and the course of recovery is prolonged.

Trivalent poliomyelitis vaccine contains live attenuated viruses. Acute paralytic disease occurs in the child or a close contact in 1/3 million doses. This vaccine should not be given to children with diseases producing immunological incompetence or who are taking immunosuppressive drugs. The vaccine also is contraindicated if a sibling or other family member has abnormalities of the immune system.

Postvaccinial neurological complications should no longer exist with the elimination of any need for smallpox vaccination. The use of human diploid cell rabies vaccine should eliminate most, if not all, of the neurological complications associated with the older vaccines which contained CNS tissue.

MULTIPLE SCLEROSIS

Multiple sclerosis is one of the disorders considered to have an immunological basis. It is quite rare in prepubertal children and young adolescents. As is the case with adults, motor impairment is the most common initial symptom. This is typically either ataxia or a myelopathy with spastic paraparesis. Optic neuritis is another early symptom. Approximately one-third of children with optic neuritis will eventually develop multiple sclerosis. The typical course of remissions and exacerbations is important diagnostically.

Laboratory studies are useful, but not definitive. There is an elevated IgG level in the CSF with oligoclonal bands. Myelin basic protein can also be demonstrated. CT scan may show hypodense lesions in the white matter, but is not very sensitive. Magnetic resonance imaging scans clearly demonstrate large numbers of plaques and show findings identical to those in adult cases.

The most frequently used treatment protocols involve administration of immunosuppressive agents or corticosteroids. Although these may shorten individual attacks, there is no evidence that the long-term course of the illness is significantly modified.

REFERENCES

1. Partin, J. C., Schubert, W. K., and Partin, J. S., 1971, Mitochondrial ultrastructure in Reye's syndrome (encephalopathy and fatty degeneration of the viscera), *N. Engl. J. Med.* **285:**1339–1343.
2. Asbury, A. K., Arnason, B. G. W., Karp, H. R., and McFarlin, D. E., 1978, Criteria for diagnosis of Guillain–Barré syndrome, *Ann. Neurol.* **6:**565–566.
3. Gracey, D. R., McMichan, J. C., Divertic, N. B., and Howard, F. M., 1982, Respiratory failure in Guillain–Barré syndrome: A six-year experience, *Mayo Clin. Proc.* **67:**742–746.
4. Guillain–Barré Syndrome Study Group, 1985, Plasmapheresis and acute Guillain–Barré syndrome, *Neurology* **35:**1096–1104.
5. Eberle, E., Brink, J., Azen, S., and White, D., 1975, Early predictors of incomplete recovery in children with Guillain–Barré polyneuritis, *J. Pediatr.* **86:**356–359.
6. Brunner, R. L., O'Grady, D. J., Partin, J. C., Partin, J. S., and Schubert, W. K., 1979, Neuropsychologic consequences of Reye syndrome, *J. Pediatr.* **95:**706–711.
7. DeLong, G. R., and Glick, T. N., 1982, Encephalopathy of Reye's syndrome: A review of pathogenetic hypotheses, *Pediatrics* **69:**53–63.

8. Hurwitz, E. S., Barrett, M. J., Bregman, D., Gunn, W. J., Schonberger, L. B., Fairweather, W. R., Drage, J. S., LaMontagne, J. R., Kaslow, R. A., Burlington, D. B., Quinnan, G. V., Parker, R. A., Phillips, K., Pinsky, P., Dayton, D., and Dowdle, D. R., 1985, Public Health Service Study in Reye's syndrome and medications: Report of the pilot phase, *N. Engl. J. Med.* **313**:849–857.
9. Shaywitz, S. E., Cohen, P. M., Cohen, D. J., Mikkelson, E., and Morowitz, G., 1982, Long-term consequences of Reye syndrome: A sibling-matched controlled study of neurologic, cognitive, academic and psychiatric function, *J. Pediatr.* **100**:41–46.

ADDITIONAL READING

Fenichel, G. M., 1982, Neurological complications of immunization, *Ann. Neurol.* **12**:119–128.

14

Trauma to the Nervous System

Head trauma is a major cause of morbidity and mortality in childhood and adolescence. Children are active and attempt to explore and master their environment, but have poorly developed motor skills and limited judgment. Although adolescents have better developed motor skills, the other factors increasing the risk of injury are still operative. When these behavioral characteristics are associated with the use of motor vehicles, and often alcohol and other drugs, the chances of suffering a serious injury obviously become greatly increased.

The importance of the problem of prevention of head and spine trauma cannot be overestimated. Accidents are the most common cause of death in children. Forty percent of serious injuries involve the head, and at least 200,000 children are hospitalized each year for treatment of such injuries. Many of these accidents can be prevented. The easiest and single most important approach is the use of seat belts or infant seats for all passengers. Other areas in which education and supervision are important are contact sports, gymnastics, the use of bicycles and motorcycles, horseback riding, and any activity involving climbing.

The consequences of trauma to the central nervous system can be devastating. Seriously injured tissue will not regenerate. Even though a certain degree of functional plasticity is apparent in some systems, recovery following severe head injuries is usually not complete.

The skull is a rather rigid structure enclosing a space filled with brain, cerebrospinal fluid, and blood which is contained within the intracranial vasculature. The system has low compliance, and brain swelling, obstruction of the flow of CSF, or the presence of a mass such as a hematoma causes a rapid rise in intracranial pressure. When intracranial pressure approaches the mean arterial pressure, vascular perfusion of the brain becomes inadequate, anoxic–ischemic damage is superimposed, additional brain swelling occurs, and a disastrous cycle is initiated.

Increased intracranial pressure also causes a shift of intracranial contents. Herniation of brain under the falx, through the tentorial notch, or into the foramen magnum results. This produces vascular compromise with infarction of the compressed tissue, and further brain swelling. Direct compression of the brain stem causes hemorrhage which leads to irreversible coma or death.

APPROACH TO THE PATIENT

The initial diagnostic approach to the patient with head trauma is to search for each of three interrelated types of injury. These are trauma to the bony skull, brain damage, and the presence of a space-occupying hematoma.

The history, the physical and neurological examinations, and knowledge of the mechanism of the injury are useful in predicting the type and severity of brain damage. Trauma produced by an object striking the head usually causes focal damage to the brain lying directly under the point of impact. An acceleration injury, caused by a force suddenly moving the head, or a deceleration injury, produced when the rapidly moving head strikes a fixed object, often causes more serious damage. Brain may be injured directly under the point of the blow, at the opposite pole (contracoup injury), or diffusely as a result of shearing forces.

Brief loss of consciousness does not necessarily indicate that a serious injury has been sustained, but prolonged coma is an adverse prognostic sign. If there are no witnesses to the accident, loss of consciousness can be suspected if post-traumatic amnesia is present. The patient will not remember the traumatic episode itself and will be amnestic for a variable period of time both before and after the accident. The period of posttraumatic amnesia correlates well with the severity of the injury and the duration of loss of consciousness. It is essential to remember, however, that a patient who does not lose consciousness at the time of the trauma still can die of the injury, either from the development of an intracranial hematoma or from cerebral edema.

The general physical examination is initially directed toward discovering other traumatic injuries which take priority in treatment. Airway, cardiac output, and circulating blood volume must be adequate before attention is turned toward the central nervous system. If the patient has effective spontaneous respirations but is hypotensive, this is almost invariably due to blood loss, externally, into a body cavity, or into soft tissues. Only if the brain stem is damaged to the extent that the patient is apneic should a central cause for the hypotension be considered and, even then, only when hypovolemic shock has been ruled out.

The neurological examination is used to define the level of consciousness (Chapter 27) and to search for focal neurological signs. If present, these indicate that there are focal areas of damage, either contusions or lacerations, or compression of brain by a hematoma. Spinal cord injury is caused by many of the same types of accidents that produce head trauma, and this possibility should always be carefully evaluated.

The major underlying principle when treating a patient who has suffered head trauma is straightforward. The secondary effects of cerebral edema and intracranial hematomas must be prevented. The ability to do this depends, of course, on the early diagnosis of these conditions.

Emergency management is the same as that for any comatose patient. Respiratory and circulatory status must be monitored and supported. Repeated neurological examinations and a systematized approach to assessing changes in the level of consciousness are the most important tools for following the patient's progress and determining the need for further diagnostic studies and intervention. Monitoring for the development of increased intracranial pressure, and its management, are discussed in Chapter 24. This is absolutely essential to assure the best possible quality of survival.

If the patient is awake and alert, there has been no significant loss of consciousness, and no focal neurological signs are present, there is no indication for further diagnostic studies. A skull fracture is rarely present in such a clinical setting and, even if found, would mandate no specific therapy.[1] Skull roentgenograms should be obtained if there is significant scalp trauma or a palpable depression of the skull, as a depressed fracture may require surgical intervention.

The initial neurodiagnostic evaluation of the comatose patient should include x-ray studies of the skull and cervical spine and computerized tomography of the head. Computerized tomography (CT) should be performed with contrast enhancement, as extravasated blood may be isodense with brain.

There is rarely any need to obtain other diagnostic studies during the acute phase following head trauma. Lumbar puncture is contraindicated unless the need to rule out an intracranial infection is overwhelming. Electroencephalography adds little at this time.

HEAD TRAUMA

Skull Injury

Injury to the skull is not always associated with injury to the underlying brain, but a skull fracture indicates that the blow to the head had considerable force and that the patient must be carefully monitored. *Linear skull fractures* occur in any portion of the cranial vault. If they cross a major venous sinus or the groove containing the middle meningeal vessels, close observation for the development of a hematoma is necessary. No specific treatment for the fracture is required, and the majority heal within a year or 2.

Leptomeningeal cyst, or "growing fracture," occurs most commonly in children under 4 years of age.[2] The fracture is typically in the temporal area, and rather than healing, it begins to enlarge. This is probably the result of herniation of arachnoid into the fracture line through a tear in the dura at the time of the original trauma. The pulsations of the brain, transmitted through the spinal fluid, erode the bony margins (Figure 14-1). Surgical treatment is required to remove the cyst and repair the dura. An underlying area of brain atrophy may lead to development of a seizure disorder.

Subgaleal hygroma presents within several days of the occurrence of a skull fracture. The child appears well but rapidly develops a soft swelling of the scalp, which is limited only by the attachment of the galea. In this case, both dura and

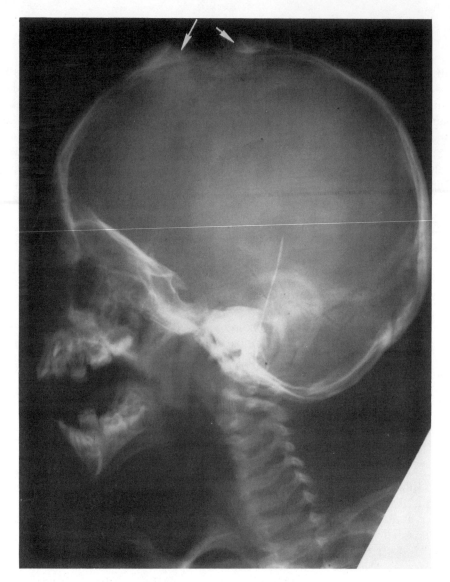

FIGURE 14-1. Leptomeningeal cyst following a skull fracture in the frontal region near the midline. The bone erosion is indicated by the arrows.

arachnoid have been torn and cerebrospinal fluid collects under the scalp. This resolves spontaneously within a few weeks and needs no specific treatment.

Depressed fractures of the skull may be difficult to diagnose unless a roentgenogram is taken tangential to the area of trauma. If the bony fragments are depressed by an amount equal to the thickness of the bone, surgical intervention is required. Surgery is generally also performed if the neurological examination gives evidence of a cerebral contusion underlying the area of injury. Finally, if there is a *compound fracture,* operative debridement is mandatory. Surgery is generally avoided if the fracture is over a major dural sinus.

It is difficult to make a diagnosis of *basilar skull fracture.* These cannot generally be seen on routine radiological examination of the skull. The most useful clinical signs are cerebrospinal fluid rhinorrhea or otorrhea and discoloration of the mastoids due to the presence of blood (Battle sign). The fluid is usually blood-tinged at first and then becomes clear. Rhinorrhea will not be obvious if the fluid drips into the back of the throat and is swallowed, although this may present as a night cough. The drainage can be distinguished from clear mucoid rhinorrhea by the higher glucose content of cerebrospinal fluid. If the leak does not spontaneously stop within a period of several weeks, surgical repair of the dura is usually attempted, although the procedure is difficult and not always successful. The major complication of a basilar skull fracture is meningitis, most frequently caused by *Streptococcus pneumoniae.* The usefulness of prophylactic antibiotics in preventing meningitis is an unresolved controversy.[3]

Brain Injury

The least serious type of brain injury is *concussion.* This is manifested by transient loss of consciousness without evidence of focal neurological signs. By definition, there is no identifiable structural damage. Recovery is rapid and complete except for the presence of a variable amount of posttraumatic amnesia. This decreases as time passes.

Patients sometimes develop a posttraumatic syndrome following a concussion. The features include irritability, difficulty concentrating, sleep disturbances, complaints of dizziness, and headache. These symptoms are self-limited, although they may persist for several months. Subtle cognitive and attention deficits can cause difficulty with schoolwork, and this should be considered if scholastic performance declines. The traumatic injury also may trigger migraine headaches in a patient who was not previously affected. The development of headaches following head trauma is always a cause for concern, however, and the patient requires careful evaluation.

Cerebral contusion, as the term implies, represents bruising of brain with damage to tissue and intraparenchymal bleeding. This is commonly seen in contracoup lesions, and most frequently involves the tips of the frontal and temporal lobes. Contusions are also found underlying the point of impact of the trauma. Focal neurological signs are always indicative of contusion, laceration, or compression of brain by an intracranial mass lesion. If the temporal lobes are involved, a defect in memory is present and may be unaccompanied by motor or sensory findings on examination. Contusions of the frontal lobes produce personality changes, often apathy and lack of motivation. Symptomatic contusions of the occipital poles are unusual; cortical blindness, diagnosed clinically by the absence of useful functional vision in the presence of normal pupillary responses, is characteristic.

Cerebral laceration is often accompanied by an *intracerebral hematoma.* This should be suspected if the patient has prolonged depression of the state of consciousness, unequivocal focal neurological signs, or increased intracranial pressure. The role of surgery in treatment is not clear, but a progressively enlarging hematoma will be evacuated by most surgeons.

Penetrating wounds combine the features of compound fracture of the skull, cerebral laceration, and intracerebral hematoma. Surgical exploration to achieve hemostasis, debride dead tissue, and remove foreign material is mandatory.

Intracranial Hematomas

The classic clinical picture of *epidural hematoma* has been well described. The patient is rendered transiently unconscious from the blow and then seems to recover. Following a latent interval of several hours, there is rapid onset of hemiparesis, a contralateral third-nerve palsy, and coma. Radiographic examination of the skull reveals a linear fracture which crosses the groove of the middle meningeal vessels.

Unfortunately, however, this scenario is rather rare in childhood. There is often no latent interval. More commonly, the child is unconscious continuously from the time of the impact and then progressively deteriorates. A fracture is observed only one-half of the time when skull roentgenograms are obtained. Epidural hematoma should, therefore, always be considered whenever a patient deteriorates following head trauma.

Diagnosis is by CT (Figure 14-2), and treatment requires surgical removal of the hematoma and coagulation of the injured vessels. If deterioration is rapid and CT or angiography is not readily available, an emergency attempt to evacuate the hematoma through twist-drill or burr-hole exploration may be lifesaving.

Subdural hematomas take two forms. *Acute subdural hematomas* are present immediately following trauma and are rarely large but are usually associated with an underlying cerebral contusion or laceration. Surgery is not indicated unless there is progressive enlargement with an increasing mass effect.

Chronic subdural hematomas are generally found in younger children, especially those under 2 years of age. If no history of significant injury can be obtained, the child should be carefully studied for other evidence of trauma or possible physical abuse.

The major clinical features are an abnormally enlarging head circumference, tense fontanelle, irritability, and lethargy. Retinal hemorrhages and focal neurological signs are frequently found. The presence of iron deficiency anemia, from blood loss into the subdural space, is common, especially in infants. CT has replaced subdural taps as the preferred diagnostic technique (Figure 14-3).

There is controversy concerning the most appropriate therapeutic intervention. It is now no longer routine to perform craniotomy and stripping of the membranes that surround the subdural hematoma. If the child is doing well clinically, is developing normally, and is not showing signs of increased intracra-

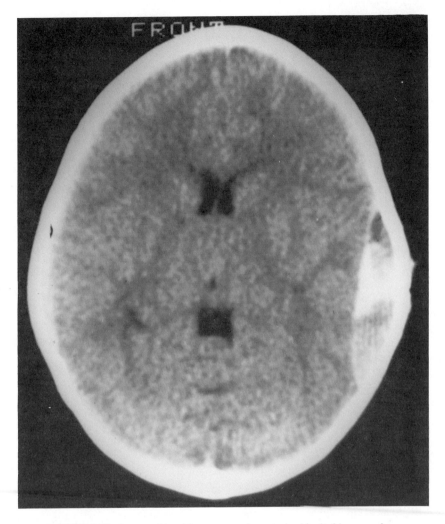

FIGURE 14-2. Acute epidural hematoma, characterized by its biconvex shape.

nial pressure or excessively rapid head growth, a conservative approach can be taken and follow-up CT obtained. If the child's progress is not optimal, or if the hematomas do not resolve or they enlarge, periodic tapping is attempted. If this is not successful, placement of a shunt from the hematoma to the peritoneal cavity is carried out.

Outcome of Head Trauma

A number of prognostic factors assist in predicting outcome following closed head injury. Negative predictors include a coma score less than 8 (Chapter 27) and the presence of signs indicating structural damage to the brain stem.

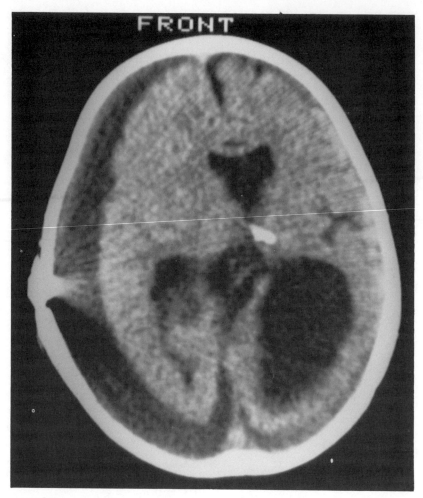

FIGURE 14-3. Large, chronic subdural hematoma with associated midline shift and ventricular enlargement.

With a coma score below 8, the mortality for children is between 5% and 10%. The prognosis for physical independence is poor if coma lasts for more than 3 months.[4] Children under 2 years of age have a worse outcome than older patients.[5]

Despite statements to the contrary, children are very susceptible to neuropsychological deficits produced by head injury.[6] School performance frequently declines, and major deficits are found in memory and motor skills. Behavior disturbances are common.

Seizures restricted to the first 24 hr following head trauma are not an index of the severity of the injury, and not necessarily a forerunner of posttraumatic epilepsy. There is no need for long-term anticonvulsant prophylaxis. If seizures appear after 24–48 hr, they should be treated vigorously, and maintenance therapy begun.

One of the least favorable outcomes of head injury is the persistent vegetative state. This is discussed in Chapter 27.

SPINAL TRAUMA

Trauma to the spinal column and spinal cord can be viewed from the same perspective as that outlined for head trauma. There may be involvement of the bony spine, injury to the spinal cord, or an extramedullary mass which compresses the cord. These can occur independently or in any combination. Although these injuries are rare in children, they have a devastating impact on the child's life.

Spinal column injury results in fracture, dislocation, or both. The mechanisms are complex and depend on whether the child suffers a penetrating wound, is struck on the back, is knocked down or thrown through the air, or falls from a height. The final result can be

- Compression of a vertebral body
- Fracture through a posterior element
- Dislocation of a vertebral body
- Dislocation of an articular facet
- Herniation of an intervertebral disc

Each of these can occur with or without involvement of the spinal cord.

Radiological evidence of injury to the spinal column is rarely found in the first few months of life. Children from the age of 6–7 months up to 7–9 years present a number of unique problems in diagnosis and manifest different types of injuries than older patients.

There are three major diagnostic problems. First, the bony elements of the spine are not completely ossified. There is some variability in the pattern of development of ossification centers, and synchondroses are often incorrectly thought to be fractures. In the physiological situation, however, the bony margins cannot be placed in apposition to "reconstruct" the bone. The rough edges of a fracture would appear to fit together as if they were pieces of a puzzle. The lack of ossification in the subdental synchondrosis, where the odontoid process attaches to the centrum of C_2, is frequently mistaken for a fracture.

The second problem arises from the normal laxity of ligaments found in young children. This permits degrees of slippage and angulation between vertebrae which are normal but would not be acceptable in an adult. The problem is most common at the C_{2-3} and C_{3-4} levels.

A useful technique for differentiating this pseudodislocation from a traumatic lesion is to construct a line between the most posterior portion of the neural canals of C_1 and C_3. The analogous point on the C_2 vertebra should fall within 1 mm of this line. Deviations of 2 mm or more are almost always abnormal.[7]

Finally, diagnosis is made difficult because the majority of injuries occur in the upper cervical spine, and this area is difficult to visualize on routine x-ray studies. If there is any doubt, tomograms or a CT scan should be obtained.

The most frequent spine fracture of the young child is through the subdental synchondrosis. Symptoms are unimpressive. Examination shows some limitation of motion and tenderness on deep palpation of the upper neck. Spinal cord injury rarely occurs. X-ray studies reveal anterior angulation of the odontoid process. Immobilization allows healing in 6–8 weeks.

Fractures through the pedicle of C_2 are also relatively common in this age group. If there is no associated damage to ligaments, immobilization for 6–8 weeks is adequate therapy. With significant anterior slippage of C_2 on C_3, however, more rigid methods of immobilization of the neck in extension for a longer period of time are necessary. Major instability mandates surgical intervention.

Disruption of the atlas (C_1) with displacement of the lateral masses occurs from blows on the top of the head. The abnormality is best seen on an open-mouth anterior–posterior x-ray study. With displacement of 3–4 mm, healing is satisfactory following 6–8 weeks of immobilization. If there is greater displacement, an initial period of skeletal traction should precede casting.

Fixed torticollis due to rotatory dislocation of the atlantoaxial joint presents with a painless head tilt. The problem usually begins following an upper respiratory infection with pharyngitis, but can be traumatic in origin. This disorder generally resolves spontaneously; if not, reduction is assisted by traction.

Atlantoaxial instability, beyond the usual physiological limits, can be congenital or can occur following inflammatory foci in the neck or pharynx. It is also found in 10–20% of all children with Down syndrome. The degree of risk of spinal cord damage following injury to the neck in these cases is not clear, but appears to be relatively low.

The major points concerning spine trauma in young children can be summarized as follows: the nature of the injury differs from that seen in older individuals, the upper cervical spine is most commonly involved, and associated spinal cord damage is rare. X-ray diagnosis is difficult because of incomplete ossification and normal ligamentous laxity. It is also important to note that when spinal cord injury does occur in children in this age group, no obvious bony injury can be identified in up to 60% of cases.

The causes and mechanisms of spinal injuries in children older than 7–9 years of age are identical to those occurring in adolescents and adults. The history is usually dramatic and suggests the possibility of spinal trauma. Bony damage occurs in the midcervical or lower cervical regions and is frequently associated with damage to the spinal cord. There are fewer diagnostic problems with x-ray studies, as ossification is largely complete and the physiological hypermobility seen in younger children is gone.

The first goal of acute management is to stabilize the spine and prevent or minimize spinal cord injury. As in the case of any serious trauma, pulse, respirations, and blood pressure must be maintained at acceptable levels. Attention is then turned to other injuries.

Definitive management depends on the architecture of the injury and whether or not the spinal cord has been damaged. If there is little or no displacement and the spinal column is stable, traction or casting allows adequate healing. With major displacement or instability, operative intervention is necessary to allow reduction of the fracture, removal of bony fragments, and fusion of unstable elements. There are many long-term complications of spinal surgery in growing children, and this step is only taken if absolutely necessary. Problems include inadequate growth of the spine, scoliosis, and disc herniation at levels above and below the area of fusion.

The major types of *spinal cord injury* are analogous to those involving the brain. *Concussion* is rare, and the diagnosis is only certain after there has been complete rapid recovery.

Contusion is associated with a varying degree of permanent deficit. Compression of the spinal cord can occur as a result of vertebral dislocation, impingement of bony fragments, or hemorrhage and is almost always associated with some degree of contusion. The final functional status cannot be determined until the compression is relieved and there has been sufficient time for maximal recovery. This takes several months. *Central cord contusion,* usually following a flexion or extension injury, is analogous to an intracerebral hematoma.

Laceration is rare, except in the case of penetrating wounds or major distraction and dislocation of bony structures. Despite intensive research and dramatic claims from other countries, there is no evidence that functional recovery is ever obtained below the level of the lesion.

Extramedullary lesions compressing the spinal cord are a frequent pathogenetic factor in spinal injuries. The mass effect can result from bony fracture or dislocation, disc herniation, or a hematoma. Significant compression is a clear indication for surgical intervention.

The signs and symptoms of spinal cord injury are dramatic. They result primarily from interruption of the conducting mechanisms of the cord, both ascending and descending, with partial or complete loss of motor and sensory function below the level of the lesion. If there is a significant longitudinal extent to the cord injury, signs of segmental denervation are found and provide useful localizing information. Damage to nerve roots in the area is associated with severe pain; this is also a good tool for determining the level of the lesion.

A careful neurological examination is required to set both the motor and sensory level. This is important for immediate care and to focus the diagnostic evaluation. Cord injury above the level of C_4 is rapidly fatal, as the diaphragm and intercostal muscles are paralyzed. Low-cervical and high-thoracic lesions impair respiratory efficiency, the severity being directly proportional to the level of the damage.

A confounding factor in the early evaluation of a patient with spinal cord injury is *spinal shock*. Immediately following the trauma there is paralysis with flaccidity and areflexia below the involved level. This state is present for a number of weeks, and as it begins to resolve, the more typical signs of spasticity develop. At that time it becomes possible to determine whether the lesion is incomplete and whether there has been any return of function.

Abnormalities of autonomic function regularly accompany spinal cord injury. These include paralytic ileus, atonic bladder, spontaneous fluctuations in blood pressure, and vasomotor disturbances. Any of these problems are serious and are more pronounced with high lesions.

Central cord contusion in the cervical region results in flaccid paralysis of the upper extremities and spasticity of the legs. The intramedullary position of the lesion allows sacral sparing, so that bladder and bowel function and perineal sensation are preserved.

Neonatal spinal cord injury is rare. The most common pathogenetic mechanism is hyperextension of the body on the head during breech delivery. This produces a fracture and dislocation at the cervicothoracic junction. The almost routine use of elective cesarean section when there is a breech presentation has now all but eliminated this complication. Spinal cord damage at the craniocervical junction has also been reported following vertex deliveries, but is rare.

X-ray studies of the spine are usually normal, despite serious damage to the spinal cord. This is probably partially due to the large amount of cartilage in the vertebrae in the first few months of life and ligamentous laxity which allows neurological damage without radiological evidence of a fracture or dislocation.

The major diagnostic tools in evaluating spinal trauma are routine x-ray studies of the spine and CT scan. The scan visualizes the bony structures and spinal cord with good resolution. If better definition is needed, metrizamide is instilled into the spinal subarachnoid space. Following this, both routine myelography and another CT scan are performed. Magnetic resonance imaging scanning appears to have great promise for defining lesions of the spinal cord, as bone does not interfere with definition of soft tissue structures. Sensory evoked potentials are useful aids in the diagnosis of partial lesions of the spinal cord.

The acute management of spinal injury requires, as noted, stabilization of the spine, support of vital functions, and treatment of other injuries. A number of pharmacological approaches have been used in an attempt to minimize damage to the cord. These include administration of naloxone[8] and large doses of dexamethasone. The efficacy of these drugs has not been fully evaluated. The role of decompression laminectomy remains controversial. If there is impingement on the cord by fragments of bone or a large hematoma, surgery is indicated.

Management and rehabilitation of patients with spinal trauma is complex and requires a specialized setting and experienced personnel. The treatment program includes physical rehabilitation, training in self-help skills, bowel and bladder care, skin care, psychological counseling, and continuation of the child's education. For older children, vocational counseling is also necessary. As soon as the patient's condition is stabilized, transfer to an appropriate center is mandatory.

PERIPHERAL NERVE TRAUMA

There are three levels of severity of trauma to peripheral nerves.[9] Temporary loss of function, typically in response to pressure on the nerve trunk, is *neurapraxia*. This is rapidly reversible and leaves no residual deficit. *Axonotmesis* implies that axons have degenerated but that the Schwann tubes and connective tissue support of the nerve remain intact. In this instance, functional recovery is usually excellent, although the course may be prolonged.

In *neurotmesis* the physical integrity of the nerve is destroyed. Degeneration of myelin (Wallerian degeneration) occurs distal to that point. Regeneration is dependent on surgical anastomosis of the nerve. Axonal regrowth is slow and often inaccurate. If the distance to be traversed is large, irreversible atrophy of the muscles occurs before innervation can take place.

The etiology of a traumatic neuropathy may be obvious or require careful exploration of the history. This is directed toward finding events that could have compressed, stretched, lacerated, or torn the involved nerve. A detailed examination of the strength of individual muscles identifies the specific nerve or nerves, roots, or portion of the plexus involved. This is possible because little variation exists in nerve–muscle relationships. Other features of nerve damage include areflexia and, eventually, atrophy. Sensory abnormalities are variable and depend on the type and degree of damage and the nerve affected.

Direct *trauma* to a nerve is relatively rare, except as part of an accident causing multiple injuries. Lacerations can occur if a limb goes through a broken window. Stab wounds are seen in adolescents with some regularity. These often involve the brachial plexus.

Nerves are in close proximity to bones in certain areas and can be injured if the bone is fractured. Most frequently involved are the radial nerve at the level of the midshaft of the humerus, the ulnar nerve at the elbow, and the common peroneal nerve at the head of the fibula.

Compression neuropathy also occurs most commonly at areas where nerves are near bones. These lesions have been reported following improper positioning during surgery, the use of restraints, and the use of splints or casts.

Injection neuropathy is usually a result of misplaced gluteal injection and involves the sciatic nerve. There is immediate severe pain and paralysis of all muscles in the sciatic distribution. This site is now rarely used for injections in children. Most injections are given in the lateral aspect of the thigh. Unfortunately, trauma to the femoral nerve has been reported when this technique is performed incorrectly.

A serious, but fortunately rare, complication of peripheral nerve injury is *reflex sympathetic dystrophy*.[10] The clinical features are burning pain, swelling, dystrophic skin and nail changes, and vasomotor phenomena in the affected extremity. Motion is limited. X-ray studies show patchy areas of bone demineralization. The condition can be severely incapacitating, and treatment is not satisfactory. Steroids and sympathectomy are most commonly used.

REFERENCES

1. Leonidas, J. C., Ting, W., Binkiewicz, A., Vaz, R., Scott, R. M., and Pauker, S. G., 1982, Mild head trauma in children: When is a roentgenogram necessary? *Pediatrics* **69:**139–143.
2. Rothman, L., Rose, J. S., Laster, D. W., Quencer, R., and Tenner, M., 1976, The spectrum of growing skull fracture in children, *Pediatrics* **57:**26–31.
3. Einhorn, A., and Mizrahi, E. M., 1978, Basilar skull fractures in children, *Am. J. Dis. Child.* **132:**1121–1124.
4. Brink, J. D., Imbus, C., Woo-San, J., 1980, Physical recovery after severe closed head trauma in children and adolescents, *J. Pediatr.* **97:**721–727.
5. Mahoney, W. J., D'Souza, B. J., Heller, J. A., Rogers, M. C., Epstein, M. H., and Freeman, J. M., 1983, Long-term outcome of children with severe head trauma and prolonged coma, *Pediatrics* **71:**756–762.
6. Fuld, P. A., and Fisher, P., 1977, Recovery of intellectual ability after closed head injury, *Dev. Med. Child. Neurol.* **19:**495–502.
7. Swischuck, L. E., 1977, Anterior displacement of C_2 in children: Physiologic or pathologic? *Radiology* **122:**759–763.
8. Faden, A. I., Jacobs, T. P., Mougey, E., and Holaday, J. W., 1981, Endorphins in experimental spinal injury: Therapeutic effect of naloxone, *Ann. Neurol.* **10:**326–332.
9. Gilliatt, R. W., 1981, Physical injury to peripheral nerves, *Mayo Clin. Proc.* **56:**361–370.
10. Kozin, F., Haughton, V., and Ryan, L., 1977, The reflex sympathetic dystrophy syndrome in a child, *J. Pediatr.* **90:**417–419.

ADDITIONAL READING

Levin, H. S., Benton, A. L., and Grossman, R. G., 1982, *Neurobehavioral Consequences of Closed Head Injury,* Oxford University Press, New York.
Singer, H. S., and Freeman, J. M., 1978, Head trauma and the pediatrician, *Pediatrics* **62:**819–825.

15

Vascular Disease

Vascular disease involving the nervous system in children is relatively rare, but often devastating when it occurs. The fundamental principles, clinical features, and laboratory findings are similar to those in adults, although there are a number of important differences. The etiological factors that are the most common in adults, arteriosclerosis and hypertension, rarely are the cause of cerebrovascular disease in children. In the pediatric age group, underlying medical disorders are more likely to be present. The pathophysiology of intracranial hemorrhage in premature infants has no counterpart in older individuals. Prognosis is also somewhat different for children, with plasticity and other developmental phenomena allowing for degrees of improvement that would be unusual in adults.

The brain is particularly sensitive to interruption of its blood supply. Cerebral blood flow in young children is approximately 100 ml/100 g per min, nearly 60% greater than that of adults. Cerebral metabolism is almost entirely aerobic with glucose used as the only substrate under ordinary conditions. There is little glycogen stored in brain, so maintenance of function depends on continuous delivery of oxygen and glucose. Cessation of the circulation also leads to accumulation of lactic acid and other metabolites, which may be an additional factor in producing cell damage.

Ischemic damage or the presence of an intracerebral hemorrhage causes breakdown of the blood–brain barrier and cerebral edema. Elevation of intracranial pressure ensues and can further compromise blood flow and compound the damage.

Arterial thrombosis produces infarction without significant hemorrhage. Edema surrounding the infarct causes temporary loss of function of nearby cerebral tissue, and it is not unusual to see improvement as the process begins to resolve. Venous thrombosis is usually associated with hemorrhage and a great deal of edema. Venous thromboses tend to propagate and involve contiguous venous structures, and progressive deterioration typically occurs with this type of stroke.

Embolism, as might be expected, presents with the acute onset of a neurological deficit. Following a delay, the embolus will often break apart and travel to more distant vessels. This produces an additional deficit and secondary deterioration due to hemorrhage into the infarcted brain. Intracranial hemorrhage also presents acutely. Signs suggesting hemorrhage are the presence of severe headache and meningeal irritation.

Intraventricular and subependymal hemorrhage (IVH/SEH) in the premature infant is the result of a complex series of events. Hypoxia and ischemia due to respiratory problems and systemic hypotension are probably the major precipitating factors. Arteriolar dilation and loss of autoregulation, the brain's ability to control cerebral blood flow, occur. Restoration of systemic circulatory integrity then causes rupture of capillaries in the damaged, highly vascular, subependymal germinal layer which is present in immature brains. This subependymal hemorrhage may then rupture into the lateral ventricles.

APPROACH TO THE PATIENT

The tasks facing the clinician when a child presents with the acute onset of a focal neurological deficit or evidence of subarachnoid hemorrhage include the following:

- Determine whether the lesion is vascular.
- Search for underlying systemic disease.
- Prevent secondary damage.

The standard neurological examination is the primary tool for determining the localization of the lesion underlying a focal neurological deficit. The examination should also be used to carefully search for signs of increased intracranial pressure and meningeal irritation.

Computerized tomography (CT) of the head now plays a central role as the initial diagnostic technique applied to patients with acute neurological disease. Early in the course of the illness, it rules out unsuspected conditions such as brain tumors or traumatic lesions, determines whether a hematoma is present, and demonstrates a shift of intracranial contents across the midline if there is a mass effect or significant cerebral edema. The area of infarction itself usually will not be clearly defined for several days, so it may be necessary to repeat the study and to use contrast enhancement.

Cerebral arteriography remains the best method for defining the vascular lesion and should be strongly considered in all patients with a stroke. Digital subtraction angiography is now being performed in children. This provides images with good resolution and obviates the need for intraarterial injections. Lumbar puncture is useful only if it is necessary to document the presence of a subarachnoid hemorrhage or there is concern that an intracranial infection is present. If CT and angiography are planned, lumbar puncture is superfluous in most cases. It should be avoided or carried out with the greatest caution if increased intracranial pressure is present.

TABLE 15-1
Medical Conditions Associated with Strokes in Children

Trauma	Collagen–vascular disease
Head	Systemic lupus erythematosus
Neck	Polyarteritis nodosa
Posterior pharynx	Hematological disorders
Fat embolism	Sickle cell disease
Infection	Leukemia
Meningitis	Thrombocytopenia
Metabolic disorders	Polycythemia
Homocystinuria	Cardiac disorders
Dehydration	Cyanotic congenital heart disease
Hyperlipidemia	Mitral valve prolapse

The remainder of the diagnostic evaluation includes a search for underlying medical conditions. Table 15-1 outlines the most important of these.

Prevention of secondary damage is largely dependent on the treatment of increased intracranial pressure. This is discussed fully in Chapter 24.

ACUTE INFANTILE HEMIPLEGIA

This term does not refer to a specific disease process, but to the sudden onset of a stroke in a child, particularly when a specific etiology cannot be defined.[1] Most commonly, a young child, previously well, develops a fever and then several convulsions, either generalized or focal. The patient presents in coma with a profound hemiplegia. A small group of children have a stroke following a single seizure. Approximately one-quarter of the patients have the sudden onset of a motor deficit in the absence of prodromal events.

Neurological examination reveals a dense hemiplegia, usually with hemianopsia and a cortical sensory deficit. Aphasia is associated if there is involvement of the dominant hemisphere.

Vascular abnormalities are visualized on angiography in 65–80% of cases. Extracranial involvement of the common or internal carotid artery is frequently found and appears to be due to a segmental area of arteritis which produces partial or complete occlusion (Figure 15-1). Intracranial vascular abnormalities are usually multiple and due to arteritis or emboli. These lesions are rarely associated with evidence of a systemic arteritis, and their etiology is unknown.

Prognosis is related to the type of clinical presentation, especially the presence of seizures. Children with multiple seizures or a single prolonged seizure are generally left with a severe motor deficit. They are also usually retarded and have a convulsive disorder that is difficult to control. If the onset is associated with a single brief seizure, or seizures do not occur, one-half of the children will make a good recovery. Younger children, in general, have a poor prognosis.

Although a residual motor deficit is common, aphasia almost always resolves, even with extensive damage to the left hemisphere. This recovery is

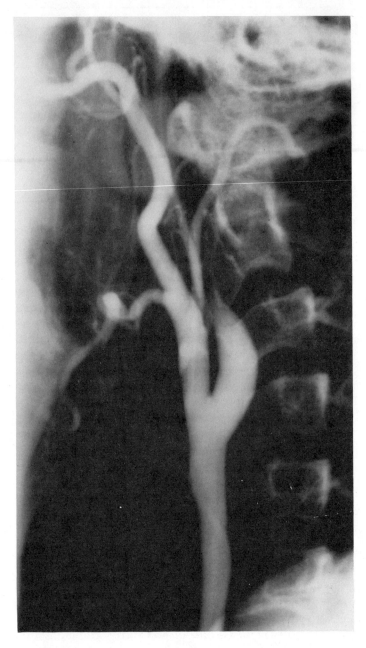

FIGURE 15-1. Complete occlusion of the internal carotid artery in the neck.

most striking in children under 4 years of age. Satisfactory functional recovery is virtually always achieved if the child is under 8 years of age, but the prognosis is less certain for older children. Obviously, a severe deficit in overall cognitive function will also be associated with poor development or recovery of language.

No specific therapy is available at the onset of the stroke, although a number of physiological approaches to attempt to limit damage are being tried. These include blood volume expanders and induced hypertension, hypothermia, and barbiturate coma. The value of these techniques is uncertain at this time.

An intensive rehabilitation effort should always be started as soon as the patient's condition is stable. Seizure control is often difficult. Some patients with a profound motor deficit, uncontrolled seizures, and a behavior disorder will benefit from hemispherectomy.

MOYAMOYA SYNDROME

The presence of transient ischemic attacks or repeated cerebrovascular accidents in children, especially if the involved side alternates, suggests the

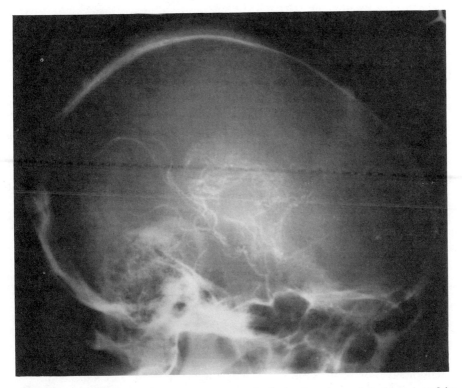

FIGURE 15-2. Moyamoya syndrome with large network of telangiectatic vessels in the region of the diencephalon.

moyamoya syndrome. Arteriography shows progressive occlusion of the vessels of the circle of Willis and a hazy blush of telangiectatic vessels in the basal ganglia (Figure 15-2). This smoky appearance has led to the use of the Japanese term "moyamoya." The condition is progressive, but may be helped by surgical construction of an extracranial–intracranial vascular anastomosis.

An occasional patient has repeated transient ischemic attacks without the development of a fixed deficit. Others have a stroke without prior warning. Seizures are common in young patients.

VERTEBROBASILAR OCCLUSION

Vascular accidents involving the posterior circulation are rare in children. The usual signs are hemiparesis, cerebellar dysfunction, and cranial nerve palsies. Vertigo is a frequent complaint. Etiological factors include cervical spine anomalies, chiropractic manipulation, and any of the factors listed in Table 15-1. One of the most severe residua of vertebrobasilar strokes is the locked-in syndrome, a state of mute quadriplegia with preserved consciousness and awareness of the environment.

Operative correction of coarctation of the aorta can be complicated by a subclavian steal syndrome. There are recurrent episodes of headache, vertigo, and hemianopia. Vertebral angiography demonstrates the abnormal hemodynamics with retrograde flow in the left vertebral and subclavian arteries. Surgical treatment is required. The approach is to ligate the left vertebral artery or construct a subclavian graft.

CAROTID TRAUMA

Trauma to the carotid artery in children can result from blunt trauma to the neck or injury to the artery in the retropharyngeal region. This occurs if the child has a stick in his mouth and falls on it. There is a latent period followed by the sudden onset of a neurological deficit. The trauma causes a tear in the intima of the vessel. Over a period of time there is thrombosis of the artery with embolization or dissection of the vessel wall followed by propagation of a thrombis. Cerebral edema may lead to rapid, and often fatal, deterioration.

SICKLE CELL ANEMIA

Cerebrovascular complications of sickle cell anemia are most frequent in young children and are an important cause of death. The stroke almost always occurs as part of a vasoocclusive crisis and may be preceded by seizures. Subarachnoid hemorrhage is common. The underlying lesion is most commonly white matter infarction secondary to thrombosis of multiple small vessels, but major arteries also can be occluded.

Angiography is associated with an increased risk of complications unless the patient receives a sufficient quantity of transfused red blood cells to reduce the level of hemoglobin S to 20% or less. The child with sickle cell anemia who has had one cerebrovascular accident is quite likely to have repeated episodes. Regular transfusions to keep the level of hemoglobin S below 25% reduce this risk, but may lead to hemosiderosis.[2] Prompt treatment of every sickle cell crisis with adequate hydration and prevention of hypoxia is most important.

CONGENITAL HEART DISEASE

The child with cyanotic congenital heart disease, especially the child under 2 years of age, is at risk for developing venous thrombosis. This problem appears to be most frequent in the face of polycythemia associated with a hypochromic, microcytic anemia. The clinical presentation is with impaired consciousness, seizures, changing neurological signs, and increased intracranial pressure.

The older child with a cyanotic lesion is more prone to have an embolic event. This can result from bacterial endocarditis or from emboli originating in the peripheral circulation and bypassing the lungs through the intracardiac shunt. Any child with cyanotic heart disease who is older than 2 years of age should always be suspected of having a brain abscess if focal neurological signs and increased intracranial pressure develop. Only when this has been ruled out should a vascular etiology be considered.

Venous Thrombosis

Infants who become dehydrated are at risk for developing cerebral venous thrombosis. This is a devastating condition, with seizures, changing neurological signs, and rapidly increasing intracranial pressure. A fatal outcome is frequent.

Older children develop purulent venous thrombosis secondary to infection of the mastoids, paranasal sinuses, scalp, or face. Nonpurulent thrombosis has been associated with the use of oral contraceptives.[3]

The clinical presentation is either with catastrophic neurological disease, as described for the infant, or with an isolated increase in intracranial pressure. If the cavernous sinus becomes involved, a typical syndrome of extraocular palsies, retinal hemorrhage, proptosis, and injection and edema of the conjunctive results. Treatment is supportive, with a vigorous attempt to prevent increased intracranial pressure.

ARTERIOVENOUS MALFORMATIONS

Arteriovenous malformations are the most frequent cause of nontraumatic subarachnoid hemorrhage in children. The most common presentation is with the sudden onset of severe headache and meningeal signs, in the absence of a focal neurological deficit. Other patients present with a convulsive disorder and have no history of subarachnoid hemorrhage. The smallest group will develop an intracerebral hematoma at the time of the bleeding and have the acute onset of focal signs.

A cranial bruit is present in one-half of cases, but the high frequency of this finding in normal preschool children makes the sign less useful in that age group. CT is an excellent diagnostic tool (Figure 15-3), although if surgery is contemplated, four-vessel angiography is still necessary.

These are serious lesions. Although an occasional patient will have repeated

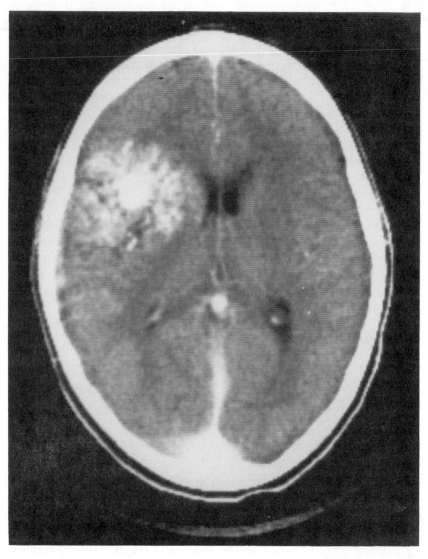

FIGURE 15-3. Large arteriovenous malformation in a 2-month-old child.

hemorrhages with no residual deficit, the long-term mortality rate is 25%, and an equal number will become severely handicapped. Microsurgical techniques have improved the operative approach, even for some of the more deeply placed lesions. Arterial embolization techniques using polymers or graded sizes of microspheres also show some promise.

Arteriovenous malformations sometimes involve the brain stem and present with the combination of cranial nerve palsies, spasticity, and ataxia. Cerebellar lesions are frequently silent, but if hemorrhage occurs, there is catastrophic collapse and rapid death unless the hematoma is evacuated.

Arteriovenous malformations of the *vein of Galen,* often incorrectly referred to as aneurysms of the vein of Galen, have three modes of clinical presentation. In the neonatal period there is cardiac failure secondary to the large vascular shunt. This should be suspected in any infant with congestive heart failure, cyanosis, a systolic heart murmur, and a loud cranial bruit. The diagnosis can be made by CT. Death occurs within 2 months in most patients due to intractable heart failure.

A second presentation, most common in later infancy, is with hydrocephalus and seizures. A loud cranial bruit is present, and there are markedly dilated scalp veins. Treatment is difficult and the prognosis is poor.

In later childhood the usual symptoms are headache and subarachnoid hemorrhage. A cranial bruit is uncommon, and the diagnosis must be made by neuroradiological studies. Surgical treatment is hazardous because of the location of the lesion, but newer techniques have allowed for some success, especially in the older patient.

Arteriovenous malformations of the *spinal cord* are quite rare. These may present as subarachnoid hemorrhage without localizing signs, but more frequently are associated with progressive involvement of spinal cord function. Back pain, bowel and bladder dysfunction, and progressive deterioration of gait are the most common symptoms. The examination shows spotty and asymmetrical abnormalities, and there often is a mixture of upper and lower motor neuron signs. A cutaneous angioma on the back, accentuated when a Valsalva maneuver is performed, and a bruit over the area are useful clinical signs. Myelography is diagnostic. Before surgery can be considered, spinal angiography is required.

INTRAVENTRICULAR/SUBEPENDYMAL HEMORRHAGE

This condition is largely restricted to the premature infant. The widespread use of CT and, more recently, real-time-sector ultrasonography, has shown that many infants have IVH/SEH without major signs or symptoms. This approaches 85% in the smallest viable infants. The frequency is inversely proportional to the infant's weight and is increased in those children who are transferred from one hospital to a special-care nursery at a different location. The risk is also greater if the child is small for gestational age or male, there are medical complications during pregnancy, or delivery is by breech or occiput posterior mechanisms.

The classical picture is seen in a premature infant with respiratory complications. The child suddenly deteriorates, developing cyanotic attacks, a high-pitched cry, opisthotonic posturing, seizures, hypotonia, and lethargy. Death is frequent. Other children have a less dramatic presentation, and this condition should be suspected in any premature infant with general deterioration, feeding problems, or an unexplained fall in the hematocrit.[4]

Treatment of the hemorrhage is conservative, although there is controversy as to whether or not multiple lumbar punctures to drain the bloody spinal fluid will prevent the development of hydrocephalus. The same controversy holds for attempts to treat hydrocephalus, the major long-term complication, with repeated lumbar punctures.

Outcome data are confusing, as most of the clinical series are not comparable, treatment modalities change constantly, and follow-up is usually brief. The most common long-term complication is spastic diplegia associated with periventricular leukomalacia. More severely involved children are quadriparetic, however, and also have seizures and mental retardation. Efforts to develop preventive measures are now being studied. The possibility that ventilatory assistance, especially the use of continuous end expiratory pressure, may be harmful is also coming under scrutiny.

REFERENCES

1. Solomon, G. E., Hilal, S. K., Gold, A. P., and Carter, S., 1970, Natural history of acute hemiplegia of childhood, *Brain* **93:**107–120.
2. Sarnaik, S., Soorya, D., Ravindranath, Y., and Lusher, J., 1979, Periodic transfusions for sickle cell anemia and CNS infarction, *Am. J. Dis. Child.* **133:**1254–1257.
3. Imai, W. K., Everhart, F. R., and Sanders, J. M., 1982, Cerebral venous sinus thrombosis: Report of a case and review of the literature, *Pediatrics* **70:**965–971.
4. Dubowitz, L. M. S., Levene, M. I., Morante, A., Palmer, P., and Dubowitz, V., 1981, Signs in neonatal intraventricular hemorrhage: A correlation with real-time ultrasound, *J. Pediatr.* **99:**127–133.

ADDITIONAL READING

Pape, K., Wigglesworth, J. S., and Avery, G. B., 1979, *Haemorrhage, Ischemia and the Perinatal Brain,* J. B. Lippincott, Philadelphia.

16

Seizure Disorders

Seizures are one of the most common serious neurological problems of child-hood. It has been estimated that 0.5% of the population has a seizure disorder. Because of the high incidence of febrile seizures, 3% of children will have at least one convulsion during their lifetime.[1]

The onset of a convulsive disorder triggers many concerns. The first is that it represents the initial presentation of a potentially life-threatening disease. If this possibility can be eliminated, a host of problems still remain. These include the possibility of long-term use of drugs that have many undesirable side effects, the fear that another seizure will occur at a time when harm can come to the child, the social stigma attached to epilepsy, and problems related to driving, participation in athletics, and vocational choice. The diagnosis of epilepsy brings about a profound change in the child's life and future and should only be made if the evidence is incontrovertible.

The neurophysiological substrate of a seizure is a sudden, pathological neu-ronal discharge. If this is brief, there may be no obvious signs or symptoms. If prolonged, there will be observable changes in cognition, behavior, conscious-ness, motor, or sensory function.

The biochemical and physiological changes associated with the neuronal discharge are complex. In general, no permanent damage results from a single, brief seizure. If the epileptic activity is prolonged, as in status epilepticus, the brain's rate of utilization of metabolites outstrips its ability to renew energy stores from circulating glucose and oxygen. The result can be severe, diffuse, permanent brain damage.

Whether or not repeated brief seizures have any permanent deleterious effect is not completely understood. The experimental phenomenon of kindling raises concern that such a situation might obtain. In an experimental model repeated electrical stimuli, below the level that produces convulsions, are pre-sented to an animal's brain. After a period of time, focal and then generalized seizures occur and continue for many months after the stimulation has been discontinued. The development of mirror foci in patients with temporal lobe spike foci suggests that a similar phenomenon may occur in the human. A spike focus develops in the contralateral temporal lobe, but is time-locked to the first and dependent on it. After a period of time, the second focus becomes independent and continues even after the original one is surgically removed.

The genetic aspects of epilepsy are complex.[2] Most forms of seizures are not inherited by simple mendelian mechanisms. The most prominent exception is absence seizures; the EEG abnormality seems to be transmitted as an autosomal dominant trait, although only 12% of first-degree relatives will actually have seizures.

The presence of any type of epilepsy in close relatives increases the risk of having a seizure. There is no clearly defined genetic mechanism, but an empirical risk of 2–5% exists. A positive family history of seizures also appears to increase the susceptibility to epilepsy following head trauma or any other encephalopathic event.

An International Classification of Seizure Disorders has been agreed upon and is most useful.[3] Seizures are classified in terms of the mode of onset of the epileptogenic discharge (focal or generalized) and the major clinical features. The classification does not speak to etiology. Table 16-1 presents the major features of the classification and also lists the older clinically oriented terms that are in common use.

TABLE 16-1
Classification of Seizures[a]

International classification	Common term
I. Partial (focal) seizures	
A. Simple partial seizures (consciousness not impaired)	
1. With motor signs	Focal motor
2. With sensory symptoms	Focal sensory
3. With autonomic signs	Autonomic
4. With psychic symptoms	Psychomotor
B. Complex partial seizures (consciousness impaired) Similar subtypes	Psychomotor
C. Partial with generalization	
II. Generalized seizures	
A. Absence	
1. Typical	Petit mal
2. Atypical	Atypical petit mal
B. Myoclonic	Myoclonic —> INFANILE SPASM
C. Clonic	Clonic
D. Tonic	Tonic
E. Tonic–clonic	Grand mal
F. Atonic	Atonic

[a]From Commission on Classification and Terminology of the International League Against Epilepsy.[3]

APPROACH TO THE PATIENT

When presented with a child who has had a sudden, unexplained episode of loss of consciousness or change in behavior, the physician must answer four questions:

- Did the patient have a seizure?
- What caused it?
- What type was it?
- What is the appropriate treatment?

The first question is often the hardest. The basic differential diagnosis can be summarized as fits, faints, falls, and fakes. Somewhat more scientifically, the clinical event could have represented

- Seizure
- Syncope
- Trauma
- Pseudoseizure

There are a number of useful diagnostic characteristics of seizures. They occur at random times without an obvious precipitating cause, except for rare types of reflex epilepsy. There are times when specific patients are more susceptible, but this does not modify the general principle; these include drowsiness, the period immediately after awakening, and, in some girls, the days immediately preceding a menstrual period.

An individual patient's seizures tend to be highly stereotyped, although the manifestations can change over time. An aura is not necessarily present, but if it is, this implies a focal onset. Incontinence and tongue biting are not required diagnostic criteria, even with generalized convulsions. Prolonged seizures are always followed by postictal confusion and lethargy, and the patient, if asked, frequently will complain of a headache.

A diagnosis of syncope can usually be made on the basis of a typical history. There is a precipitating event such as pain, an emotional stimulus, or suddenly standing upright. The patient will remember blacking out of vision and may have vertigo immediately prior to the loss of consciousness. Witnesses report pallor and diaphoresis. Convulsive movements are rare, the episode resolves rapidly when the patient is placed in a recumbent position, and any postictal confusion or drowsiness is brief. Unless the cause of the syncope is clear, evaluation should include a search for a cardiogenic basis. Basilar artery migraine can produce syncope, especially in adolescence.

The episode of loss of consciousness could have been produced by trauma, either accidental or sustained for other reasons. In this case the patient may be able to supply important historical details unless there is significant posttraumatic amnesia. Findings of head trauma on physical examination do not resolve the issue, as this could be the result of a fall due to a seizure.

Pseudoseizures, often referred to as hysterical epilepsy, are not rare in childhood and adolescence. Diagnosis is difficult, and to further complicate the issue, patients with a convulsive disorder may also have pseudoseizures. Diagnostic clues include seizures that occur only in certain locations or interpersonal situations, bizarre clinical manifestations, a prolonged episode without postictal confusion or somnolence, and the use of the situation for obvious secondary gain. It may be necessary to record the EEG for a prolonged period while simultaneously monitoring the patient's behavior on videotape. The occurrence of an episode without concurrent EEG changes is very strong evidence for a psychogenic etiology. A normal interictal EEG cannot be used to rule out a seizure disorder.

Following the decision that the patient did have a seizure, the cause must be defined. The first step is to eliminate the possibility of a generalized systemic or metabolic disorder, such as encephalitis, meningitis, shigellosis, hypoglycemia, or hyponatremia. A patient who does not regain consciousness following a seizure requires the same diagnostic approach as that directed toward any comatose patient.

If the patient appears well following the postictal phase, and the neurological examination is normal, laboratory evaluation has a limited role. Measurement of serum electrolytes, glucose, calcium, and phosphorus is rarely of value if the sample is not obtained during the seizure. Even then, the diagnostic yield is low. The only neuroradiological study that need be considered is a computerized-tomography (CT) scan. Skull x rays provide little information that cannot also be obtained from a CT scan and do not visualize the brain itself. Reasonable indications for CT include focal seizures, focal findings on neurological examination, a focal EEG discharge, or evidence of increased intracranial pressure. Even using these criteria, in only 2% of cases will there be a lesion, such as a tumor, that is amenable to direct therapeutic intervention.[4]

The EEG is an important diagnostic tool and assists accurate classification of the seizure. This is especially true if a seizure has a focal EEG onset and secondary generalization, but there are no clinical manifestations to suggest the focal origin. Proper classification of seizure type helps guide the choice of the initial drug.

The major diagnostic criteria are clinical. Normal EEG recordings can be found in as many as 20% of patients with seizures and so do not rule out the diagnosis. This can occur because of sampling error (no seizure discharges during the recording) or the presence of a deep focus that is not reflected by the scalp electrodes. There should always be some changes on the EEG if it is recorded during the seizure, although these may only be observed in the background activity. False positive records are not common. Although 20% of children have mild nonspecific abnormalities on their EEG, it is rare to find a well-defined epileptogenic focus in an otherwise normal child. Such an individual must be followed closely, although therapy is usually not initiated unless a seizure actually occurs.

SPECIFIC DISORDERS

Simple partial seizures present with motor, somatosensory, or autonomic signs, but with no impairment of consciousness. There may occasionally be abnormalities in higher cognitive function such as aphasia. The EEG, if abnormal, reveals a focal epileptogenic discharge over the contralateral hemisphere.

Any portion of the body can be involved. Among the most common manifestations is repetitive twitching of the thumb and the corner of the mouth on the same side. The eyes deviate to the side away from the EEG focus during the seizure and toward the focus during the postictal state. Sensory signs are usually described as an unpleasant tingling or burning. There may be visual or auditory experiences, but these are generally not formed hallucinations. Consciousness is maintained, and the patient can describe the episode in detail. Communication during the seizure is possible unless aphasia occurs.

A typical focal seizure may demonstrate a jacksonian march with spread of the motor activity up the affected limb. At that point the seizure becomes generalized and consciousness is lost. Secondary generalization can also occur without a preceding jacksonian march. Transient paralysis of the involved limb, Todd paresis, often occurs. If this has not disappeared within 24 hr, the presence of a structural lesion must be suspected.

The recent onset of focal seizures usually triggers an intensive evaluation because of the possibility of focal cerebral pathology. Although this is often found, it is rarely progressive and usually has no therapeutic or prognostic significance. In general, the younger the child, the less likely is a progressive lesion to be found.

Benign focal epilepsy of childhood (Rolandic seizures) is characterized by hemifacial seizures preceded by a somatosensory aura. Nocturnal seizures also occur and frequently become generalized. The EEG shows a centrotemporal spike focus, most prominent during sleep. Treatment with anticonvulsants is effective, and the prognosis is excellent, with disappearance of seizures by the end of adolescence.[5]

Complex partial seizures have the same clinical manifestations as simple complex seizures, but consciousness is impaired, either from the onset or after the other symptoms have begun. Automatisms are common. The seizures also may present as lapse attacks, clinically indistinguishable from absence seizures. Unilateral or bilateral seizure discharges are present on the EEG, most commonly in the temporal or frontotemporal regions.

As with other focal seizures, evaluation including CT scan is generally carried out although the yield of treatable conditions is low. With bilateral spike discharges, the chances of finding a focal lesion are even further decreased.

Absence seizures are a form of generalized epilepsy. The classical clinical presentation is a brief lapse of consciousness, lasting several seconds, and then clearing with no postictal confusion. If the child is speaking, the sentence may be interrupted and then continued with no loss of content. Simple clonic movements, such as eye blinking, are commonly present, and more complex automatisms may also be seen. The majority of patients have generalized 3-Hz spike-and-wave discharges on the EEG. These also occur interictally. If a burst lasts more than 1–3 sec, a clinical seizure will occur.

The patient who has large numbers of unrecognized absence seizures each day can present with a complaint of school failure. This is the result of multiple episodes of disruption of consciousness which interfere with sustained attention. Continuous spike-and-wave discharges are associated with a state of lethargy and confusion termed spike–wave stupor. Drug ingestion or encephalitis is often considered in these patients. The diagnosis should be suspected if eye blinking or other automatisms are present, but must be confirmed by obtaining an EEG.

Atypical absence seizures present in the preschool child. The clinical features often are a mixture of lapse attacks, atonic seizures, myoclonic seizures, and focal seizures. The association of this mixed seizure pattern with a slow (2–2.5 Hz) spike-and-wave EEG and mental retardation is referred to as the Lennox–Gastaut syndrome. Seizures are virtually impossible to control in approximately 60% of these patients.

Myoclonic seizures, appearing after the first year of life, are associated with a large number of familial, metabolic, and degenerative neurological disorders. They also are seen following diffuse encephalopathies such as those caused by hypoglycemia or hypoxia. Some of the most important causes are listed in Table 16-2.

TABLE 16-2
Selected Causes of Myoclonic Seizures[a]

Metabolic	Infection
Primary	Meningitis
PKU	Encephalitis
Maple syrup urine disease	Subacute sclerosing panencephalitis
Hyperammonemia	Congenital
Wilson disease	Structural defects of cerebral cortex
Trichopoliodystrophy	Porencephaly
Pyridoxine dependency	Anencephaly, hydranencephaly
Subacute necrotizing encephalomyelitis	Toxic
Lipidoses	CNS stimulants
Leukodystrophies	CNS depressants
Lafora body disease	Neurotoxins
Huntington chorea	Other
Secondary	Trauma
Hypoglycemia	Sturge–Weber syndrome
Hypocalcemia	Tuberous sclerosis
Hypernatremia	
Water intoxication	
Hypoxia	
Uremia	

[a]Modified from Myers.[6]

TABLE 16-3
Treatable Causes of Infantile Spasms[a]

Phenylketonuria
Maple syrup urine disease
Pyridoxine dependency
Hyperammonemia
Hypoglycemia
Hypoxia
Lead encephalopathy
Meningitis
Syphilis
Neonatal polycythemia
Subdural hematoma

[a]From Myers.[6]

In infancy, the most common type of myoclonic seizures are *infantile spasms.* This term refers to a clinical syndrome of massive myoclonic jerks which produce flexion or extension of the neck, arms, and legs, in any combination. These spasms occur in flurries many times each day and are especially prominent after the child has awakened from sleep. Following each series of seizures, the infant is often irritable for a period of time.

The most commonly associated EEG pattern is hypsarrhythmia. The record is markedly abnormal with a slow, disorganized background and spikes, polyspikes, and spike-and-wave discharges occurring asynchronously from all areas. There is an 85% concordance between infantile spasms and hypsarrhythmia.

An etiology can be determined in approximately 60% of cases. The most common are static encephalopathy, from perinatal trauma or hypoxia, and congenital malformations of the central nervous system. A careful search for the depigmented nevi of tuberous sclerosis should be carried out and a CT scan performed on all patients for whom no biochemical cause can be found. The typical subependymal calcifications of tuberous sclerosis can be present at birth in the absence of any cutaneous stigmata. There is also an increased incidence of infantile spasms in patients with Down syndrome. Screening studies for metabolic disorders will rule out the presence of phenylketonuria and other less commonly associated conditions. An intensive evaluation is most important, as there are a number of potentially treatable causes of infantile spasms (Table 16-3).[6]

If no specific treatable cause is found, the drug of choice is ACTH, which is given intramuscularly as the gel, 80 units every other day.[7] Other treatment schedules have been used, but none has any clear advantage. After several weeks, the dose is tapered and the medication discontinued. A good response is associated with rapid cessation of seizure activity. If ACTH is ineffective, valproate or clonazepam is sometimes useful.

The prognosis of this condition is poor. Seizures frequently recur, and the child may develop the Lennox–Gastaut syndrome. Mental retardation is associated with infantile spasms in 80–85% of cases. The features of a restricted age of onset (almost always under 1 year), multiplicity of etiological factors, and rather uniformly poor outcome suggest that infantile spasms is not a specific disorder but represents the end result of a severe insult to an immature brain.

Attempts have been made to define the small group of children with a good prognosis.[8] The most useful predictors appear to be absence of a definable etiology and normal development prior to the onset of the spasms. A rapid response to therapy is also a positive indicator.

Generalized *tonic–clonic, tonic,* or *clonic* seizures are dramatic events. There is no aura, the first manifestation being loss of consciousness. The patient may cry out, and he falls to the ground. There should not be a major focal component to the seizure, and the neurological examination shows no focal signs. Following the seizure, which may last several minutes, there is postictal somnolence and confusion, and the patient will sleep briefly if left undisturbed. Complaints of headache and backache are often offered when alertness is regained.

The typical EEG correlate is diffuse spike-and-wave or polyspike-and-wave discharges. Diagnostic studies can be limited if no focal features are present on the neurological examination or EEG. With onset in late adolescence, performance of a CT scan is reasonable, as a tumor is more likely than in younger patients.

Febrile seizures are also generalized. Diagnostic criteria and appropriate treatment for febrile seizures have long been sources of controversy. In an attempt to resolve differences and make useful recommendations, a Consensus Development Conference was held at the National Institutes of Health in 1980.[9] Available evidence supports the viewpoint that brief generalized seizures occurring with fever in neurologically normal children between the ages of 1 and 5 years are, in fact, benign. They are not associated with subsequent mental retardation, cerebral palsy, or other neurological deficits.[10] Status epilepticus is rare. The risk for the development of other seizure disorders is slightly increased over that of the general population, however.

The risk of epilepsy increases significantly if the child is neurologically abnormal, the seizures are prolonged, focal, or followed by a transient or permanent neurological deficit, or there is a family history of epilepsy.[11] A family history of febrile seizures is a positive prognostic sign. The number of seizures does not seem to affect the outcome.

It is clear that maintenance therapy with phenobarbital in doses that assure a therapeutic blood level can reduce the risk of further febrile seizures from approximately 24% to 3%. There seems to be no other effect on outcome. The intermittent use of phenobarbital is not effective. Unfortunately, behavior or sleep problems occur in up to 40% of treated patients. For this reason, the current recommendation is that treatment is not necessary in the absence of the high-risk criteria listed earlier. It should be considered if these risk factors are present and may also be instituted if there are multiple febrile seizures or if they occur in a child under 12 months of age.

Rectal administration of diazepam when the child's temperature exceeds 38.5°C can significantly reduce the recurrence of febrile seizures.[12] Unfortunately, the convulsion is often the first sign that the child is ill and has developed fever, and so no preventative technique can be completely effective.

Neonatal seizures present a difficult diagnostic problem. Manifestations are often subtle, and seizures should be suspected with any unusual change in the infant's behavior or status, especially if it is stereotyped. Apneic episodes may be the only manifestation. A complete evaluation, including metabolic studies and either a CT scan or ultrasonography, is indicated in this age group. EEG is a useful aid but is often difficult to interpret, as focal abnormalities occur even in the presence of metabolic disease.

Seizures in the neonatal period are associated with a mortality as high as 35%. Of the survivors, approximately 70% are normal. Mental retardation, cerebral palsy, and epilepsy are the most common residua.[13]

Status epilepticus is an acute medical emergency. It is defined as a continuous seizure that does not stop spontaneously or seizures repeated so frequently that consciousness is not regained between episodes. The most frequent cause is sudden discontinuation of anticonvulsant medication, but status epilepticus can also be the presenting sign of any diffuse encephalopathy. As already noted, the brain is unable to continue to meet its metabolic requirements in the face of continuous seizure activity, and serious damage can result.

The principles of treatment are initially the same as those of any emergency. Attention must be paid to the status of the airway, respirations, pulse, and blood pressure. At that point a vigorous attempt should be made to stop the seizures. The recommended drugs are listed in Table 16-4. If status continues despite a maximum therapeutic effort, general anesthesia may be necessary. Cerebral edema often follows prolonged status epilepticus. As this can be destructive, therapy must be promptly instituted.

TABLE 16-4
Treatment of Status Epilepticus

Initial drugs to stop seizures
    Diazepam, 0.1–0.2 mg/kg i.v. *or*
    Lorazepam, 0.05–0.2 mg/kg i.v.
Secondary drugs to stop seizures if the initial drugs fail *and*
Maintenance drug to be given after seizures stop
    Phenobarbital, 20 mg/kg i.v. *or*
    Phenytoin, 18 mg/kg i.v.
Drugs that can be used if secondary treatment fails
    Paraldehyde (4%), 20 mg/kg per hr i.v. by slow drip *or*
    Lidocaine, 2–3 mg/kg i.v. (single dose) *or*
    Lidocaine, 6–10 mg/kg per hr i.v. by slow drip *or*
    Valproate, 10 mg/kg rectally *or*
    General anesthesia

TREATMENT OF SEIZURES

The first management decision is whether or not drug therapy should be initiated. Following the first afebrile seizure, only one-half of children will have a recurrence.[14] Risk factors for recurrence include the presence of an abnormal neurological examination, focal spikes on the electroencephalogram, and partial complex seizures. The lowest risk is for patients with a generalized tonic–clonic seizure, normal EEG, and normal neurological examination. Although administration of an anticonvulsant does not significantly alter the risk of a recurrence, most clinicians would institute therapy for the high-risk patient.

The treatment of seizure disorders depends on the use of medication, except in cases where a definable metabolic abnormality can be found and corrected. There are a number of basic principles of therapy. The drug most likely to be effective is chosen first and the dosage increased until a therapeutic effect is obtained or toxic side effects supervene. If the patient does not respond, a second drug should be added and the first one discontinued. Regimens using more than one drug should not be used until several drugs have each been tried individually.[15]

Recent studies have shown that all anticonvulsants can have an adverse effect on cognitive function, even in the absence of clinical signs of toxicity.[16] This is most apparent with sedative anticonvulsants (barbiturates and diazepates), and there is now a tendency to limit the use of these substances as drugs of first choice. It also appears that in many instances, the patient will function at a more optimal level if the balance between drug and toxicity and seizure control is weighted toward minimizing side effects.[17]

Serum concentrations of all the commonly used anticonvulsants can now be measured. It is important to remember that the published therapeutic range and toxic levels are only statistical statements concerning those concentrations that are most likely to be beneficial or to cause untoward side effects. If the patient is doing well, there is little to be gained by performing routine anticonvulsant level determinations.

Anticonvulsant levels should be obtained if the patient does not respond to an appropriate medication, as rapid metabolism or excretion of the drug can keep the blood level lower than expected. They are also helpful if an additional drug is added to the patient's regimen, as metabolic interactions can cause the level of the original drugs to change markedly. Finally, if the patient is taking more than one medication and develops symptoms of toxicity, determination of blood levels will help differentiate which drug is causing the symptoms.

The most frequently used anticonvulsants in pediatric practice are listed in Table 16-5, as are the usual pediatric dose range and recommended serum concentrations.

Phenobarbital is still the most commonly prescribed drug for generalized tonic–clonic and partial seizures. It is the preferred drug for prophylaxis of febrile convulsions. There are few serious side effects, except for occasional hypersensitivity reactions. Adverse behavioral effects can occur in up to 40% of

TABLE 16-5
Anticonvulsant Drugs

Drug	Dose (mg/kg per day)	Blood level (μg/ml)
Phenobarbital	4–8	15–40
Primidone	10–25	6–12
Phenytoin	4–7	10–20
Carbamazepine	20–30	6–12
Valproic acid	30–60	50–100
Ethosuximide	20–30	40–100
Clonazepam	0.01–0.2	0.013–0.072
Chlorazepate	0.4–3.0	—

young children when phenobarbital is first introduced. These include restlessness, irritability, short attention span, and difficulty sleeping. Other children appear sedated. Many of these problems resolve in time, but there is now movement away from the use of potentially sedating drugs.

The claim has been made that *mephobarbital* does not share the behavioral side effects of phenobarbital but is equally effective in controlling seizures. There is little documentation in the literature, however, and the drug is rapidly converted into phenobarbital. *Primidone* is metabolized into phenobarbital and phenylethylmalonylamide, both of which are effective anticonvulsants. This drug is most useful for tonic–clonic and partial seizures. Treatment must be initiated at low dose levels, or severe sedation and ataxia will occur.

Phenytoin has the same therapeutic spectrum as the barbiturates, but is less sedating. Toxic effects of high dose levels include ataxia, nystagmus, and slurred speech. Approximately one-third of patients develop gingival hyperplasia. Rare side effects include megaloblastic anemia and rickets, mainly in institutionalized, nonambulatory, retarded patients. If a morbilliform rash occurs, the drug should be stopped, as the patient is at risk for developing Stevens–Johnson syndrome and acute hepatic necrosis.

Carbamazepine is now considered by many neurologists to be the drug of choice for partial seizures. It is not sedating, and studies have shown less impairment of cognitive abilities than with barbiturates or phenytoin. The major serious side effects, bone marrow suppression and hepatic toxicity, are rare in children. The drug must be started at low dose levels, or lethargy and ataxia will occur.

Valproic acid is useful for absence seizures, myoclonic seizures, and atonic seizures. A number of cases of fatal acute hepatic necrosis have been reported. Patients at highest risk seem to be children less than 2 years of age, those with brain damage, and those taking multiple drugs. This complication is most likely to occur during the first 6 months of treatment. Slight elevations of SGOT and SGPT levels are frequently found in patients taking valproic acid, but this does not seem to predict serious hepatic disease. Other side effects include hyperammonemia with lethargy, thrombocytopenia, alopecia, and loss of appetite.

The drug causes an increase in phenobarbital levels and may cause a decrease in phenytoin levels.

Ethosuximide is still the primary drug for the treatment of uncomplicated absence seizures. Gastrointestinal problems, lethargy, and leukopenia are the major untoward effects.

Various benzodiazepines have been used in the treatment of myoclonic and atonic seizures. The most useful is *clonazepam,* although it produces lethargy and hypersalivation. *Clorazepate* has been recommended for treatment of partial seizures. Many centers now use *lorazepam* as the drug of choice in status epilepticus. A general problem with this class of drugs is the development of tolerance, which necessitates periodic increases in dose.

The prognosis of seizure disorders is a function of the type of seizure and the rapidity with which treatment brings the seizures under control.[18] A long duration of uncontrolled seizures, abnormalities on the neurological examination, and jacksonian or mixed seizures are the factors most closely associated with a relapse (Table 16-6). The EEG does not appear to have major prognostic value.

Other workers found that the presence of spikes on the electroencephalogram was a negative prognostic indicator, as was worsening of the record.[19] Complex partial seizures, atypical febrile seizures, and older age at occurrence of the first seizure were associated with a relapse when therapy was discontinued.

The IQ of children with seizure disorders is no different from that of their siblings, if the condition is not due to an acute neurological illness. On long-term follow-up, however, a subgroup of approximately 10% of these children will show a persistent decrease in IQ, averaging 10 points. This change correlates with a higher incidence of episodes of drug toxicity, the number of drugs to which the patient became toxic, and the age of onset of the seizures. There is a much weaker relationship to the total number of seizures and complete seizure control. This suggests that drug toxicity should be avoided, even if seizure control is not perfect.[20]

TABLE 16-6
Recurrence Risk for Seizures[a]

Seizure type	Relapses (%)
Grand mal	14
Jacksonian	58
Psychomotor	31
Simple febrile	12
Petit mal	12
Combination	43
Total	28

[a]From Thurston *et al.*[18]

SEIZURES NOT REQUIRING THERAPY

It has already been stated that anticonvulsant therapy is not useful if the seizures have a treatable metabolic cause or occur as part of an acute illness that does not primarily involve the CNS. In addition, most patients with febrile seizures do not require medication.

A child may have a brief generalized convulsion immediately following head trauma. This *contact seizure*, if unassociated with other evidence of head injury, is benign and requires no treatment. A seizure that occurs after a delay is very different, however, and implies an underlying brain injury.

Cyanotic breath-holding spells occur when a child cries, holds his breath in inspiration, and loses consciousness. A few clonic jerks of the limbs may be seen. These spells can start in the first 6 months of life and resolve during the preschool years. There is no need for anticonvulsants, and no specific treatment is effective. The episodes do no harm, and they are not a forerunner of a convulsive disorder.

Pallid breath-holding spells are not due to anoxia but are a type of syncope associated with bradycardia or transient asystole. The child, following a sudden fright or painful stimulus, becomes pale, loses consciousness, and often assumes an opisthotonic posture. Clonic jerking may occur in this syndrome also. Here again, treatment is neither effective nor indicated, and the prognosis is excellent.

Shuddering attacks may be confused with seizures, but are not associated with electroencephalographic abnormalities.[21] The children have brief episodes of shuddering or shivering, often associated with flexion of the head, trunk, elbows, and knees. These can occur hundreds of times each day. Some of these patients develop essential tremor in later life.

REFERENCES

1. Baumann, R. J., Marx, M. B., and Leonidakes, M.G., 1978, Epilepsy in rural Kentucky: Prevalence in a population of school age children, *Epilepsia* **19**:75–80.
2. Jennings, M. T., and Bird, T. D., 1981, Genetic influences in the epilepsies, *Am. J. Dis. Child.* **135**:450–457.
3. Commission on Classification and Terminology of the International League Against Epilepsy, 1981, Proposal for revised clinical and electroencephalographic classification of epileptic seizures, *Epilepsia* **22**:489–501.
4. Bachman, D. S., Hodges, F. J., and Freeman, J. M., 1976, Computerized axial tomography in chronic seizure disorders in childhood, *Pediatrics* **58**:828–832.
5. Loiseau, P., Pestre, M., Dartigues, J. F., Commenges, D., Barberger-Gateau, C., and Cohadon, S., 1983, Long-term prognosis in two forms of childhood epilepsy: Typical absence seizures and epilepsy with rolandic (centrotemporal) EEG foci, *Ann. Neurol.* **13**:642–648.
6. Myers, G. J., 1975, The therapy of myoclonus, in: *Myoclonic Seizures* (M.H. Charlton, ed.), Excerpta Medica, Princeton, NJ, pp. 121–160.
7. Singer, W. D., Rabe, E. F., and Haller, J. S., 1980, The effect of ACTH therapy upon infantile spasms, *J. Pediatr.* **96**:485–489.
8. Matsumoto, A., Watanabe, K., Negoro, T., Sugiura, M., Iwase, K., Hara, K., and Miyazaki, S.,

1981, Long-term prognosis after infantile spasms: A statistical study of prognostic factors in 200 cases, *Dev. Med. Child. Neurol.* **23:**51–65.

9. National Institute of Neurological and Communicative Disorders and Stroke, 1980, Consensus Development Conference on Febrile Seizures, *Pediatrics* **66:**1009–1012.
10. Nelson, K. B., and Ellenberg, J. H., 1978, Prognosis in children with febrile seizures, *Pediatrics* **61:**720–727.
11. Hauser, W. A., Annegers, J. F., Anderson, V. E., and Kurland, L. T., 1985, The risk of seizure disorders among relatives of children with febrile convulsions, *Neurology* **35:**1268–1273.
12. Knudsen, F. U., 1985, Effective short-term diazepam prophylaxis in febrile convulsions, *J. Pediatr.* **106:**487–490.
13. Holden, K. P., Mellits, E. D., Freeman, J. M., 1982, Neonatal seizures. I. Correlation of prenatal and perinatal events with outcomes, *Pediatrics* **70:**165–176.
14. Camfield, P. R., Camfield, C. S., Dooley, J. M., Tibbles, J. A. R., Fung, T., and Garner, B., 1985, Epilepsy after a first unprovoked seizure in childhood, *Neurology* **35:**1657–1660.
15. Forsythe, W. I., and Sills, M. A., 1984, One drug for childhood grand mal: Medical audit for three-year remissions, *Dev. Med. Child. Neurol.* **26:**742–748.
16. Committee on Drugs, American Academy of Pediatrics, 1985, Behavioral and cognitive effects of anticonvulsant therapy, *Pediatrics* **76:**644–647.
17. Theodore, W. H., and Porter, R. J., 1983, Removal of sedative–hypnotic antiepileptic drugs from the regimens of patients with intractable epilepsy, *Ann. Neurol.* **13:**320–324.
18. Thurston, J. H., Thurston, D. L., Hixon, B. B., and Keller, A. J., 1982, Prognosis in childhood epilepsy, *N. Engl. J. Med.* **306:**831–836.
19. Shinnar, S., Vining, E. P. G., Mellits, E. D., D'Souza, B. J., Holden, K., Baumgardner, R. A., and Freeman, J. M., 1985, Discontinuing antiepileptic medicine in children with epilepsy after two years without seizures, *N. Engl. J. Med.* **313:**976–980.
20. Bourgeois, B. F. D., Prensky, A. L., Palkes, H. S., Talent, B. K., and Busch, S. G., 1983, Intelligence in epilepsy: A prospective study in children, *Ann. Neurol.* **14:**438–444.
21. Holmes, G. L., and Russman, B. S., 1986, Shuddering attacks: Evaluation using electroencephalographic frequency modulation radiotelemetry and videotape monitoring, *Am. J. Dis. Child.* **140:**72–73.

ADDITIONAL READING

Gomez, M. R., and Kless, D. W., 1983, Epilepsies of infancy and childhood, *Ann. Neurol.* **13:**113–124.

17

Metabolic Disorders

Metabolic disorders are those conditions in which there is an abnormality in one or more metabolic pathways, producing disease or impaired function. The central nervous system can be primarily involved by such a process or affected secondary to a severe generalized metabolic disturbance. The great majority of these disorders are hereditary; most are transmitted by autosomal recessive mechanisms.

These diseases are relatively rare, but are important to understand for a number of reasons. First, many are a threat to life or normal development. Second, the hereditary nature of most of these conditions brings with it important implications for genetic counseling. Finally, some of the metabolic diseases can be treated by dietary manipulation or other management strategies. The new techniques of molecular genetics and genetic engineering will almost certainly provide a permanent cure for many of these conditions.

The pathogenesis of the metabolic disorders is complex and depends on the specific metabolic pathways involved. This is discussed in detail by Stanbury *et al.*[1] A number of basic mechanisms, at the molecular level, can be defined. These are outlined in Table 17-1.

Prenatal diagnosis is now possible for many of the conditions in which understanding of the basic biochemical defect has been obtained. The usual strategy is to obtain fetal cells by amniocentesis or chorionic villus biopsy, grow the fibroblasts in tissue culture, and investigate the pertinent enzymatic pathways. Newer techniques have expanded the possibilities, and abnormalities in structural proteins and even DNA can be documented. In most instances the only option, if the fetus is affected with a serious condition, is termination of the pregnancy. The next step, in some disorders, will be the development of prenatal treatment techniques.

Some conditions can be detected in newborn screening programs. These are legally mandated in most states. Blood samples are taken from the neonate before discharge from the nursery and are sent to a designated laboratory. The sample is then analyzed for evidence of one of a number of relatively common metabolic disorders. Although the metabolic diseases being sought are uncom-

TABLE 17-1
Pathogenesis of Genetic Disorders[a]

Altered DNA structure
Disturbed protein function
Disrupted cell and organ function
  Altered flux through metabolic pathways
  Disordered feedback regulation of synthetic pathways
  Disordered membrane function
  Disordered intracellular compartmentalization

[a]From Stanbury *et al.*[1]

mon, these programs are cost-effective as many of the disorders for which screening is carried out can be treated, helping assure the child's normal development.

Any screening program has two potential sources of error. False negative tests occur, and so definitive diagnostic studies must still be carried out if there is any clinical suspicion that a metabolic disorder is present. The second issue is that a positive screening test is not diagnostic. It does mandate prompt referral to a center where a detailed metabolic evaluation can be performed. Treatment should not be started on the basis of a screening examination alone.

The results of one state's screening program are presented in Table 17-2.[2] Although the number of infants with confirmed metabolic diseases is not great, the majority of these children can expect to have normal development if adequate treatment is instituted.

Treatment of children with metabolic disorders depends on the nature of the specific condition, the availability of a useful treatment strategy, and the child's condition at the time the diagnosis is made. Table 17-3 lists some of the possible approaches to therapy.[1] The most common treatment methods for the classical inborn errors of metabolism are restriction of substrate and replacement of deficient end products, in various combinations. Amplification of enzyme activity is the basis for treatment of the vitamin-responsive disorders.

TABLE 17-2
Results of Texas Newborn Screening Program (1981)[a,b]

Disorders	Abnormal screen	Infants diagnosed	Incidence
Phenylketonuria	174	6	1:47,000
Homocystinuria	32	0	—
Galactosemia	58	3	1:94,000
Hypothyroidism	6008	87	1: 3,300

[a]A total of 283,000 infants were screened during this period.
[b]From Therrell *et al.*[2]

TABLE 17-3
Treatment of Metabolic Diseases[a]

Dietary restriction of the substrate	Replacement of the mutant protein
Replacement of the deficient end product	Modification of the mutant protein
Depletion of the storage substance	Organ transplantation
Use of metabolic inhibitors	Surgical removal
Amplification of enzyme activity	Genetic engineering

[a]From Stanbury et al.[1]

APPROACH TO THE PATIENT

Metabolic disorders should be suspected in a number of clinical situations. The most important of these are

1. Unexplained metabolic abnormalities such as acidosis or hyperammonemia
2. Repeated episodes of serious metabolic derangement
3. Intolerance to specific classes of food
4. Severe mental retardation with no other acceptable explanation
5. Familial clustering of mental retardation
6. Clinical features characteristic of a specific metabolic disorder

If it appears reasonable to pursue this diagnostic possibility, it is mandatory to obtain consultation with someone actively working in the area of metabolic diseases or to refer the child to a center where the studies can be carried out. It is completely unacceptable to send a blood or urine specimen to a laboratory for "metabolic screening tests" and discount this class of diseases if the studies are negative.

The metabolic disorders are traditionally classified on the basis of the substrate affected by the abnormal metabolism (e.g., amino acids, carbohydrates, mucopolysaccharides). This is a useful approach, as there are similarities between the disorders in each group and the metabolic pathways are interrelated. At the bedside, however, the first step in differential diagnosis is more dependent on clinical features. This allows the laboratory search to be more efficient and clearly focused.

General Features

When there is suspicion of a metabolic disorder, two features assist in the initial classification:

1. Apparent age of onset. The majority of these conditions are present at birth. If the only manifestation is delayed development, this will probably not be recognized until 6–12 months of age or later. Some disorders,

TABLE 17-4
Metabolic Disorders Inherited by X-Linked
Recessive Mechanisms

Lesch–Nyhan syndrome
Lowe syndrome
Mucopolysaccharidosis II (Hunter syndrome)
Ornithine transcarbamylase deficiency
Trichopoliodystrophy

such as Wilson disease, do not become symptomatic until later in life, when there has been sufficient accumulation of an endogenous product or an environmental substance.

2. Family history. Although the majority of the metabolic disorders are inherited by an autosomal recessive mechanism, some are X-linked (Table 17-4). This information can best be obtained from a detailed analysis of the pedigree.

Course of Illness

This provides extremely important diagnostic information. Conditions representative of each group are listed in Table 17-5.

1. Static disability. The most common presentation of these metabolic disorders is developmental delay, with or without motor abnormalities, mimicking a static encephalopathy. This possibility should always be con-

TABLE 17-5
Course of Illness of Selected Metabolic Disorders

Static disability	Severe acute metabolic illness
Phenylketonuria	Maple syrup urine disease
Histidinemia	Carbamyl synthetase deficiency
Hyperphenylalanemia (DHPR or BH_2	Propionic acidemia (ketotic hyperglycinemia)
deficiency)	Methylmalonic aciduria
Nonketotic hyperglycinemia	Ornithine transcarbamylase deficiency (male)
Lesch–Nyhan syndrome	Intermittent acute symptoms
Lowe syndrome	Isovaleric acidemia
Glycogenoses (certain types)	Ornithine transcarbamylase deficiency
Normal development followed by deterioration	(female)
Homocystinuria	Hartnup disease
Subacute necrotizing encephalomyelopathy	Glycogenoses (certain types)
Mucopolysaccharidoses	Carnitine deficiency
Mucolipidoses	Maple syrup urine disease (later-onset
Galactosemia	variants)
Glycogenoses (certain types)	Subacute necrotizing encephalomyelopathy
Trichopoliodystrophy	Arginosuccinic aciduria
Citrullinemia	

sidered if there is no good alternative explanation for the mental retardation.

2. Normal development followed by deterioration. This group broadly overlaps the disorders in the first group and those discussed in Chapter 18. The distinction is somewhat arbitrary.

3. Severe acute metabolic illness. These conditions generally present in infancy and are life-threatening illnesses. If they are triggered by specific nutritional or environmental substances, the age of onset is delayed until such an exposure takes place.

4. Intermittent acute symptoms. These disorders also can be fatal unless treatment is rapidly instituted. An important diagnostic clue for the conditions in this group and group 3 is the unexplained death of siblings.

Physical Signs

Some of these conditions are associated with stigmatizing physical features or unusual findings such as a characteristic urinary odor. Table 17-6 highlights important representative conditions which are suggested by findings on examination.

The specific conditions discussed in the following sections are some of the more common of the metabolic disorders. They have also been chosen to illus-

TABLE 17-6
Specific Features on Examination

Urinary odor	Mucopolysaccharidoses
Maple syrup urine disease	Dependent on type
Maple syrup	Corneal clouding
Isovaleric acidemia	Bony abnormalities
Sweaty feet	Hepatosplenomegaly
Physical signs	Mucolipidoses
Phenylketonuria	Dependent on type
Fair hair and skin	Resembles mucopolysaccharidoses
Eczema	Galactosemia
Homocystinuria	Jaundice
Marfanoid stature	Hepatosplenomegaly
Arachnodactyly	Glycogen storage diseases
Dislocated lenses	Dependent on type
Lesch–Nyhan syndrome	Hepatosplenomegaly
Self-mutilation	Macroglossia
Choreoathetosis	Trichopoliodystrophy
Hartnup disease	Hair abnormalities
Pellagralike rash	Arginosuccinic aciduria
Intermittent ataxia	Friable hair
Lowe syndrome	
Rickets	
Cataracts	
Glaucoma	

trate many of the biological principles concerning pathophysiological mechanisms, diagnosis, and treatment.

DISORDERS OF AMINO ACID METABOLISM

Phenylketonuria (PKU) is the prototypic disorder of amino acid metabolism, the most common, and the best understood. In classical PKU, the child appears normal at birth but demonstrates increasingly severe developmental delay through the first year of life. Fair skin, blue eyes, eczema, irritability, and a mousy urinary odor are characteristic, but none of these are absolutely reliable clinical features. If the children are not treated, mental retardation is invariable and usually is in the severe range. Behavioral abnormalities are also common, and some of the children present with the clinical picture of autism. Seizures, especially infantile spasms, are a frequent concomitant.

PKU is transmitted by an autosomal recessive gene, which is rare in blacks and Jews. The majority of neonatal screening programs include a test that detects increased serum levels of phenylalanine. This finding mandates immediate referral to a center where definitive metabolic studies can be carried out and treatment instituted promptly. Diagnosis requires demonstration of a persistently elevated serum phenylalanine level, low serum tyrosine levels, and the excretion of abnormal urinary metabolites (phenylpyruvic acid and *o*-hydroxyphenylacetic acid). It is these metabolites which are detected by the urinary ferric chloride test.

It is important to remember that as many as 10% of infants with PKU will not be detected by the neonatal screening program, as serum phenylalanine levels take some time to reach the threshold of detection for these tests. This is becoming more of a problem with the trend toward early discharge of obstetrical patients from the hospital. All children should have urinary testing performed at the time of the first health maintenance visit.

A rational approach to treatment requires some knowledge of the biochemistry of the disorder. Phenylalanine hydroxylase is a complex enzyme system which requires two cofactors, each of which is involved in its own metabolic cycle. These are tetrahydrobiopterine (BH_4) and dihydrobiopterin (BH_2). In the classical form of the disorder, phenylalanine hydroxylase activity is absent. Conversion of phenylalanine to tyrosine is blocked, serum levels increase, and abnormal metabolites are formed and excreted in the urine. The mechanism of brain damage has not been clearly defined, but probably involves abnormalities in the synthesis of proteins or biogenic amines.

Treatment is accomplished by limiting the intake of phenylalanine so that serum levels remain in the normal range. This then halts production of abnormal metabolites. It is also necessary to provide additional tyrosine, as the deficiency of phenylalanine hydroxylase activity makes this an essential amino acid. All these requirements are met by severely limiting dietary protein intake and supplementing the diet with a product containing all the necessary amino acids except phenylalanine. This formula also contains supplemental tyrosine. Controlled intake of food provides sufficient phenylalanine to meet the needs of protein synthesis and growth. This treatment protocol requires frequent monitoring of serum levels and constant consultation with a knowledgeable nutritionist. Overtreatment causes poor growth, anemia, and hypoglycemia.

The results of dietary treatment are excellent; on follow-up evaluation many of the children have normal intelligence and behavior, and the seizure disorder usually resolves. It appears that early treatment and consistently good control are important factors. There is some controversy concerning the age at which discontinuation of the special diet is possible. This is being intensively studied.[3] Behavioral abnormalities and declining school performance are seen following discontinuation of the diet in some children.

Many children with successfully treated PKU are entering the reproductive years. If a woman carries an elevated phenylalanine level during her pregnancy, the fetal brain will be damaged and the child will be mentally retarded. This syndrome of *maternal PKU* is of great biological interest. The child, although obviously an obligatory heterozygote, does not share the metabolic defect but suffers because of the abnormal intrauterine environment. The woman should be stabilized on dietary therapy before the pregnancy is begun and then be carefully controlled during the entire prenatal period.[4] If no cause for severe mental retardation can be found during the evaluation of any child, it is important to test for maternal PKU, especially if the mother's intelligence is not normal.

There are a number of other metabolic disorders which present with elevated serum phenylalanine levels and are detected by the neonatal screening program. Most of these conditions are benign, but two are associated with serious neurological disease and mental retardation. These involve the cofactors required by the phenylalanine hydroxylase enzyme complex and are *dihydropteridine reductase deficiency* and *biopterin synthesis deficiency*.[5] These should be suspected if the usual good response to dietary restriction does not occur and progressive neurological deterioration continues in the face of biochemical evidence of good control. Only a few centers are capable of carrying out the required studies to prove the diagnosis. Treatment with dietary restriction of phenylalanine and supplementation with tryptophan and L-dopa has been attempted, but the neurological problems have remained severe.

Histidinemia is another condition caused by absence of activity of an enzyme (histidase), which is needed for the metabolism of an amino acid, and the production of abnormal metabolites, which can be detected in the urine. There is lack of agreement as to whether this is a benign disorder or is associated with mild mental retardation, speech defects, and behavioral abnormalities. There is no evidence that dietary treatment is effective. Histidinemia is an autosomal recessive disorder.

Nonketotic hyperglycinemia is characterized by high concentrations of glycine in blood, urine, and CSF. Symptoms begin in the neonatal period with spasticity, seizures that are difficult to control, and growth failure, and some children will progressively deteriorate and die. Survivors are severely damaged neurologically. Treatment with a low-protein diet and administration of sodium benzoate partially corrects the biochemical abnormalities, but there is no clear evidence that the clinical course is modified.

Homocystinuria was initially described as a syndrome associated with a marfanoid habitus, dislocated lenses, and repeated episodes of thromboembolism. Increased plasma and urinary levels of homocystine are present. It is now known that there are at least three distinct metabolic defects that produce similar clinical and laboratory findings. Their distinction is most important, as some of these are amenable to treatment.

The classical form of the disorder is caused by *cystathionine synthase deficiency*. There are increased levels of homocystine, homocysteine, and methionine in blood and urine and decreased cystathionine concentrations. There may be two subtypes of this disorder, one of which is responsive to treatment with large doses of pyridoxine. This is administered in conjunction with a diet low in methionine. In addition to manifesting the typical physical features of homocystinuria, children with this disorder are mentally retarded.

Elevated serum homocystine and homocysteine levels and decreased methionine levels are found in *methyltetrahydrofolate methyltransferase deficiency*. The biochemical abnormalities are reversed by administration of vitamin B_{12}. The condition is rare, and the clinical outcome of this therapy has not been well documented.

Normal or decreased serum levels of methionine are also present in *5,10-N-methylene-tetrahydrofolate reductase deficiency*. The biochemical deficit responds to administration of folic acid, but the clinical benefit is not clear. Various patients with this disorder have been reported to have, in addition to the classic symptoms of homocystinuria, myopathy, behavioral disturbances, and psychotic episodes.

Maple syrup urine disease (MSUD) is caused by a defect in the ability to decarboxylate the branched-chain amino acids valine, leucine, and isoleucine and the presence of an increased level of their branched-chain keto-acid metabolites. These are excreted in the urine, and the odor lends the condition its picturesque name. The classical clinical pattern is dramatic, with seizures, spasticity, and respiratory irregularities beginning in early infancy. Many of these children die, and the survivors are severely mentally retarded. Treatment consists of restricting the intake of branched-chain amino acids. Although this has met with some success, it is difficult to sustain.

A number of variants of MSUD have been reported. One form presents as an intermittent metabolic illness in late infancy. These children are seriously ill with a depressed state of consciousness, ataxia, and seizures. Biochemical studies have shown that there is some residual enzyme activity, although it is far below normal levels. A second variant associated with a reduced level of enzyme activity presents with mental retardation and episodes of acidosis with seizures and coma.

A related condition, *isovaleric aciduria*, results from the inability to decarboxylate only leucine. The abnormal metabolites produce a characteristic odor, which is said to resemble the odor of sweaty feet. The children have repeated episodes of critical illness precipitated by infections or excessive ingestion of protein and consisting of acidosis, vomiting, coma, anemia, leukopenia, and thrombocytopenia. The mortality rate is high, especially in the first month of life, and survivors are left with mental retardation. Treatment with glycine, which appears to detoxify the abnormal metabolites, has been reported to be effective.

Lowe syndrome (oculocerebrorenal syndrome) is an X-linked disorder of amino acid transport. The symptom complex is characteristic, with mental retardation, cataracts, glaucoma, and renal rickets. There is laboratory evidence of renal tubular acidosis and a generalized aminoaciduria starting early in infancy. Treatment of the renal disease can prolong life, but does not ameliorate the neurological deficits.

Hartnup disease is due to a defect in the renal tubular reabsorption of neutral amino acids and presents with intermittent episodes of ataxia and a rash resembling that of pellagra. Headache is also common. Approximately one-half of these patients are mentally retarded. Treatment with nicotinic acid has been recommended.

ORGANIC ACIDURIAS

The disorders in this group present with severe metabolic disease which is characterized by acidosis and the excretion of excessive amounts of organic acids in the urine. Analysis of serum shows a large anion gap. There is obviously some overlap with certain of the aminoacidopathies, such as MSUD and isovaleric aciduria, which share these metabolic abnormalities.

Propionic acidemia, also referred to as ketotic hyperglycinemia, produces vomiting, ketosis, coma, neutropenia, and thrombocytopenia. Symptoms begin in early infancy. The children develop permanent neurological disability with mental retardation, spasticity, and a seizure disorder. These symptoms are triggered by the intake of protein and often resolve when the child is given intravenous fluids. Extreme protein restriction prevents attacks, but the children suffer from the effects of protein deficiency. *Methylmalonic acidemia* is also associated with protein intolerance and characterized by episodes of ketoacidosis and hypoglycemia. Survivors are mentally retarded.

DISORDERS OF CARBOHYDRATE METABOLISM

Galactosemia presents in the first week of life with jaundice. Levels of both conjugated and unconjugated bilirubin are elevated. Galactose is present in the urine; tests for reducing sugar are positive, but those specific for glucose are negative. The diagnosis is made by demonstrating absence of galactose-1-phosphate uridyl transferase activity. If the diagnosis is delayed, and treatment not instituted, the child goes on to develop hepatic cirrhosis, aminoaciduria, cataracts, and mental retardation. Treatment involves removal from the diet of the only source of galactose, milk and milk products. Many of the symptoms regress if treatment is begun early, and development is normal.

The *glycogen storage diseases* vary greatly in their manifestations. Several of them involve the central nervous system or muscle. The prototypical disorder in this group is *glucose-6-phosphatase deficiency* (von Gierke disease). Glycogen cannot be converted to glucose and accumulates in the liver and kidneys. Hepatomegaly is present in the neonatal period. The stored glycogen is structurally normal. Inability to mobilize glycogen from the liver leads to severe, sustained hypoglycemia, lactic and pyruvic acidosis, and hyperlipemia. Seizures and mental retardation are a result of the hypoglycemia. Various treatment strategies have helped ameliorate the metabolic abnormalities with modest success. These include frequent small feedings of glucose and the use of medium-chain triglycerides to reduce the hyperlipemia.

Acid maltase deficiency is associated with storage of normal glycogen in skeletal muscle. There are several clinical variants. The *infantile form* presents in the first 6 months of life with marked hypotonia and weakness. There are difficulties with swallowing and respiration. Cardiomegaly, hepatomegaly, and an enlarged tongue are present. Subcutaneous fat is extremely sparse. The children die in the first year of life from cardiac and respiratory problems.

The *late-infantile form* of acid maltase deficiency does not become symptomatic until the second year of life. The children then develop a progressive myopathy which resembles that of Duchenne dystrophy. There is no hepatomegaly, cardiomegaly, or macroglossia.

An *adult form,* also associated with a progressive myopathy, has been reported. Symptoms begin in mid- to late life. It does not appear to be hereditary, unlike the early-onset forms, which are autosomal recessive conditions.

McArdle disease results from deficiency of muscle phosphorylase activity. The inability to convert muscle glycogen to glucose causes severe muscle weakness and pain following exercise. If attempts to exercise vigorously are pursued, rhabdomyolysis and myoglobinuria result. Symptoms do not appear before adolescence.

A clinical diagnosis can be made by the ischemic work test. A tourniquet is applied to the arm to impair the arterial supply, and the patient is asked to exercise the limb. Normally, there should be a sharp rise in venous lactate levels. The patient with McArdle disease has a reduced capacity to exercise under these conditions, rapidly develops severe pain, and demonstrates no rise in venous lactate levels. The diagnosis should be confirmed by histochemical staining or biochemical studies of muscle obtained at biopsy, as other defects in glycolysis can produce similar findings. These include *phosphohexose isomerase deficiency* and *phosphofructokinase deficiency.* The only effective management is for the patient to learn the limits of his exercise tolerance.

DISORDERS OF AMMONIA METABOLISM

Hyperammonemia can be caused by an enzymatic defect at any point in the urea cycle. The general symptoms of these disorders are poor development and episodes of vomiting and depressed consciousness which are often triggered or worsened by protein ingestion. Seizures may also occur. Placing the child on intravenous glucose-containing fluids then leads to temporary improvement.

Transient hyperammonemia can occur in newborn infants and must be differentiated from the urea cycle disorders.[6] The children with transient hyperammonemia have lower birth weights and earlier onset of respiratory distress, the need for ventilatory support, lethargy, and coma than those with enzyme defects. Onset of respiratory distress within the first 24 hr of life is characteristic of transient hyperammonemia; after 30 hr, the urea cycle disorders.

These disorders are rare, and the majority are inherited as autosomal recessive traits. *Ornithine transcarbamylase deficiency* differs in that it is an X-linked recessive condition which can produce mild clinical abnormalities in heterozygous females. The male is severely involved, with typical symptoms of ammonia intoxication and early death. Some girls present with a clinical picture of migraine and elevation of blood ammonia during the attacks.

Carbamyl phosphate synthetase deficiency is associated with the severe classical symptoms of hyperammonemia. Even small amounts of protein cause serious metabolic crises.

Citrullinemia is also a cause of the severe form of hyperammonemia and can produce death in infancy. Other children do not become symptomatic until the second half of the first year of life. Development regresses and severe mental retardation results. The attacks of vomiting and metabolic derangement are less severe.

Arginosuccinic aciduria has several clinical types. The neonatal form presents as a severe metabolic disorder with seizures, depressed consciousness, and respiratory distress. A diagnostic clue is the presence of friable hair. In the subacute form the symptoms are severe, but are not present in the neonatal period. In addition to protein intolerance and the typical hair abnormalities, hepatomegaly occurs. The late form also shares in the hair abnormalities. The children are mentally retarded and have intermittent episodes of ataxia.

Treatment strategies are complex and include nitrogen restriction and the use of supplements of sodium benzoate, arginine, citrulline, and sodium phenylacetate. Survival rates of 92% are now possible.[7] Morbidity is still high, however, with 79% of children having at least one developmental disability; the mean IQ of the study group was 43. The IQ is inversely correlated with the duration of neonatal coma and the peak ammonia level.

MUCOPOLYSACCHARIDOSES

The number of types and variants of the mucopolysaccharidoses has expanded greatly in recent years. Several of them affect the central nervous system and present as progressive degenerative diseases. *Hurler syndrome* (MPS I H) is the best known. Mental retardation and the typical somatic features become apparent during the first year of life. The face has a coarse appearance, which led to the use of the older term gargoylism. Skeletal abnormalities are prominent with hyphosis, lumbar lordosis, joint flexion contractures, and short, broad hands. Characteristic changes in the long bones (Figure 17-1) and vertebral bodies are present on x-ray examination. Corneal clouding and deafness

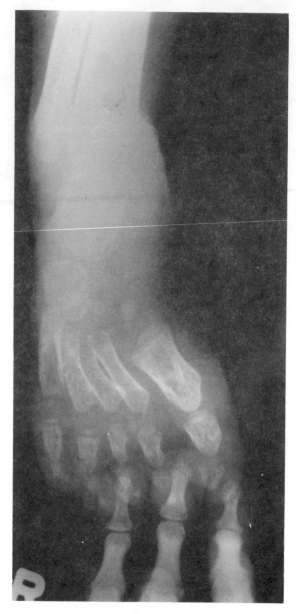

FIGURE 17-1. Expansion and distortion of metacarpal bones and phalanges in a patient with Hurler syndrome.

occur. Death in late childhood is usually from cardiac disease, owing to involvement of the coronary arteries and heart valves.

This condition and the others in this group can be detected by simple urine screening tests, but sophisticated biochemical studies are required to fully define the disorder. The specific enzymatic defect is absence of α-L-iduronidase. Dermatan sulfate and heparan sulfate accumulate in the brain and other organs and are excreted in large quantities in the urine. Transmission is as an autosomal recessive. Prenatal diagnosis is possible, but requires specialized techniques. There is no satisfactory treatment.

Hunter syndrome (MPS II) is an X-linked condition. The symptoms and signs are similar to those of Hurler syndrome, although less severe. There is no corneal clouding. Life-span is longer. A variant form allows survival into adult life and is not associated with severe mental retardation. The deficient enzyme is sulfoiduronate sulfatase. Prenatal detection is possible.

Sanfilippo syndrome (MPS III) is associated with even less prominent physical signs, but marked intellectual deterioration begins at age 2–3 years. Three different biochemical varieties have been defined.

MUCOLIPIDOSES

This is a complex group of rare hereditary disorders. There is tissue storage of mucopolysaccharides, but no excessive excretion of these compounds in the urine. Somatic features resemble those of the mucopolysaccharidoses, and there is usually mental retardation. Most of these disorders are progressive, and life-span is limited.

OTHER METABOLIC DISORDERS

Lesch–Nyhan syndrome is dramatic because of the unusual characteristic of self-mutilation. This begins in childhood or adolescence. These children compulsively bite at their lips and fingers, destroying tissue. They will do everything possible to break out of restraints to continue this activity. The patients are also mentally retarded and have choreoathetosis. Hyperuricemia is due to a deficiency in the activity of hypoxanthine–guanine phosphoribosyltransferase. The elevated uric acid level leads to crystalluria, renal calculi, and death from renal failure. Treatment with allopurinol can delay the onset of the renal disease. Genetic transmission is X-linked.

Subacute necrotizing encephalomyelopathy (Leigh disease) is associated with variable signs and symptoms. The onset is in infancy or childhood. The major features suggest involvement of the brain stem and include ophthalmoplegias, difficulty swallowing, irregular respirations, ataxia, and visual abnormalities. There is also mental retardation and seizures. Peripheral neuropathy has been described.

The disorder may present acutely with death rapidly ensuing. Other patients remain ill but survive for many months. Spontaneous remissions have also been reported.

A tremendous amount of biochemical research has not provided a single reproducible metabolic abnormality. The most consistent findings point to the presence of an inhibitor of the enzyme systems involved in the metabolism of lactate and pyruvate. Because of this, there have been numerous attempts to treat the condition with thiamine and some of its derivatives, but without consistent success. Transmission is as an autosomal recessive trait.

Menkes kinky-hair syndrome (trichopoliodystrophy, steely-hair syndrome) is another X-linked metabolic disorder. The children become symptomatic in early infancy and present with seizures and profound developmental failure. The hair is distinctly abnormal, with beading (monilethrix), twisting (pili torti), and breakage of the hair shaft (trichorrhexis nodosa). There appears to be an abnormality in the absorption of copper from the gastrointestinal tract and low serum copper and ceruloplasmin levels. Attempts at treatment with the intravenous administration of copper have not given dramatic results.

Carnitine deficiency presents with progressive muscle weakness. There is also a generalized form, which produces repeated episodes of hepatic and central nervous system dysfunction, clinically and biochemically resembling Reye syndrome.[8] These attacks are often precipitated by illness or caloric deprivation. Intravenous administration of glucose rapidly corrects the abnormalities. This syndrome should also be considered in any familial case of what appears to be Reye syndrome.

Biotinidase deficiency presents with seizures in infancy. Other clinical features then develop and include hypotonia, ataxia, alopecia, skin rash, optic atrophy, hearing loss, and developmental delay.[9] Laboratory studies reveal metabolic acidosis with increased levels of ketoacids and lactic acid, organic aciduria, and, in one-third of patients, hyperammonemia. There is decreased activity of biotinidase, which can be increased by administration of biotin. Some children improve dramatically with therapy.

Rett syndrome is characterized by dementia, ataxia, seizures, and behavior similar to that in infantile autism.[10] The patients also stop using their hands for purposeful behavior and they develop characteristic stereotyped hand movements. The disorder begins between 1 and 4 years of age and is progressive. It is restricted to girls. Studies of the cerebrospinal fluid show decreased levels of HVA and MHPG, metabolites of dopamine and norepinephrine.

REFERENCES

1. Stanbury, J. B., Wyngaarden, J. B., Fredrickson, D. S., Goldstein, J. L., and Brown, M. S., 1983, *The Metabolic Basis of Inherited Disease*, 5th ed., McGraw-Hill, New York.
2. Therrel, B. L., Brown, L. O., Dziuk, P. E., and Peter, W. P., 1983, The Texas Newborn Screening Program, *Texas Med.* **79:**44–46.
3. Koch, R., Azen, C. G., Friedman, E. G., and Williamson, M. L., 1982, Preliminary report on the effects of diet discontinuation in PKU, *J. Pediatr.* **100:**870–875.
4. Levy, H. L., Kaplan, G. N., and Erickson, A. M., 1982, Comparison of treated and untreated pregnancies in a mother with phenylketonuria, *J. Pediatr.* **100:**876–880.
5. Berlow, S., 1980, Progress in phenylketonuria: Defects in the metabolism of biopterin, *Pediatrics* **65:**837–839.
6. Hudak, M. L., Jones, M. D., and Brusilow, S. W., 1985, Differentiation of transient hyperammonemia of the newborn and urea cycle enzyme defects by clinical presentation, *J. Pediatr.* **107:**712–719.
7. Msall, M., Batshaw, M. L., Suss, R., Brusilaw, S. W., and Mellits, E. D., 1984, Neurologic outcome in children with inborn errors of urea synthesis, *N. Engl. J. Med.* **310:**1500–1505.

8. Rebouche, C. J., and Engel, A. G., 1983, Carnitine metabolism and deficiency syndromes, *Mayo Clin. Proc.* **58:**533–540.
9. Wolf, B., Heard, G. S., Weissbecker, K. A., McVoy, J. R. S., Grier, R. E., and Leshner, R. T., 1985, Biotinidase deficiency: Initial clinical features and rapid diagnosis, *Ann. Neurol.* **18:**614–617.
10. Zoghbi, H. Y., Percy, A. K., Glaze, D. G., Butler, I. J., and Riccardi, V. M., 1985, Reduction of biogenic amine levels in the Rett syndrome, *N. Engl. J. Med.* **313:**921–924.

ADDITIONAL READING

Horwitz, A., 1979, The mucopolysaccharidoses: Clinical and biochemical correlations, *Am. J. Ment. Def.* **84:**113–123.
Koch, R. (ed.), 1981, Urea cycle symposium, *Pediatrics* **68:**271–279, 446–462.
Rosenberg, R. N., 1981, Biochemical genetics of neurologic disease, *N. Engl. J. Med.* **305:**1181–1193.

18

Degenerative Disorders

The hallmark of degenerative disorders of the nervous system is the progressive loss of previously acquired abilities. In young children, deceleration in the rate of development is often the first sign of degeneration. The patient falls progressively behind other children, and subsequently there is actual loss of previously acquired achievements. This is quantitated as a declining developmental quotient. By definition, this deterioration is not due to an exogenous agent or event, or to secondary involvement of the nervous system by a generalized systemic disease. Most of the degenerative disorders are hereditary, although the biochemical basis of many of these conditions is not fully understood.

The degenerative disorders can be conveniently divided into three groups:

- Gray-matter diseases
- White-matter diseases
- System diseases

The gray-matter diseases are manifested by primary involvement of neurons. This occurs with or without histological evidence of storage of abnormal metabolic products and leads to neuronal death and secondary degeneration of axons. In the white-matter disorders myelin is disrupted. This can be the result of destruction of normal myelin or the production of biochemically abnormal myelin. The system diseases form a heterogeneous group of conditions in which there is progressive degeneration of anatomically defined systems, such as the dorsal columns, pyramidal tracts, or cerebellar nuclei. Typically, both neurons and myelin are lost in these disorders.

There is some overlap of the degenerative diseases, the metabolic disorders (Chapter 17), and conditions due to storage of toxic levels of a dietary constituent, such as copper in Wilson disease or phytanic acid in Refsum disease. Inclusion in this chapter is somewhat arbitrary and more a function of custom than of biological distinction.

APPROACH TO THE PATIENT

The first clinical task is to document that the child has lost previously acquired abilities or has a decelerating developmental quotient. This second diagnostic criterion must be used cautiously, as a child with a severe static encephalopathy will make so little developmental progress that there is an apparent progressive drop in the developmental quotient. The most important diagnostic tool is repeated developmental evaluations. Older children, especially those with slowly progressive disorders, should be referred to a psychologist for full cognitive assessment and periodic follow-up testing.

The major clinical features differentiating gray-matter diseases from those of white matter can be predicted from an understanding of the functional roles of neurons and myelin. Neuronal involvement causes the early onset of dementia, the progressive loss of cognitive abilities. Seizures are common, and myoclonic seizures are especially characteristic. The basal ganglia and cerebellar nuclei are collections of neurons, and so extrapyramidal and cerebellar signs commonly occur. Ganglion cells of the retina are affected in many of the neuronal storage disorders, producing pigmentary degeneration of the retina which may be associated with a cherry-red spot.

The earliest sign of most of the white-matter degenerations is spasticity. Dementia and seizures tend to occur later. Extrapyramidal signs are rare, but involvement of cerebellar pathways causes ataxia. Optic atrophy is the most characteristic ocular change. Some patients have cortical blindness due to demyelination of the optic pathways in the cerebral hemispheres.

Each of the system diseases has its own characteristics, depending on the particular anatomical pathways involved. The spinocerebellar degenerations are discussed in Chapter 25, and Huntington disease and juvenile Parkinson disease in Chapter 21.

GRAY-MATTER DISEASES

Alper disease is a disorder manifested only by progressive loss of neurons without evidence of storage. The condition is rare, and there is controversy concerning its existence as a specific clinical and pathological entity.

The majority of the gray-matter diseases are associated with storage of abnormal material in neurons and subsequent neuronal degeneration. Those neuronal storage disorders which become symptomatic in infancy are generally characterized by definable abnormalities in lysosomal enzymes. Specific diagnosis is possible by assaying the level of enzyme activity in leukocytes or in fibroblasts grown in tissue culture. The patient's cells have absent activity or levels that are extremely low; prenatal diagnosis is possible using fetal cells obtained by amniocentesis. Heterozygotes generally have enzyme levels approximately one-half of normal, allowing carriers to be detected.

Tay–Sachs disease is the prototype of the neuronal storage disorders. The disease manifests itself in the first 6 months of life with irritability and a prominent startle response to sounds. It soon becomes evident that developmental milestones are not being met, and that the child does not see. Myoclonic and generalized seizures appear. The child, who was initially hypotonic, becomes spastic and loses all responsiveness to the environment. Death occurs in the first few years of life from malnutrition, pneumonia, and other infections.

The classical feature found on neurological examination is a cherry-red spot in the ocular fundus. Storage of lipid in retinal ganglion cells makes the perifoveal area appear gray and opaque. The fovea contains no ganglion cells and appears red by contrast. The remainder of the examination confirms blindness and the failure of development. There is no hepatosplenomegaly.

The biochemical abnormalities are absence of hexosaminidase A and S and storage of Gm2 ganglioside in neurons. These cells are swollen, and the brain is larger and heavier than normal. As the condition progresses, neurons are lost and there is secondary degeneration of white matter.

Genetic transmission is as an autosomal recessive trait; the majority of parents are of Eastern European (Ashkenazi) Jewish background. Population studies have traced many of these families back to several small villages in Eastern Europe. Genetic screening programs, based on measurement of serum hexosaminidase A levels, in the group at high risk have been very successful in reducing the incidence of this condition. Prenatal diagnosis by amniocentesis is also possible.

Sandhoff disease has a clinical presentation and course virtually indistinguishable from those of Tay–Sachs disease except for the presence of hepatosplenomegaly. Hexosaminidase A and B are both absent, and there is storage of Gm2 and a related metabolic product in the brain and peripheral organs.

Generalized gangliosidosis presents at birth with abnormal features on physical examination. The child has the coarse dull facies and hepatosplenomegaly reminiscent of Hurler syndrome. Development progresses very slowly, vision and hearing are lost, and seizures begin by the end of the first year. Somatic features become more pronounced with the passage of time, and the diagnosis is aided by characteristic changes on x-ray studies of the vertebral column and long bones. The lumbar vertebrae have a beaked appearance, and long bones are expanded in the center and taper toward the ends.

The disease is defined biochemically by absence of β-galactosidase and storage of Gm1 ganglioside. It is transmitted as an autosomal recessive disorder and is found in all ethnic and racial groups. Prenatal diagnosis can be established by amniocentesis.

A variant of this disease is associated with absence of β-galactosidase in the brain and Gm1 storage restricted to the central nervous system. Symptoms begin in the school-age period, and the course is protracted as compared to the congenital form. This illustrates an important concept. As more cases of degenerative disorders are studied, and as biochemical techniques become more sophisticated, variants of almost all of the classical disorders are being described.[1,2]

Niemann–Pick disease is another example of a condition with several variants. These are all characterized by absence of sphingomyelinase and storage of sphingomyelin in tissue. They differ, however, in the organ systems involved in this storage, the clinical features, and the rate of progression of the illness. The infantile form (type A) presents in the first year of life with progressive developmental and motor deterioration, spasticity, and hepatosplenomegaly. Some patients have a cherry-red spot. Death occurs early. Other variants of this disorder have a later onset and slower progression than the infantile form. They are all associated with hepatosplenomegaly. Each type is produced by a distinct autosomal recessive gene.

Specific biochemical diagnosis is possible. An additional diagnostic aid is the presence of characteristic cells which can be found in biopsy specimens of liver or bone marrow. These are large and vacuolated, owing to storage of sphingomyelin.

There are also several distinct variants of *Gaucher disease*. Glucocerebrosidase is deficient in the involved organs in each form. Whether or not glucocerebroside is stored in increased quantities in the brain is a matter of controversy at this time. The acute infantile type presents early in the first year with spasticity, dysphagia, and seizures. Deterioration is rapid, and death occurs in early infancy.

A subacute form presents later in childhood with myoclonic seizures. There are no neurological problems associated with the adult-onset chronic form of the disorder. Hepatosplenomegaly occurs in all variants, and biochemical and histological diagnosis is possible.

The term *neuronal ceroid lipofuscinosis* refers to a clinically heterogeneous group of disorders, all of which manifest progressive degeneration of the central nervous system. They share similar histopathological features consisting of cerebral atrophy and neuronal storage of abnormal pigmentary material. This substance has been referred to as ceroid-lipofuscin. Differences in the ultrastructural characteristics of this material allow some consistent histological correlations with clinical subgroups.

Certain clinical features are common to most variants of this disorder. These are progressive dementia, loss of vision owing to pigmentary degeneration of the retina, and seizures, typically myoclonic. Any of the other features characteristic of gray-matter diseases can be found. The variations are mainly in the prominence of any specific sign or symptom, the rate of progression of the illness, and the age of clinical onset and death.

There are no consistent biochemical markers for this group of conditions. A specific diagnosis can now be made in most cases without resorting to brain biopsy. Electroretinography is characteristic of generalized retinal degeneration and confirms the ophthalmoscopic findings. Specific abnormal inclusions of several types can be identified by ultrastructural study of skin biopsies.[3] Similar findings have been reported in leukocytes. All forms of this disorder are transmitted as autosomal recessive traits. The role of skin biopsy in defining the carrier state and in prenatal diagnosis has not been determined.

A number of experimental types of treatment are in use. These are largely based on the administration of antioxidants such as vitamin E. No dramatic changes in the clinical course have been documented.

WHITE-MATTER DISEASES

Demyelination refers to the destruction of normal myelin in the white matter of the brain, spinal cord, or peripheral nerve. The *postinfectious encephalopathies* appear to attack normal myelin and are the most common of the demyelinating conditions in childhood. These are discussed in Chapter 13. Multiple sclerosis, rare in childhood, is probably an immunologically mediated disorder and is also discussed in the same chapter.

Central pontine myelinolysis, destruction of myelin in the central portion of the pons, is usually a postmortem diagnosis, although some patients present with pseudobulbar palsy, spastic paraparesis, and ataxia. The lesion can be visualized on magnetic resonance imaging scans. It has been described in malnourished children and also may be produced by overly vigorous replacement of sodium in hyponatremic patients.

The majority of the degenerative diseases of white matter result from biochemical defects which cause the formation of abnormal myelin. This does not function normally and rapidly breaks down. These conditions are referred to as the dysmyelinating disorders, or leukodystrophies.

The classic form of *adrenoleukodystrophy* is a condition beginning in the early school years and characterized by progressive dementia and abnormal behavior. This is associated with optic atrophy, hearing loss, spasticity, ataxia, and seizures. Visual field defects and cortical blindness are frequently present. Brain stem involvement causes difficulty with swallowing, and extraocular palsies can also occur.

Adrenal insufficiency is usually present in this condition. Even if this is not clinically apparent, there are characteristic ultrastructural abnormalities in the adrenal cortex. Pathological changes in the brain consist of large areas of destruction and loss of myelin, the presence of lipid containing macrophages, perivascular infiltration by mononuclear cells, and gliosis. Changes in peripheral nerves have been used as a diagnostic tool.[4]

The disorder is transmitted as an X-linked recessive trait and rarely occurs in girls. No specific enzymatic marker has been defined, but an increase in very-long-chain fatty acids is found in fibroblasts. This assay can confirm the diagnosis and also be used for carrier detection.[5] Prenatal diagnosis is possible through studies of lipids in cultured amniocytes.[6]

A condition related to adrenoleukodystrophy has been described. *Adrenomyeloneuropathy* is also an X-linked recessive disorder. Young adult men present with progressive stiffness and weakness of the legs and evidence of peripheral neuropathy. Changes in the adrenal glands and plasma fatty acids are identical to those in adrenoleukodystrophy.

Neonatal adrenoleukodystrophy is inherited by an autosomal recessive mechanism and becomes symptomatic in the first year of life. The most prominent features are severe psychomotor retardation, hypotonia, and seizures.[6] Additional clinical findings, present in some patients, are hepatomegaly, retinopathy, and dysmorphic features.

Schilder disease has always been the subject of confusion, as the author probably described three different conditions. It is now generally accepted that most, if not all, cases of Schilder disease are really adrenoleukodystrophy. An occasional girl seems to be affected, but this probably represents another demyelinating disorder, such as multiple sclerosis or metachromatic leukodystrophy.

Spongy degeneration of Canavan presents in early infancy with hypotonia, failure to achieve developmental milestones, and optic atrophy. The child later becomes spastic and develops seizures. Head circumference is abnormally large in many cases. There is no biochemical marker that can be used diagnostically, but the neuropathological changes are characteristic. Marked vacuolization of the cortex and subcortical white matter are found. Ultrastructural studies show the vacuoles to be within the myelin and also demonstrate changes in mitochondria. The disease is transmitted as an autosomal recessive and has increased incidence among patients of Ashkenazi Jewish origin.

Several variants of *Pelizaeus–Merzbacher disease* have been described. The classic form is transmitted by an X-linked recessive gene. The male infant manifests nystagmus and delayed development. This is later followed by ataxia, spasticity, and choreoathetosis. Survival is often prolonged. No specific biochemical findings have been reported. Characteristic pathological changes include severe demyelination with preservation of myelin in perivascular areas.

Metachromatic leukodystrophy is the most common white-matter degeneration in which a specific enzymatic abnormality has been described. There is absent cerebroside sulfatase activity. The late-infantile form presents in the preschool years with ataxia and hypotonia. Motor function deteriorates, and there is a combination of spasticity and peripheral neuropathy; the patient demonstrates Babinski signs and absent deep-tendon reflexes. Loss of cognitive skills follows, and the child becomes vegetative and quadriplegic. Death results from pneumonia or other infections.

The juvenile form begins at a later age and has a longer course. Behavioral and cognitive changes are an early symptom. An adult form shows an even slower rate of progression. Each of the three variants is inherited by a different autosomal recessive gene. Carrier identification and prenatal detection can be accomplished by measuring the level of cerebroside sulfatase in fibroblasts or leukocytes.

The activity of the enzyme is absent; this leads to storage of sulfatide and the formation of abnormal myelin. Microscopic studies show abnormal staining characteristics (metachromasia) of the stored material. Myelin loss is extensive. Neurons in the basal ganglia and thalamus store some abnormal material, and so the disorder is a bridge between the white-matter and gray-matter diseases.

Krabbe disease begins in the middle of the first year of life with extreme irritability. Severe spasticity and opisthotonos become evident, and previous developmental achievements are lost. The child also develops optic atrophy and peripheral neuropathy. There is no hepatosplenomegaly. The disorder is transmitted as an autosomal recessive condition.

Diagnosis depends on demonstration of absent galactocerebrosidase activity, which can be assayed in fibroblasts. Carrier ascertainment and prenatal detection of the disorder are possible. Neuropathological changes consist of loss of myelin and cortical atrophy. The classic feature is the presence of globoid cells, large cells containing PAS-positive material, in the central nervous system. There is also demyelination in peripheral nerves.

Neuraxonal dystrophy presents after the first year of life with signs suggesting motor unit involvement (weakness and atrophy) and corticospinal tract involvement (Babinski signs). Optic atrophy and seizures also develop. Degeneration is progressive, and death occurs within a few years. The disease is transmitted as an autosomal recessive trait.

There is degeneration and loss of myelin and abnormal swellings (spheroids) in axons. It is not clear whether the primary pathogenetic process involves axons, myelin, or both. Identical findings are present in a number of other conditions, some of which may be related to vitamin E deficiency and include malnutrition, cystic fibrosis, and congenital biliary atresia.

Myelin loss and axonal spheroids are found in *Hallervorden–Spatz disease.* This degenerative disorder presents a picture of dementia, dystonia, rigidity, and choreoathetosis. It is genetic, with an autosomal recessive mode of inheritance. The condition is relentlessly progressive, beginning in the first decade and leading to death in early adulthood. Despite the many shared histopathological features, it appears to be genetically distinct from neuraxonal dystrophy. In addition, Hallervorden–Spatz disease is associated with accumulation of iron in the globus pallidus and substantia nigra. This can often be visualized on CT scan, which provides some diagnostic assistance.

TREATMENT

None of these disorders can be treated at this time, although most are theoretically amenable to the strategies listed in Table 17-3. One problem is that in some conditions, such as Tay–Sachs disease, there is a good deal of neurological damage in fetal life, at a time before the diagnosis can be made. In addition, correcting the enzymatic defect peripherally will not necessarily correct the central nervous system abnormalities.[7]

Vitamin E has been administered to patients with neuronal ceroid lipofuscinosis, neuraxonal dystrophy, and Hallervorden–Spatz disease with no obvious benefit. Attempts to remove iron from the CNS using deferoxamine in patients with Hallervorden–Spatz disease have also not met with success.

REFERENCES

1. Farrell, D. F., and Ochs, U., 1981, G_{M1} gangliosidosis: Phenotypic variation in a single family, *Ann. Neurol.* **9:**225–231.
2. Farrell, D. F., and MacMartin, M. P., 1981, G_{M1} gangliosidosis: Enzymatic variation in a single family, *Ann. Neurol.* **9:**232–286.
3. Miloy, C. E., Gilbert, E. F., France, T. D., O'Brien, J. F., and Chun, R. W. M., 1978, Clinical and extraneural histologic diagnosis of neuronal ceroid-lipofuscinosis, *Neurology* **28:**1008–1012.

4. Martin, J. J., Centerick, C., and Libert, J., 1980, Skin and conjunctival nerve biopsies in adrenoleukodystrophy and its variants, *Ann. Neurol.* **8:**291–295.
5. Moser, H. W., Moser, A. E., Trojak, J. E., and Supplee, S. W., 1983, Identification of female carriers of adrenoleukodystrophy, *J. Pediatr.* **103:**54–59.
6. Moser, H. W., Moser, A. E., Singh, I., and O'Neill, B. P., 1984, Adrenoleukodystrophy: Survey of 303 cases: Biochemistry, diagnosis, and therapy, *Ann. Neurol.* **16:**628–641.
7. von Specht, B. U., Geiger, B., Arnon, R., Passwell, J., Keren, G., Goldman, B., and Padeh, B., 1979, Enzyme replacement in Tay–Sachs disease, *Neurology* **28:**848–854.

ADDITIONAL READING

Dyken, P., and Krawiecki, N., 1983, Neurodegenerative diseases of infancy and childhood, *Ann. Neurol.* **13:**351–364.

19

Neoplasms

Accidents, nearly one-half involving motor vehicles, are the leading cause of death in children beyond the neonatal period. Malignancies are second, with only leukemia and lymphomas surpassing brain tumors in frequency. The average annual incidence rate for CNS neoplasms is between 2 and 5 cases/100,000 population per year.[1]

The origin of brain tumors is unknown, and no specific carcinogenic or genetic factors have been determined. The incidence rate is greater in the white population than in the black, and greater in boys than in girls.

Approximately 60% of brain tumors in preadolescent children are infratentorial. Many of the supratentorial tumors do not involve the cerebral hemispheres, but are suprasellar extraaxial neoplasms. During adolescence, there is an even higher incidence of tumors in this region.

The most common histological type of intraaxial tumor is medulloblastoma, followed by astrocytoma and glioblastoma. Craniopharyngioma is the most common of the suprasellar tumors; dysgerminomas and teratomas are next in frequency.

APPROACH TO THE PATIENT

The signs and symptoms of brain tumors result from their effects as space-occupying mass lesions and from direct involvement of neural structures that are compressed or destroyed by the neoplasm. The mass effect produces increased intracranial pressure, with symptoms of headache, lethargy, irritability, personality change, diplopia, and transient obscurations of vision. Clues that differentiate the headache of brain tumor from that of other headache syndromes include a change in pattern of severity, prolonged headache, pain that awakens the patient from sleep, and associated vomiting, often without nausea.[2]

Neurological examination documents papilledema and may also show third- or sixth-nerve palsies. Young children will have excessive head growth and may have dilated veins over the scalp. In infants, a bulging fontanelle and separation of the cranial bones at the suture lines will be found.

The history and examination allow localization of the tumor in most cases. Several clinical patterns can be defined.

Hemispheric tumors present with progressive hemiparesis. Other symptoms and signs depend on the exact location of the tumor and include homonymous hemianopsia, aphasia, personality changes, and declining cognitive performance. Some children develop an attention deficit disorder or behavior problems. Seizures, either focal or generalized, are the initial problem in approximately one-quarter of children and occur at some time in two-thirds of those with hemispheric tumors.

Deep tumors, located in the thalamus, often have an insidious course with only a slowly progressive hemiparesis.[3] When CSF pathways are compromised, intracranial pressure then rapidly increases. One-half of these children will have ataxia of the limbs or gait, due to involvement of cerebellar pathways.

Suprasellar tumors involve the optic chiasm, anterior and posterior pituitary, hypothalamopituitary connections, hypothalamus, and third ventricle. If there is no increase in intracranial pressure, many of the symptoms and signs are subtle, and there are often long delays in diagnosis. Impingement on the optic chiasm typically produces a bitemporal hemianopsia. As the condition progresses, optic atrophy with loss of visual acuity ensues. Involvement of the chiasm and one optic nerve will produce blindness in one eye and a temporal field defect in the other. Early diagnosis is difficult, as individuals with field cuts are often unaware of their presence, and young children rarely complain of slowly progressive visual loss. In addition, examination of the visual fields in young children is a problem, although some of the new techniques using computer-averaged visual evoked responses may prove to be useful. Parents' complaints of abnormal visual behavior in a child should always be taken seriously.

Hypothalamic–pituitary involvement most frequently presents as growth failure. A properly maintained growth chart is the most powerful tool for early diagnosis, and a suprasellar neoplasm should be considered when any child's growth rate decelerates and the growth curve falls through several percentiles. Diabetes insipidus often has a more dramatic onset with polyuria, polydipsia, and, in young children without free access to water, severe dehydration and hypernatremia. Precocious puberty is also common.

Invasion of the hypothalamus by a suprasellar tumor or, more commonly, a glioma primary to this region can present with the *diencephalic syndrome.* The children are severely emaciated but have an alert appearance and may even appear to be hyperkinetic. Vomiting, optic atrophy, and nystagmus are often present. Impingement on the third ventricle produces hydrocephalus.

Infratentorial tumors can be clinically differentiated into those that involve the brain stem primarily and those arising within the cerebellum. The latter neoplasms differ somewhat in presentation, depending on whether they are situated in the cerebellar hemispheres or vermis. Intraaxial *brain stem tumors* present with a combination of pyramidal tract, cerebellar, and cranial nerve signs. Spasticity is generally bilateral, and ataxia of both gait and limbs is present. The most common cranial nerves involved initially are the seventh, with facial diplegia, and the sixth, with bilateral abducens palsies. Lower cranial nerves then become compromised and produce drooling, difficulty swallowing, and nasal regurgitation of liquids as the palate becomes involved. Clinical involvement of higher cranial nerves is unusual until late in the course.

Tumors of the *cerebellar vermis* are associated with severe gait ataxia and inability to maintain the head and trunk steady in space. This produces titubation, a tremulousness of the body and head when the patient is in the upright position. Dysarthria is common. Pathological nystagmus, especially on upward gaze, is generally present. Some neoplasms in a midline location do not involve the vermis, but invade the floor of the fourth ventricle. Cerebellar signs are lacking. The predominant symptoms are vomiting and those associated with increased intracranial pressure.

Tumors arising in the *cerebellar hemispheres* present with limb ataxia on the ipsilateral side of the body. As the tumor grows, distortion of midline structures will superimpose the findings associated with a vermal syndrome.

Primary neoplasms of the *cranial nerve* are unusual in children, except those who have neurofibromatosis. Optic gliomas are initially associated with unilateral visual loss. Children rarely complain of this problem, but a change in visual behavior is often reported by the parents. As the tumor spreads posteriorly, the optic chiasm becomes involved, and the syndrome of a suprasellar tumor will evolve.

Acoustic neuromas are associated with hearing loss, but, as is the case with decreasing visual acuity, young children rarely complain of this symptom. If the tumor is unilateral, the child is often completely unaware of the problem. Involvement of the vestibular portion of the eighth nerve rarely causes symptoms. As the tumor grows, the brain stem and cerebellum are distorted, and a host of neurological signs referable to posterior fossa structures develops.

As in many areas of diagnostic neurology, the development of computerized tomography (CT) has been revolutionary. The definition of the lesion with this study is generally superior to that possible with older neuroradiological techniques, and it can be obtained with less morbidity and at lower cost.[4] The CT scan, carried out with and without the administration of a contrast agent, is the primary diagnostic technique if brain tumor is suspected.

Magnetic resonance imaging (MRI) scanning has higher resolution than CT scans and is especially useful for detecting low-grade astrocytomas. These are often difficult to define with CT scans. This technique is especially useful for the diagnosis of brain stem gliomas and for any lesions lying close to bone.

X-ray studies of the skull have limited usefulness. They may add diagnostic information when tumors are in the suprasellar region, by defining bony destruction of the pituitary fossa. In addition, CT scans still are not useful for visualizing small lesions close to dense bone. MRI scanning will probably supplant skull x rays for this indication, however.

Stereotactic biopsy allows histological diagnosis to be obtained without the risks inherent in craniotomy. This technique can also be applied to regions, such as the brain stem, that have limited surgical accessibility.

The general principles for *treatment* of brain tumors are relatively simple. Increased intracranial pressure must be promptly relieved. The most direct approach is surgical removal of as much of the tumor as possible without damaging intact neural tissue and producing a greater deficit. In emergency situations, especially if the increased intracranial pressure is due to blockage of CSF pathways and obstructive hydrocephalus, ventriculostomy with CSF drainage is required. This is not without hazard, as upward herniation of posterior fossa contents through the tentorial notch and brain stem compression can occur.

The surgical approach to tumors rarely allows removal of all of the neoplastic tissue, because of the obvious impossibility of radical resections, and because many tumors infiltrate into surrounding brain tissue and are without clear demarcation. Radiotherapy supplements surgery in most cases. The doses used (5000–6000 rads) are close to the radiation tolerance of surrounding brain. Higher doses are associated with a risk of radionecrosis, which presents as a progressive encephalopathy. This may mimic tumor regrowth. Secondary neoplasms, such as dural sarcomas, have also been reported following higher doses. There are a number of regional and national study protocols investigating the role of chemotherapy in brain tumor treatment. This modality may prove to be important in the treatment of specific neoplasms.

Survival rates depend on the specific tumor type and location. Overall, 50% of children will survive 5 years without evidence of tumor recurrence.

SPECIFIC DISORDERS

Tumors of the cerebral hemispheres are primarily glial in origin. Thirty-five percent of all brain tumors are *benign gliomas,* and an additional 5% are classified as *malignant* gliomas. Prognosis of hemispheric tumors relates to both the cellular characteristics and the location. Even with radical resection, most malignant gliomas can be expected to recur. Radiation therapy rarely is curative. If more benign grades of astrocytoma are restricted to the frontal, occipital, or temporal poles, surgical cure is a reasonable goal.

One-quarter of *ependymomas* in children arise in the lateral ventricles. The most common presentation is with increased intracranial pressure, although some are aggressive and produce a typical syndrome of hemispheric involvement. Occasionally, they will seed throughout the neuraxis, and multiple areas of tumor involvement will develop. The risk of recurrence is very high, despite appropriate surgical intervention and radiotherapy. *Choroid plexus papilloma* is the least common of the intraventricular tumors in children and also presents primarily with signs and symptoms of intracranial hypertension.

Craniopharyngiomas account for almost 10% of CNS neoplasms in children and are the most common supratentorial tumor (Figures 19-1 and 19-2). They are probably congenital in origin and arise from ectodermal cell remnants of Rathke's pouch. There is a mixture of solid tissue, consisting of well-differentiated epithelium with whorls of keratinized cells, and cysts containing fluid and cholesterol crystals. Attempts at radical surgical removal put the patient at high

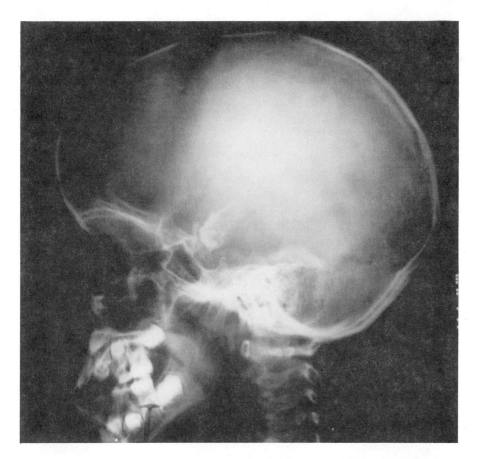

FIGURE 19-1. Suprasellar calcifications in a patient with a craniopharyngioma.

risk for damage to the hypothalamus and upper brain stem, and it is most difficult to retrieve every portion of the tumor from the many irregularities in the base of the skull. One additional hazard of surgery is rupture of a cyst and spilling of the contents into the subarachnoid space. This leads to a severe chemical meningitis. Although the risk of recurrence of craniopharyngioma is still high, gross total surgical removal followed by radiation is now the approach used in most centers.

Dysgerminomas, histologically indistinguishable from those occurring in the gonads, are the second most common of the nonglial suprasellar tumors. They are highly radiosensitive, and cures are possible.

Brain stem gliomas have classically been described as having a benign histilogical appearance (spongioblastoma polare), prolonged course, and good response to radiotherapy. It now appears that these tumors very frequently contain areas of glioblastoma and present with rapid evolution of symptoms and signs. Those with malignant changes do not show any appreciable response to

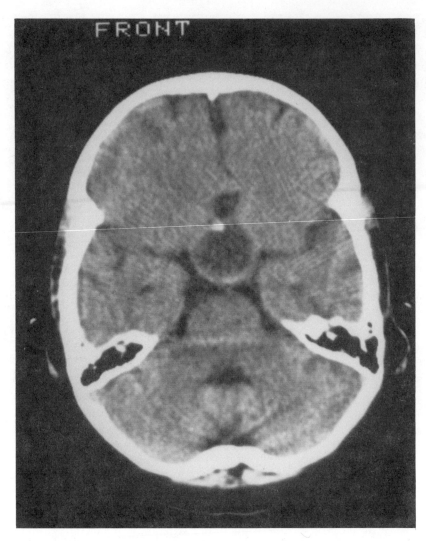

FIGURE 19-2. Computerized-tomography scan demonstrating a large cystic suprasellar craniopharyngioma.

radiation, and life expectancy is measured in months. There have been isolated reports of cysts within these tumors and improvement of the patient following surgical intervention, but for all practical purposes, this is rarely useful and is potentially associated with a good deal of morbidity.

The most common tumor found in the posterior fossa, and the neoplasm most frequently associated with a vermal syndrome, is *medulloblastoma* (Figure 19-3). It is probably of congenital origin and arises from cells in the fetal external granular layer of the cerebellum. The tumor is malignant and seeds rapidly throughout the subarachnoid space, producing implants on the spinal cord and over the cerebral hemispheres. Standard treatment at this time is surgical removal of as much of the primary tumor as possible and radiotherapy to the tumor bed and the entire remainder of the neuraxis. The spinal cord has lower radiation tolerance than the rest of the nervous system, so it is imperative that the radiation ports do not overlap significantly. On the other hand, recurrences are frequently found in areas not included in the radiation field, so full coverage must be assured. There is a good deal of current interest in the use of chemotherapeutic agents for the treatment of medulloblastoma. Long-term survival is approximately 30%. Evidence is accumulating that this may be substantially higher with the aggressive use of chemotherapy.

Two-thirds of *ependymomas* arise within the fourth ventricle. Typically, they present with obstruction to the flow of CSF, but can invade the brain stem or grow through the foramina of Luschka and Magendie into the posterior fossa and seed the subarachnoid space with tumor implants. Vomiting is a frequent

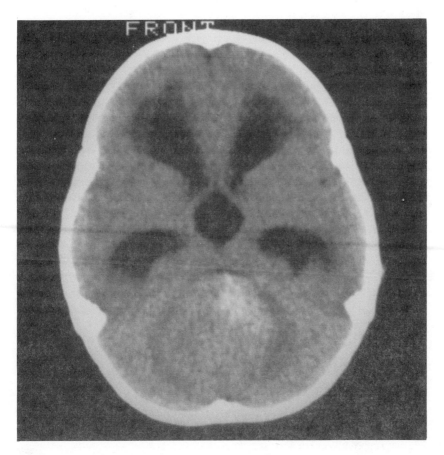

FIGURE 19-3. Computerized-tomography scan demonstrating a large medulloblastoma which is distorting the fourth ventricle and producing hydrocephalus.

early sign, due to involvement of the floor of the fourth ventricle. The current approach to treatment is surgical removal followed by radiotherapy. If seeding is suspected, or if there is histological evidence of malignancy, radiation of the entire neuraxis is warranted. The role of chemotherapy is still being investigated. Even with vigorous treatment, the recurrence rate is extremely high.

Cystic cerebellar astrocytomas occur in the cerebellar hemispheres. Surgical exploration reveals a cyst with a tumor nodule on its wall. This tumor is histologically benign, and long-term survivals have been reported, even with incomplete surgical removal and no radiotherapy. Radiation is not used in most centers at this time. Other forms of astrocytoma, both benign and malignant, can also occur in this region and are treated as they would be in any other location.

Acoustic neuromas in children always raise the suspicion of neurofibromatosis. Bilateral tumors are virtually diagnostic of this condition. This is important because of the implications for a large number of other complications and for genetic counseling. The prognosis for these lesions is good, especially with early diagnosis and removal. The use of the operating microscope now allows the seventh nerve to be spared if it is not already seriously involved.

Optic glioma should also raise suspicion of neurofibromatosis. Some workers have attempted to differentiate a "central" form of the disorder, with tumors of the neuraxis but little in the way of peripheral manifestations. A thorough evaluation of the entire family is warranted. Treatment relies mainly on radiotherapy.

The features of *intracranial neoplasms* in infants under 18 months of age are similar to those found in older children.[5] Sixty percent are also in the posterior fossa, and medulloblastoma is the single most common histological type. Ependymomas in the lateral ventricles and choroid plexus papillomas occur more frequently than gliomas of the cerebral hemispheres. There is a lower incidence of suprasellar tumors. The 5-year survival is only 25%, unlike the situation in older children. The most frequent clinical presentation of brain tumors in this age group is with vomiting, lethargy, and increasing head circumference. Seizures and abnormalities on motor examination are less common.

CNS involvement in *leukemia* occurs both as a function of the presence of leukemic cells and as a complication of treatment.[6] Now that prolonged survival of children with leukemia is common, the incidence of meningeal involvement has increased, reaching 50–75% in different series. This also has great importance for another reason; the central nervous system is felt to represent a "privileged site" where leukemic cells are protected from systemic chemotherapeutic agents that do not cross the blood–brain barrier. These cells can then reenter the circulation and produce a relapse. For this reason, most treatment protocols call for prophylactic use of intrathecal methotrexate or radiation of the neuraxis.

Meningeal leukemia presents with signs and symptoms of increased intracranial pressure in the absence of focal neurological abnormalities. Cranial nerves are rarely involved. Parenchymal involvement by a mass of leukemic cells occasionally occurs and follows the course of any brain tumor. In those forms of leukemia with an extremely high leukocyte count, especially acute myelogenous leukemia, diffuse hemorrhagic infarction can result from plugging of smaller blood vessels with abnormal cells. Hemorrhage into the brain or subarachnoid space can also occur as a consequence of the hemorrhagic diathesis associated with thrombocytopenia.

The child with leukemia is at risk for developing opportunistic infections of the CNS. These include fungal infections, chronic viral infections, and disorders such as multifocal leukoencephalopathy.

Generalized cerebral atrophy has been reported following the use of intrathecal methotrexate, radiotherapy, or a combination of the two. There may be no clinical signs, although learning disabilities and a decreased IQ may occur following prophylactic radiation to the cerebral hemispheres. This is most apparent with children under 4 years of age and appears to be dose dependent.

Metastatic tumors to the central nervous system are less common in children than in adults, because of the biological differences of the type of neoplasms found in the two age groups.[7] Wilms tumor, osteogenic sarcoma, and rhabdomyosarcoma metastasize most frequently. In almost all cases, metastases to the lungs precede involvement of the brain. The cerebral hemispheres are the usual intracranial site for the metastic tumors, and the signs and symptoms are appropriate to that location. Recommended treatment includes surgery followed by radiotherapy.

Although *extraneural metastases* of brain tumors have been considered to be a rare phenomenon, a recent study found such lesions in 5 of 36 children treated with surgery, radiotherapy, and chemotherapy.[8] The tumors involved were medulloblastoma, glioma, ependymoma, and a primitive neuroectodermal tumor. It is not clear whether this phenomenon results from an increased length of survival as a result of treatment or is an effect of the therapy itself. Extraneural metastases also occur in patients with shunts from the ventricles to a body cavity. Some of these patients have had varying combinations of surgery and radiotherapy, and others had received no prior treatment.

SPINAL CORD TUMORS

Tumors involving the spinal column, meninges, and spinal cord are not common in childhood. There is no preponderance by sex, and older children are involved most frequently.

Back pain is the most frequent and most important symptom. This complaint should always be taken seriously; the differential diagnosis is more limited than in adults. Nonneoplastic lesions presenting with back pain include infections of the vertebrae or intervertebral discs, discitis, and herpes zoster. Herniated discs are rare, although they do occur in obese adolescents.

The next most common symptoms are leg weakness and gait disturbance. Young children stumble and fall frequently, but generally voice few complaints. Older patients are more aware of their declining abilities. Progressive scoliosis is an early sign in some patients and must be differentiated from idiopathic scoliosis in adolescents. Bladder dysfunction presents as secondary enuresis or day-

TABLE 19-1
Lesion Types and Symptoms

Extramedullary lesion	Cauda equina lesion
Radicular pain	Severe radicular pain, multiple roots
Sharp sensory level	Saddle anesthesia, often asymmetrical
Saddle anesthesia	Asymmetrical weakness and atrophy
Segmental lower motor neuron involvement	Flaccid weakness
Severe spastic paraparesis	Bladder dysfunction late
Bladder dysfunction early	Conus medullaris lesion
Intramedullary lesion	Minimal pain
Diffuse burning pain	Saddle anesthesia, symmetrical
Patchy sensory changes	Mild symmetrical motor loss
Sacral sparing	Ankle jerks lost
Widespread lower motor neuron involvement	Bladder dysfunction early
Mild spastic paraparesis	
Bladder dysfunction late	

time incontinence; rarely, acute urinary retention occurs. There are usually few complaints of sensory abnormalities.

The history and neurological examination can assist in differentiating intramedullary lesions of the spinal cord from extramedullary tumors that compress the cord (Table 19-1). This is important, as the presumptive localization provides a clue to the most likely tumor type. All tumors above the region of the cauda equina produce spasticity. Sensory abnormalities are almost always present below the level of the lesion.

Lumbar puncture is rarely necessary and is associated with some hazard. This procedure can precipitate a shift in intraspinal contents and sudden cord transection. X-ray studies of the spine provide information about bony destruction, loss of disc spaces, and widening and destruction of the pedicles. This aids in ascertaining the longitudinal extent of the tumor.

The most definitive diagnostic procedure is CT scan of the spine; the usefulness of the study is enhanced by the injection of metrizamide into the spinal subarachnoid space. This is supplemented by routine myelography after the contrast medium is administered. If CT scan cannot be performed because an appropriate machine is not available, routine myelography will still provide a good deal of information. MRI scanning appears to provide excellent resolution of these tumors.

Intramedullary tumors are primarily glial or ependymal. Astrocytomas are usually benign and extend over several spinal segments. Treatment is not satisfactory, as complete surgical removal is not practical and radiotherapy is not highly effective.

Ependymomas can often be surgically removed with good results. At times, however, they involve the central region of the cord throughout its entire length.

The most common *extramedullary tumor* is a neurofibroma. Many of these patients have neurofibromatosis. These tumors can involve many nerve roots and become very large. In addition to compressing the cord, they sometimes extend through the intervertebral foramen and present as a thoracic or abdominal mass. Less common neoplasms include lipomas and dermoid tumors. These are often congenital and are frequently associated with cutaneous malformations over the midline of the back. Typical lesions are hemangiomas, nevi, skin pits, and tufts of hair.

REFERENCES

1. Schoenberg, B. S., Schoenberg, D. G., Christine, B. W., and Gomez, M. R., 1976, The epidemiology of primary intracranial neoplasms in childhood, *Mayo Clin. Proc.* **51:**51–56.
2. Honig, P. J., and Charney, E. B., 1982, Children with brain tumor headaches, *Am. J. Dis. Child.* **136:**121–124.
3. Hirose, G, Lombroso, C. T., and Eisenberg, H., 1975, Thalamic tumors in childhood, *Arch. Neurol.* **32:**740–744.
4. Winston, K. R., 1978 Neurodiagnostic tests in children with brain tumors: Changing patterns of use and impact on cost, *Pediatrics* **61:**847–852.
5. Farwell, J. R., Dohrmann, G. J., and Flannery, J. T., 1978, Intracranial neoplasms in infants, *Arch. Neurol.* **35:**533–537.
6. Crosley, C. J., Rorke, L. B., Evans, A., and Nigro, M., 1978, Central nervous system lesions in childhood leukemia, *Neurology* **28:**678–685.
7. Vannucci, R. C., and Baten, M., 1974, Cerebral metastatic disease in childhood, *Neurology* **24:**981–985.
8. Duffner, P. K., and Cohen, M. E., 1981, Extraneural metastases in childhood brain tumors, *Ann. Neurol.* **10:**261–265.

ADDITIONAL READING

Cohen, M. E., and Duffner, P. K., 1984, *Brain Tumors in Children: Principles of Diagnosis and Treatment*, Raven Press, New York.
Duffner, P. K., Cohen, M. E. and Freeman A. I., 1985, Pediatric brain tumors: An overview, *CA* **35:**287–301.
Gjerris, F., 1976, Clinical aspects and long-term prognosis of intracranial tumours in infancy and childhood, *Dev. Med. Child. Neurol.* **18:**145–159.
Shapiro, W. R., 1982, Treatment of neuroectodermal brain tumors, *Ann. Neurol.* **12:**231–237.

20

Neuromuscular Disorders

Neuromuscular disorders are those conditions primarily involving the motor unit: the anterior horn cell, peripheral nerve, neuromuscular junction, and muscle. Although there are a number of clinical similarities among these diseases, they are extremely diverse pathologically and in terms of treatment, prognosis, and genetics.

Hypotonia and weakness are the critical common features of the neuromuscular disorders. As these signs can also occur with damage to the central nervous system, especially in the young infant, the first clinical task is to seek other features of motor unit involvement, and to rule out cerebral injury.

Additional signs assist in making a more accurate clinical localization of the process. The most useful include the following:

1. Fasciculations are random contractions of groups of muscle fibers innervated by single anterior horn cells and indicate damage primarily to these cells. They are often difficult to see in infants except on the tongue, the surface of which appears to shimmer.
2. Fibrillations are spontaneous contractions of single denervated muscle fibers. They are not clinically visible, but can be detected on electromyographic studies.
3. Muscle atrophy occurs with involvement of any portion of the motor unit, but is rare in disorders of the neuromuscular junction unless they are severe and prolonged.
4. Areflexia is most commonly present in conditions affecting the anterior horn cell or peripheral nerve. It is less common with involvement of the neuromuscular junction, unless paralysis is complete, and is variable in muscle diseases.
5. Abnormalities in the sensory examination are limited to diseases of the peripheral nerves.
6. Muscle weakness that increases with exercise and improves with rest suggests abnormalities of the neuromuscular junction. If the onset of weak-

215

ness is delayed for a period of an hour or more following cessation of exercise, a metabolic myopathy is more likely.

7. Abnormally firm or "woody" muscles suggest muscular dystrophy. Muscle tenderness is seen in some patients with inflammatory myopathies. Acute muscle pain occurring during or immediately following exercise is most commonly associated with metabolic myopathies, as is postexercise myoglobinuria.

APPROACH TO THE PATIENT

A detailed history is directed toward determining the patient's age at the onset of the symptoms, whether they are static or progressive, and the rate of progression. The presence of associated features is important. These include systemic illness, fever, rash, and muscle pain; involvement of vision and hearing; and bladder dysfunction. Some of these abnormalities can be confirmed on the general physical examination.

The neurological examination is the best tool for determining the severity and distribution of the weakness and setting the anatomical location of the lesion. Traditional manual muscle testing is extremely difficult with young children, so reliance on functional tests of strength becomes important. Careful observation of the child while he is walking, running, and standing on his toes and having him attempt to climb several flights of stairs provide adequate assessment of lower-extremity function. The arms can be evaluated by having the child play games or perform tasks with his arms held over his head, or seeing whether he can support his full weight on his arms and "walk" on his hands.

When cranial nerve function is assessed, special attention should be paid to the pharyngeal muscles. A nasal voice, pooling of secretions in the pharynx, difficulty swallowing, and nasal regurgitation when swallowing indicate pharyngeal weakness and put the patient at high risk for aspiration, pneumonia, and problems in maintaining adequate nutrition. Respiratory function and reserve capacity must be carefully evaluated in any child with significant weakness. A semi-quantitative approach is to determine the child's ability to count after taking one deep breath. This can be recorded and periodically reevaluated.

Laboratory evaluation can provide a good deal of assistance. Electrodiagnostic studies (nerve conduction velocity, electromyography, evoked potentials) are discussed in Chapter 8. A number of different enzymes are released into the circulation from abnormal muscles, and elevated levels are a sign of some myopathic conditions. The most useful enzyme is creatinine phosphokinase. It is usually not necessary to obtain a determination of the isoenzymes, but this may be important in selected cases. Ultimately, most children with neuromuscular disease will come to diagnostic muscle biopsy.

ANTERIOR HORN CELL DISEASES

Progressive infantile spinal muscular atrophy, or Werdnig–Hoffmann disease, is the prototype of anterior horn cell diseases in childhood. In the classic form of the disorder, a history of decreased fetal movements may be obtained, and the child is obviously weak and hypotonic at birth. The facial and extraocular musculature is spared, and the child gives every appearance of being bright and alert. There is difficulty sucking and swallowing, and secretions pool in the pharynx. Examination of the tongue reveals almost constant fasciculations. It is important to make this determination when the infant is quiet, as the tongue of every crying infant will appear to have fasciculations.

There are few spontaneous movements, although some strength may be preserved in the distal extremities. Deep-tendon reflexes are absent. The child appears to perceive painful stimuli. Scoliosis develops early and progresses. Diaphragmetic or "paradoxical" respirations are present because of weakness of the intercostal muscles. During inspiration the abdomen rises while the chest appears to collapse; during expiration the abdomen falls and the chest expands.

In a typical case the weakness prevents achievement of any motor milestones. Intellectual development appears to progress normally, however, as indicated by the age-appropriate use of language. Progressive involvement of bulbar musculature necessitates the use of a nasogastric tube or gastrostomy for feeding. Respiratory therapy is important, but the disease is inexorably progressive, and the majority of children die of pulmonary infections before the third birthday.

There are a number of related disorders in which degeneration of the anterior horn cells begins somewhat later, progression is less rapid, and life-span longer.[1] These children become hypotonic and weak, but this is not evident at birth. Deep-tendon reflexes are present initially, but disappear as the weakness progresses. There is variable development of motor skills. In general, the highest level of motor function achieved varies inversely with the apparent age of clinical onset. The disorder is progressively disabling in all affected children, however.[2]

Definitive diagnosis depends on muscle biopsy. There are groups of small, angulated, atrophic fibers, interspersed with areas of muscle containing fibers of normal size and morphology (Figure 20-1). Each group of abnormal fibers represents the loss of innervation resulting from dysfunction or death of an anterior horn cell.

There is no effective treatment. Supportive nutritional and respiratory care can prolong life. Physical therapy is useful in preventing contractures and decubitus ulcers. Adaptive devices will allow older patients to maintain some self-help skills.

Genetic counseling is of major importance as the condition is transmitted as an autosomal recessive trait. The clinical course is stereotyped for each affected member in a family.

Juvenile spinal muscular atrophy, or Kugelberg–Welander disease, has a clinical onset between early childhood and late adolescence. There is progressive development of weakness in the hip and shoulder girdles following a period of normal development; this led to use of the term "pseudomuscular dystrophy." Progression is slow, and motor abilities may not be lost until the early- or mid-adult years. Neither extraocular movements nor swallowing is impaired. Deep-tendon reflexes are present initially but are eventually lost.

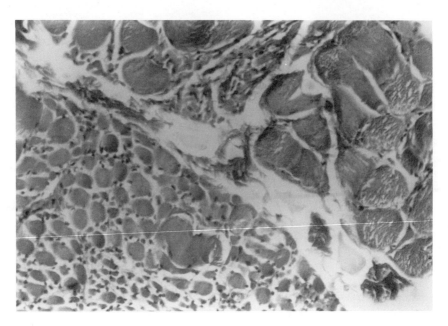

FIGURE 20-1. Muscle biopsy from a patient with Werdnig–Hoffmann disease. There is a group of small angular atrophic fibers next to a group of muscle fibers of normal size and shape.

Both autosomal recessive and autosomal dominant modes of transmission are seen in different families. Muscle biopsy reveals group lesions. No specific treatment has been proven to be useful.

PERIPHERAL NEUROPATHIES

Peripheral neuropathies in infants are rare, except for those due to birth trauma. As the child grows older, however, there are innumerable diseases and environmental agents that can damage the peripheral nerves.[3]

Many hereditary neuropathies have their clinical onset during childhood. Exact diagnosis is most important, as treatment, prognosis, and genetic counseling depend on knowledge of the underlying disease. This frequently requires specialized metabolic and histological studies. These disorders have been classified as the hereditary motor and sensory neuropathies (HMSN), based on age of onset, genetic pattern, clinical features, and pathological abnormalities.[4] The original eponyms are still broadly used in clinical practice, however.

A detailed history allows ascertainment of whether the condition is congenital or acquired, static or progressive, and of acute or subacute onset. Table 20-1 lists some of the most important neuropathies.

Peroneal muscular atrophy (Charcot–Marie–Tooth disease, HMSN I) is the most common of the hereditary neuropathies. This disorder begins in childhood or adolescence and is manifested by progressive weakness, most prominent in

TABLE 20-1
Major Causes of Neuropathy

Hereditary	Traumatic
Peroneal muscular atrophy (HMSN I)	Injection neuropathy
Hypertrophic interstitial neuritis (HMSN III)	Postfracture
Spinocerebellar degeneration	Penetrating wound
Familial dysautonomia	Birth trauma
Metabolic	Associated with systemic illness
Metachromatic leukodystrophy	Diabetes
Acute intermittent porphyria	Leukemia
Toxic	Collagen vascular disease
Heavy metals	Vitamin deficiency
Glue sniffing	Idiopathic
Hydrocarbons	Bell palsy
Vincristine	Guillain–Barré syndrome
Infectious	
Diphtheria	
Osteomyelitis	
Herpes zoster	

the legs. Pes cavus and hammertoe deformities are generally present and may also be seen in clinically unaffected family members. Deep-tendon reflexes progressively disappear. The most useful diagnostic feature is prominent muscle atrophy involving especially the anterior compartment muscles of the legs, those of the lower portion of the thigh, and the intrinsic muscles of the hands and feet. Cranial nerves are spared. Careful examination often shows some sensory signs, and autonomic dysfunction may be present. The majority of cases are inherited as an autosomal dominant trait.

Hypertrophic interstitial neuropathy (Dejerine–Sottas disease, HMSN III) is an autosomal recessive disorder of early onset. There is delayed gross motor development, but the child eventually is able to ambulate independently. Motor and sensory loss then become progressive. All sensory modalities are impaired. The hallmark of this condition is easily palpable hypertrophied nerves. Biopsy shows loss of myelin and axons and replacement by an "onion-skin" layering of fibrous tissue. Nerve conduction velocities are extremely slow.

Familial dysautonomia (Riley-Day syndrome) primarily involves the autonomic nervous system, but is also associated with changes in sensory nerves and dorsal root ganglia. The children are small for gestational age at birth. A number of difficulties are evident during early infancy, the most prominent being dysphagia with choking, vomiting, recurrent pulmonary infections, and excessive irritability.

As the child becomes older, new signs include growth failure, delayed development, breath-holding spells, and hypotonia. Autonomic instability is a major problem. The manifestations are diverse and include absence of tears when crying, excessive sweating, skin blotching, poor temperature regulation, hypertensive episodes, and postural hypotension. Sensory dysfunction causes decreased responsiveness to pain, hyporeflexia, and reduced corneal sensation.

Findings on physical and laboratory examinations assist in making a diagnosis. Fungiform papillae of the tongue are absent. Intradermal injection of 0.05 ml of 1:1000 histamine does not produce the expected flare. Instillation of 2.5% methacholine into the conjunctival sac produces miosis in children with familial dysautonomia, but not controls. These three findings, if present, are diagnostic.

The condition is inherited by an autosomal recessive mechanism and is largely, but not entirely, restricted to Ashkenazi Jews. Prenatal detection is not possible. There is no specific treatment, but attention must be paid to all of the associated medical problems. Survival into the adult years is now possible. The major causes of death are pneumonia, respiratory arrest during sleep, hypotensive crises, sepsis, and renal failure.[5]

Acute intermittent porphyria is rarely symptomatic before adolescence. During an attack, the patient may present with a serious, life-threatening, flaccid quadriplegia, resembling Guillain–Barré syndrome. The patient with porphyria has more sensory abnormalities and is more likely to have urinary retention, however. Mental changes, psychiatric abnormalities, and colicky abdominal pain are also common in this disorder.

Other patients have a mixed sensory and motor neuropathy with a spotty distribution. Barbiturates may trigger attacks of porphyria. The condition is inherited by an autosomal recessive gene. The diagnosis is confirmed by demonstrating increased urinary excretion of porphobilinogen and δ-aminolevulinic acid.

Many *toxins* can produce a peripheral neuropathy. *Hydrocarbon* compounds, especially hexacarbons, seem to be especially toxic. A mixed motor and sensory neuropathy is characteristic of *arsenic* poisoning. Diagnostic clues are the characteristic desquamating rash and white lines transversely across the nails. *Lead* rarely causes neuropathy in childhood. Children with hemoglobinopathies appear to be at increased risk, however. Large doses of pyridoxine can produce a severe neuropathy.

Vincristine commonly causes neuropathy, especially as the total dose of the drug increases. Most children being treated with vincristine become areflexic. The condition generally is reversible when the drug is discontinued.

Although *diptheria* has become rare in most parts of this country, it is still an important problem in regions with a large number of immigrants from less developed nations. The disorder results from absorption of the toxin from a persistent pharyngitis. The initial neurological symptoms are almost always nasal speech and difficulty swallowing. The course of the disease is insidious, and several weeks later there is blurred vision, diplopia, and weakness. The diagnosis is made by isolating the organism from the pharyngeal exudate. Following treatment with diphtheria antitoxin and penicillin, there is slow recovery.

Herpes zoster, in contrast to diphtheria, is produced by direct viral infection of the nerve. The organism, identical to that causing varicella, remains latent in the nerve for long periods of time. In most cases, the cause of the viral reactivation is not known, although it is frequently associated with lymphoreticular neoplasms.

The patient initially develops pain in the distribution of the affected nerve. Several days later, the typical vesicular rash appears, and there may be paralysis of the muscles innervated by that nerve. More widespread weakness can result from myelitis or the development of the Guillain–Barré syndrome.

Zoster frequently involves the ophthalmic division of the fifth nerve (Ramsay Hunt syndrome). If the eye is involved, vision can be lost as a result of corneal damage.

Brachial neuritis presents with severe burning pain in the arm, shoulder, and neck, on one or both sides. This is followed within a day or 2 by paralysis of muscles of the shoulder girdle on the affected side. There are no sensory deficits. The etiology is unknown, but an infectious or postinfectious mechanism is supported by the simultaneous occurrence of several cases in a restricted geographical area. There is no specific treatment, and the prognosis is good.

DISEASES OF THE NEUROMUSCULAR JUNCTION

Three different forms of *myasthenia gravis* are found in childhood. Juvenile myasthenia gravis is virtually indistinguishable from the adult form. The most common presentation is with ptosis and ophthalmoplegia; this may occur suddenly and not resolve or may change in severity over time. The limbs then become involved, with variability in the degree of weakness and the muscle groups affected. Increasing weakness toward the end of the day is common, and symptoms improve temporarily after a period of rest.

Findings on examination depend on the degree of involvement on any given day. Weakness can usually be demonstrated by having the patient contract the affected muscle forcibly for a short period of time. For instance, if the patient is asked to maintain upward gaze, ptosis will quickly become evident. Deep-tendon reflexes remain intact, and there are no sensory abnormalities.

Electrodiagnostic studies are useful. Rapidly repeated stimuli applied to a nerve produce a muscle response that gradually decreases in amplitude. The most reliable clinical test makes use of edrophonium, a short-acting acetylcholinesterase inhibitor. Intravenous injection produces a short-lived recovery in the strength of the muscle being tested. A saline control should always be used to rule out a placebo response or malingering.

Myasthenia gravis appears to result from an immune response directed against postsynaptic nicotinic acetylcholine receptors. The number of functional receptor sites is thereby reduced. This mechanism does not easily explain the spotty distribution and variability of the weakness, however.

Treatment is based on the use of drugs that inhibit acetylcholinesterase; this slows the degradation of acetylcholine released at the neuromuscular junction and allows it to have an enhanced effect. One problem in regulating therapy is that excessive quantities of acetylcholine at the neuromuscular junction can produce a depolarization block and weakness. It is often difficult to find the level of medication that maximizes muscle strength. The situation is further complicated by the fact that at any drug level, a given muscle may be inadequately

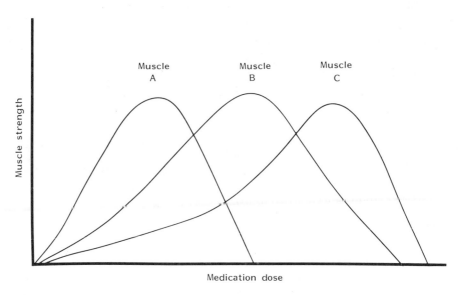

FIGURE 20-2. Graph illustrating the dose–response curve of three muscles in a patient with myasthenia gravis.

treated, another muscle optimally treated, and another one overtreated (Figure 20-2). Changing the dose can strengthen some muscles while weakening others. Frequent detailed evaluations and adjustment of medication are required to optimize therapy.

Patients sometimes suddenly become extremely weak, often with associated respiratory insufficiency. This can represent a myasthenic crisis or a cholinergic crisis, the latter due to an excess of acetylcholinesterase inhibitors. The first step in emergency management is support of respirations. A test dose of edrophonium will improve strength in a myasthenic crisis, but will produce no change or weakening if the episode represents a cholinergic crisis.

Other treatment approaches have been designed to attack the underlying immune disorder.[6] Thymectomy in patients without a thymoma is clearly useful in some patients, but the indications, based on severity and duration of disease, sex, and response to medication, are the subject of a good deal of controversy. Obviously, surgery is required if a thymoma is present. Corticosteroids are sometimes helpful, but increased weakness often occurs initially and their long-term use is associated with many complications. Plasmapheresis and immunosuppressive drugs are being used in some centers, but the results and criteria for patient selection are not clear. Remission occurs in up to one-quarter of patients.

Transient neonatal myasthenia gravis is present in a small percentage of infants born to mothers who have myasthenia gravis. The child is hypotonic and weak, feeds poorly, and may have ventilatory compromise. Although spontaneous remission occurs in a few weeks, it is necessary to treat some infants with acetylcholinesterase inhibitors while waiting for the condition to run its course.

Congenital myasthenia gravis is the least common form of the disorder and is not associated with maternal myasthenia gravis. The major problems are ptosis and difficult swallowing, and the children often have generalized weakness. This persists and requires treatment with acetylcholinesterase inhibitors. Unlike the other form of myasthenia, this condition is often familial.

Botulism can occur at any age and is due to ingestion of food contaminated with a toxin produced by *Clostridium botulinum.* The symptoms initially resemble those of any food poisoning. These are then followed by blurred vision, due to paralysis of accommodation, and diplopia. Other cranial nerves become involved, and then progressive generalized weakness occurs, often associated with respiratory insufficiency.

Electrodiagnostic studies can help confirm the diagnosis showing low-amplitude muscle potentials and a decremental response to repeated stimulation. Newly developed techniques are sensitive enough to detect the toxin in serum.

Treatment utilizes the same approach to the paralyzed patient as outlined for the Guillain–Barré syndrome. If ventilatory assistance is required, it is often necessary to continue it for a prolonged period of time. The toxin appears to inhibit the release of acetylcholine from the synapse. Guanidine has been used to stimulate release, but with variable therapeutic effects. Specific antitoxin, given early, may modify the severity of the illness.

Infant botulism appears to have a different pathophysiology. Contaminated food is not involved, but the organism appears to grow in the child's gastrointestinal tract and the toxin is absorbed from that site. Infants between 1 and 5 months of age are affected. Severe constipation is the most common early sign and is followed by hypotonia, weakness, and feeding difficulty. Pupillary abnormalities are often present. The course of the illness is several weeks in duration. Most children need no specific treatment other than special attention to feedings to ensure adequate nutrition and prevent aspiration of food. There is now evidence that some children are asymptomatic carriers of the organism and that the condition can vary greatly in severity.[7] Other children have a clinical picture resembling sudden infant death syndrome.

Tick paralysis is a dramatic condition that results from a toxin produced by certain species of dog or wood ticks. The clinical picture is that of ascending paralysis which is difficult to distinguish from Guillain–Barré syndrome. Differences include the presence of pain and the absence of an elevated cerebrospinal fluid protein concentration in tick paralysis. Respiratory insufficiency may require ventilatory assistance. Removal of the tick produces a rapid and complete recovery.

MUSCULAR DYSTROPHIES

The muscular dystrophies comprise a group of hereditary progressive diseases which primarily involve muscle. Each specific condition has a rather stereotyped clinical pattern although, as with many neurological disorders, variants are being regularly described.

Progressive muscular dystrophy (PMD, Duchenne dystrophy) is the best known and most common form presenting in childhood. It is transmitted as an X-linked recessive trait; the rare occurrence in girls is probably due to predominant inactivation of the normal X chromosome. The child's early development is normal, although there may be slight delay in independent walking. By age 2 years he appears to stumble and fall more than other children and frequently walks on his toes.

Weakness of the lower extremities begins to become obvious by age 4 years. This progresses rapidly, and by age 8 years most of the children have difficulty in independent ambulation and begin to require a wheelchair for mobility. The majority of patients are nonambulatory by age 12 and have lost almost all strength, except in the hands, by age 16 years.

A clinical sign found in many patients is "pseudohypertrophy" of the muscle, the appearance of large muscle bulk due to replacement by fat and fibrous tissue. This is most easily seen in the calves (Figure 20-3), but is often present in the deltoids and quadriceps. Palpation of the muscles gives a typical "woody" feeling. Muscle contractures, especially shortening of the gastrocnemius, occur, and progressive scoliosis develops. Death is usually the result of respiratory insufficiency and infection. Cardiomyopathy is frequently found pathologically and in some cases becomes clinically significant and contributes to early death. In the past, most of the children with PMD did not live past age 20 years, but with improvement in the techniques of pulmonary care, a few live into their thirties.

Mental retardation accompanies PMD in approximately 30% of cases. This seems to be specific to certain families, so that every child with PMD in a given family is either mentally retarded or is normal. Other types of cognitive abnormalities also can be present.[8]

Creatinine phosphokinase (CPK) levels in the serum are extremely high, even before clinical weakness is prominent. These decline late in the course of the illness when muscle wasting is extreme. Muscle biopsy is required for absolute diagnostic certainty. The specimen must be removed isometrically and rapidly frozen for histochemical studies. The diagnosis of muscle diseases requires these specialized procedures, as well as the standard histological techniques. The biopsy shows marked degeneration of muscle fibers with replacement by fat and connective tissue. Large basophilic fibers represent an ineffective attempt at regeneration.

No specific treatment is available. Recent studies of protein abnormalities in muscle and erythrocyte membranes may provide a clue to the molecular pathology of the condition and permit the development of biochemical treatment strategies. At this time, management is limited to the use of physical and occupational therapy to maintain function at the maximum level possible, slow the progression of joint contractures, and provide adaptive aids to enhance mobility and self-care activities. Surgical release of contractures may improve ambulation initially and ease nursing care. Any operative procedure should be carefully planned, and carried out by a technique that will limit the period of bed rest, as many children will be unable to resume walking if put to bed for a substantial period of time. If scoliosis becomes severe and significantly limits

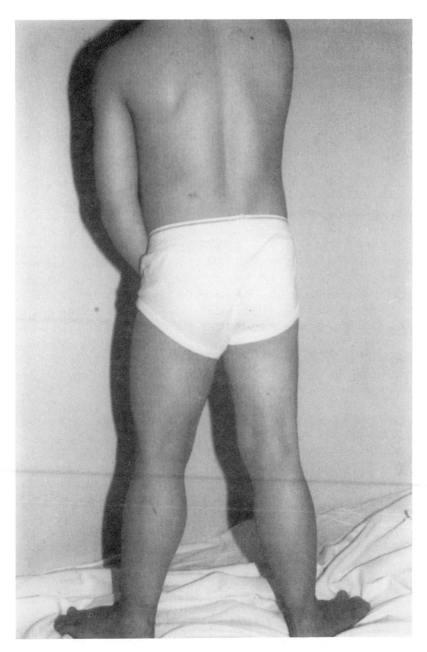

FIGURE 20-3. Psuedohypertrophy of the calf muscles in a child with Duchenne muscular dystrophy.

vital capacity, newer surgical techniques using instrumentation with flexible rods can be considered. The most important aspect of management is respiratory care. A vigorous home program should be developed and followed faithfully.

Genetic counseling is mandatory. The affected child's mother is a definite carrier if she has an affected brother or one of her sisters has a son with PMD. A probable carrier is any woman with more than one affected son. If the child with PMD is the firstborn in a family, his mother is a possible carrier. In this case, her actual carrier status must be ascertained if at all possible.[9] Determination of several serum CPK levels taken from the mother, her sisters, and her daughters is useful. If any of these are clearly elevated, the individuals should be considered to be carriers. Prenatal detection is not yet possible, although some families will elect selective termination of pregnancies with a male fetus. They should understand, however, that half of the female children will be carriers of PMD.

Myotonic muscular dystrophy typically presents in young adulthood with progressive weakness and muscle wasting, myotonia, cataracts, frontal baldness, and psychiatric abnormalities. The condition is occasionally seen at birth, however. The infant is hypotonic, has facial diplegia with difficulty sucking, and often has orthopedic deformities such as clubfeet.[10] Death from respiratory insufficiency can occur. Weakness becomes apparent in the preschool years, and the classic features of the condition develop as the child approaches adulthood. Myotonia is present but difficult to demonstrate clinically until the child can cooperate with the examination. It can be brought out by any maneuver requiring the child to suddenly relax a muscle group following sustained contraction; the inability to quickly relax the muscle is characteristic. Percussion of a muscle produces contraction and a "mound" at the point where it was struck.

CPK levels are elevated, and electromyography shows characteristic abnormalities with high-frequency repetitive discharges. Muscle biopsy is diagnostic.

No specific treatment is available, but the same management principles as outlined for PMD apply. If myotonia is disabling, phenytoin may provide some relief. The genetic pattern is clearly that of an autosomal dominant, but if the infant is affected, it is always the mother who carries the condition. There is no good explanation for this phenomenon. Prenatal detection is not possible at this time.

Fascioscapulohumeral dystrophy is rare, but the signs and symptoms are highly characteristic. Weakness of the facial muscle begins in the preschool years and produces difficulty in closing the eyes and pursing the lips. There may be weakness of extraocular muscles. During the school years or adolescence, striking weakness and atrophy of the muscles of the shoulder girdle become evident and progress. The facial appearance is characteristic, and the atrophy of the scapular muscles produces a sloped appearance to the shoulders which actually represents the upper portion of the rib cage appearing above the scapulae. Hip girdle weakness develops, and occasionally the anterior tibial muscles are involved, producing footdrop.

The characteristic clinical findings and elevated CPK levels assist diagnosis. Inheritance is by an autosomal dominant mode; there are no prenatal diagnostic tests.

Limb–girdle dystrophy is a term referring to a group of hereditary progressive myopathies, all of which have predominant involvement of the shoulder and hip girdles. Each of the involved families shares these basic characteristics, but varies in other details of the clinical course. In most instances there is an autosomal recessive mechanism of inheritance.

CONGENITAL MYOPATHIES

The child who presents with weakness and hypotonia is always a complex diagnostic problem. Muscle biopsy, combined with increasingly sophisticated histochemical and ultrastructural techniques, has allowed the definition of a

TABLE 20-2
Congenital Myopathies

Central core disease
    Weakness at birth or later childhood
    Nonprogressive
    Mild
    Skeletal anomalies
    Malignant hyperpyrexia
    Dominant or sporadic
Multicore (minicore) disease
    Weakness at birth
    Nonprogressive
    Most patients males
    Recessive or sporadic
Myotubular myopathy
    Weakness at birth or later childhood
    Nonprogressive or slowly progressive
    Extraocular palsies, ptosis
    Seizures
    Recessive, dominant, or X-linked
Nemaline myopathy
    Weakness at birth
    Nonprogressive
    Mild
    Dysmorphic features
    Dominant
Congenital fiber–type disproportion
    Weakness at birth
    Progressive in first year, then nonprogressive
    Short stature
    Skeletal deformities, dislocated hips
    Recessive or dominant
Pleioconial myopathy (mitochondrial)
    Weakness at birth
    Episodic weakness (?normokalemic periodic paralysis)
Megaconial myopathy (mitochondrial)
    Onset late infancy or adulthood
    Progressive

number of disorders than can be differentiated on the basis of clinical and histopathological features. Some of these conditions lead to progressive weakness and disability, but others appear to remain static. Although these conditions are uncommon and no treatment is available, specific diagnosis is important for genetic counseling and determination of the prognosis. Table 20-2 lists important features of some of the more common of these rare conditions.

INFLAMMATORY MYOPATHIES

The inflammatory myopathies are nonhereditary conditions associated with progressive muscle weakness. Histological examination of muscle demonstrates atrophy, necrosis of muscle cells, and an infiltration of inflammatory cells. Prompt diagnosis of the inflammatory myopathies is important, as early treatment will, in many cases, induce a remission and limit disability. Weakness and inflammatory changes in muscle can accompany any of the systemic collagen vascular diseases, and these must be excluded as part of the evaluation.

Polymyositis occurs at any age, but is most common during adolescence. The cardinal feature is progressive muscle weakness, often of fairly rapid onset and involving predominantly the muscles of the limb girdles and flexors of the neck. Muscle pain and tenderness are not reliably present, and there is no skin rash. CPK levels are elevated, and muscle biopsy is diagnostic. Treatment relies on high doses of corticosteroids, starting with prednisone, 2 mg/kg body weight daily, or twice that amount every second day. When muscle strength begins to improve and the CPK becomes normal, the dose of medication is gradually reduced. Recurrence of weakness is common, and it may take several attempts before treatment can be discontinued. If there is no response to steroids, immunosuppressive drugs are sometimes used.[11]

Dermatomyositis presents at a younger age than polymyositis. There is a characteristic rash which produces a heliotrope discoloration of the eyelids. Progressive muscle weakness and muscle tenderness are prominent. Systemic signs such as fever and weight loss are common, and gastrointestinal signs and symptoms may occur because of the presence of a diffuse vasculitis. Calcium deposits develop under the skin of some patients, and the overlying tissue ulcerates with extrusion of gritty material. The course of the disease may be monocyclic, chronic polycyclic, or continuous.[12] The approach to diagnosis and treatment is the same as for polymyositis. In both conditions, physical therapy is an important adjunct to pharmacological treatment.

Early and vigorous treatment with high doses of corticosteroids for an adequate length of time is associated with the best functional outcome and minimal calcinosis.[13] Patients who do not respond well to initial therapy with corticosteroids have a poor prognosis and are candidates for immunosuppressive therapy.

PERIODIC PARALYSIS

A number of disorders associated with abnormalities in the physiology of potassium and sodium present with episodic paralysis of muscles. These conditions are generally inherited by autosomal dominant mechanisms, although the clinical and biochemical features of each type are different.

Hypokalemic periodic paralysis typically begins in the second decade of life. Attacks are triggered by a meal high in carbohydrates or by a period of rest following exercise. They often occur when the patient awakens from sleep. In severe attacks, there is flaccid quadriplegia although the muscles of respiration and those innervated by the cranial nerves are spared. Deep-tendon reflexes are absent during an attack, and myotonia of the eyelids may be demonstrated. Serum potassium levels are markedly depressed, and an electrocardiogram shows the characteristic changes of hypokalemia.

If a blood specimen cannot be obtained during an episode, an attempt can be made to precipitate an attack under careful supervision. This can be done either by making use of the factors that usually trigger the patient's symptoms or with an intravenous infusion of glucose and insulin. An attack can be aborted by the cautious administration of potassium chloride. Prophylaxis with daily administration of acetazolamide or spironolactone will usually decrease the frequency and severity of the episodes.

Hyperkalemic periodic paralysis presents in the first decade of life. The attacks, triggered by rest following exercise, are brief, usually lasting less than 1 hr. They occur much more frequently than those of the hypokalemic form of the disorder. Symptoms are usually less severe, but are accompanied by paresthesias. The serum potassium level is typically only slightly elevated or in the upper portion of the normal range during an episode. Electrocardiographic evidence of hyperkalemia provides useful corroborating evidence. Precipitation of an attack by the administration of potassium chloride may be necessary to confirm the diagnosis. Patients can often abort an attack by exercising when the paresthesias begin. Salbutamol inhalation will also prevent the majority of attacks in most patients. Prophylaxis with acetazolamide also may be effective.

Normokalemic periodic paralysis is poorly understood and may actually be a clinical manifestation of pleoconial myopathy.

OTHER NEUROMUSCULAR DISORDERS

Myoglobinuria, the urinary excretion of myoglobin, results from any condition causing rhabdomyolysis. This always indicates that there has been severe damage to muscle. The child complains of intense muscle pain, and tenderness is prominent. Weakness is also present. Chills, fever, malaise, and abdominal pain accompany the illness. The characteristic feature of the condition is the passage of reddish-brown urine.

Laboratory studies provide documentation that the urinary pigment is myoglobin. Serum haptoglobin levels, which are depressed in hemoglobinuria, remain normal. Serum CPK levels are markedly elevated.

There are many causes of myoglobinuria. In some, historical data provide an obvious diagnosis. These include trauma, infections, and vascular occlusion. If no cause can be found, or if there is a family history of myoglobinuria, the possibility of a metabolic myopathy must be investigated. Other etiological agents include diabetic ketoacidosis, hypokalemia, narcotic abuse, and carbon monoxide poisoning.

Malignant hyperthermia occurs in children and adolescents following administration of inhalation anesthesia. There is a rapid rise in body temperature to levels of 40°C or higher. Aggressive management is required and includes discontinuation of anesthesia, hyperventilation with oxygen, infusion of large amounts of fluid that contains sodium bicarbonate, administration of dantrolene, and rapid cooling by packing the patient in ice. Despite heroic efforts, the mortality rate is quite high.

Familial cases have been reported, and patients with central core disease are at risk for this complication. Diagnosis can be made *in vitro* with the halothane–caffeine contracture test. This requires a muscle biopsy specimen. Administration of dantrolene before and during anesthesia may reduce the risk in susceptible patients.

Benign congenital hypotonia is a diagnostic term applied to infants who are hypotonic at birth, have no definable neuromuscular disorder after complete diagnostic evaluation, and gradually improve during the first few years of life. As diagnostic tests become more sophisticated, some of these children are found to have either a congenital myopathy or a metabolic disorder involving muscle. The variability in the rate and degree of recovery also suggests that this is not a homogeneous diagnostic group.

A reasonable diagnostic approach is to determine initially whether a hypotonic infant has signs suggesting anterior horn cell disease such as areflexia and fasciculations of the tongue. If so, muscle biopsy is mandatory at that point. If no such signs are present, the child should be followed carefully. Muscle biopsy should be considered by 1 year of age if there is no clear evidence of improvement in muscle tone or strength, motor skills remain delayed, and it is certain that the problem is not due to a static encephalopathy. If the histology of the muscle is normal, a tentative diagnosis of benign congenital hypotonia can be made, with the understanding that this may be revised as new clinical evidence is obtained.

Möbius syndrome presents in infancy as facial diplegia, usually associated with inability to abduct either eye. The children have great difficulty sucking. This condition can be differentiated from myotonic dystrophy by the absence of generalized hypotonia or other evidence of muscle weakness. In *Duane syndrome,* the abducens palsy is present without associated facial diplegia.

Arthrogryposis multiplex congenita refers to a condition of muscle atrophy and joint contractures, present at the time of birth. It may result from a number of pathophysiological mechanisms including anterior horn cell diseases and myopathies.

Bell palsy usually follows an upper respiratory infection. The child presents with the sudden onset of weakness of one side of the face; the eye cannot be closed, and liquids run out of the corner of the mouth. Food may get stuck between the teeth and the buccal mucosa. The eye appears to tear excessively. A major controversy regarding the use of corticosteroids in treatment has raged for a long time and is still unresolved. The most important aspect of management is protecting the cornea of the eye on the affected side from becoming abraded or drying out. The use of methylcellulose drops or ophthalmic ointments is usually required. The eyelid can be carefully taped closed at night. Prognosis in children is good.

REFERENCES

1. Benady, S. G., 1978, Spinal muscular atrophy in childhood: Review of 50 cases, *Dev. Med. Child. Neurol.* **20:**746–757.
2. Russman, B. S., Melchreit, R., and Drennan, J. C.. 1983, Spinal muscular atrophy: The natural course of the disease, *Nerve Muscle* **6:**179–181.
3. Evans, O. B., 1979, Polyneuropathy in childhood, *Pediatrics* **64:**96–105.
4. Dyck, P. J., 1975, Inherited neuronal degeneration and atrophy affecting peripheral motor, sensory, and autonomic neurons, in: *Peripheral Neuropathy*, Vol II (P. J. Dyck, P. K. Thomas, and E. H. Lamber, eds.), WB Saunders, Philadelphia.
5. Axelrod, F. B., and Abularrage, J. J., 1982, Familial dysautonomia: A prospective study of survival, *J. Pediatr.* **101:**234–236.
6. Rodriguez, M., Gomez, M. R., Howard, F. M., and Taylor, W. F., 1983, Myasthenia gravis in children: Long-term follow-up, *Ann. Neurol.* **13:**504–510.
7. Thompson, J. A., Glasgow, L. A., Warpinski, J. R., and Olson, C., 1980, Infant botulism: Clinical spectrum and epidemiology, *Pediatrics* **66:**936–942.
8. Karagan, N. J., 1979, Intellectual functioning in Duchenne muscular dystrophy: A review, *Psychol. Bull.* **86:**250–259.
9. Roses, A. D., Roses, M. J., Metcalf, B. S., Hull K. L., Nicholson, G. A., Hartwig, G. B., and Roe, C. R., 1977, Pedigree testing in Duchenne muscular dystrophy, *Ann. Neurol.* **2:**271–278.
10. Sarnat, H. B., O'Connor, T., and Byrne, P. A., 1976, Clinical effects of myotonic dystrophy on pregnancy and the neonate, *Arch. Neurol.* **33:**459–465.
11. Fischer, T. J., Rachelefsky, G. S., Klein, B., Paulus, H. E., and Stiehm, E. R., 1978, Childhood dermatomyositis and polymyositis, *Am. J. Dis. Child.* **133:**386–389.
12. Spencer, C. H., Hanson, V., Singsen, B. H., Bernstein, B. H., Kornreich, H. K., and King, K. K., 1984, Course of treated juvenile dermatomyositis, *J. Pediatr.* **105:**399–408.
13. Bowyer, S. L., Blane, C. E., Sullivan, D. B., and Cassidy, J. T., 1983, Childhood dermatomyositis: Factors predicting functional outcome and development of dystrophic calcification, *J. Pediatr.* **103:**882–888.

ADDITIONAL READING

Dubowitz, V., 1978, *Muscle Disorders in Childhood*, W.B. Saunders, Philadelphia.
Fenichel, G. M., 1978, Clinical syndromes of myasthenia in infancy and childhood, *Arch. Neurol.* **35:**97–103.
Thomas, P. K., 1983, Inherited nueropathies, *Mayo Clin. Proc.* **58:**476–480.

Movement Disorders

Movement disorders in children share the unifying characteristics of abnormalities of movement, posture, and tone, but encompass a broad range of conditions. The underlying pathophysiological processes involve the extrapyramidal system, and by custom this category excludes diseases primarily manifesting ataxia, spasticity, and muscle atrophy.

The extrapyramidal system consists of the basal ganglia, certain brain stem structures (subthalamic nucleus, red nucleus, substantia nigra), and the brain stem reticular formation, as well as their interconnections. This system is responsible for establishing appropriate posture and tone so that voluntary movements, arising predominantly from the cerebral cortex, can be carried out accurately, efficiently, and rapidly. Certain automatic and highly overlearned motor activities may originate primarily from the basal ganglia and are performed without obvious involvement of the motor cortex.

Research using standard neurochemical approaches and fluorescence histochemistry, a technique allowing the visualization of chemically specific neuronal pathways, has provided important information concerning the neurotransmitters involved in the function of the extrapyramidal system. Much of the research has focused on dopamine, norepinephrine, serotonin, acetylcholine, and GABA (γ-aminobutyric acid). More recently, the role of endorphins has come under scrutiny. Many of the current therapeutic strategies are based on attempts to modify the levels of these compounds or change their interactions with specific receptor sites.

APPROACH TO THE PATIENT

A specialized vocabulary is used to describe the movement disorders, and agreement on definitions is important. The major terms used are the following:

- Akinesia. Few spontaneous movements and difficulty in initiating and carrying out voluntary movements. Associated movements are decreased.

- Athetosis. Slow, forceful, writhing movements along the axis of the limb. They are irregular and associated with fluctuating muscle tone.
- Ballism. Large-amplitude, violent, flinging movements, originating at the shoulder or hip.
- Chorea. Rapid, random, fleeting, irregular movements, more prominent distally. They are not stereotyped.
- Dyskinesia. Any movement disorder.
- Dystonia. Slow, forceful, sustained contractions of both agonist and antagonist muscles, so that limbs are moved into an abnormal position, which is maintained for varying periods of time.
- Myoclonus. Sudden, shocklike contraction of a single muscle or muscle group. This occurs at random intervals, but in some patients may be triggered by environmental stimuli such as touch, sound, or a light flash.
- Rigidity. Marked uniform increase in muscle tone through the entire range of motion of the joint.
- Tic. Sudden, rapid, random, inappropriate, highly stereotyped movements. They may be quite simple or rather complex. Tics can be manifested as repetitive, stereotyped sounds.
- Tremor. Highly regular, rhythmical, oscillating movements at a joint or several joints.

The initial approach to diagnosis depends on analyzing three major features of the disorder:

1. What are the characteristics of the abnormalities in tone, posture, and movement?
2. Are there any other associated neurological abnormalities?
3. Is there any evidence of underlying systemic disease?

Figure 21-1 provides an approach to the first question.[1] The second two points will be discussed under the specific disease entities.

CHOREA

Sydenham chorea can follow a streptococcal infection and is one of the major diagnostic criteria of acute rheumatic fever. The onset is insidious or subacute, and it presents with adventitious movements of the limbs and face. This often is mistaken for clumsiness, and the child is punished for spilling and dropping things or for constantly fidgeting. The motor abnormalities may be restricted to one side of the body, hemichorea. Emotional lability is prominent and may be the feature that brings the child to medical attention.

The diagnosis is clinical, and it is important to rule out other causes of chorea. Serological evidence of a recent streptococcal infection is useful; studies may not help if the pharyngitis occurred many weeks previously, however.

If the movement disorder is incapacitating, haloperidol in doses of 2–5 mg/

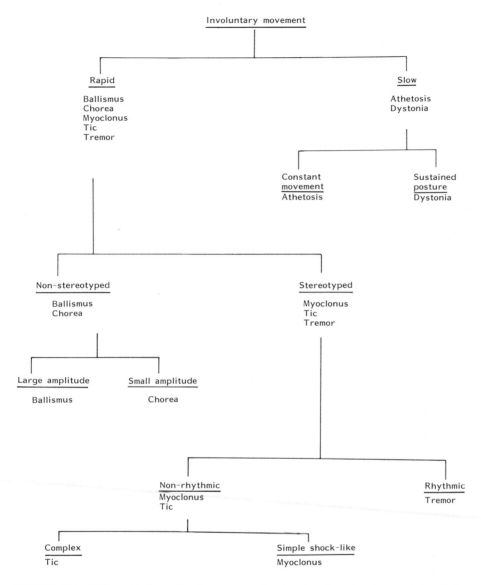

FIGURE 21-1. Differential diagnosis of movement disorders based on the characteristics of the dyskinesia. (Reprinted with permission from Golden.[1])

day is useful. The response to phenothiazines and sedatives is less consistent, and there is no indication for the use of antiinflammatory agents or corticosteroids. The patient with Sydenham chorea should be begun on the same regimen of antistreptococcal prophylaxis as any child with rheumatic fever, since a significant number of these children will have evidence of rheumatic valvular disease on long-term follow-up.

Improvement is gradual, may take many months, and can be incomplete, leaving the child with behavior problems and difficulties with fine motor coordination. Recurrences are seen, either spontaneously or during pregnancy *(chorea gravidarum)*.

Chorea associated with the use of *oral contraceptives* occurs in patients with a previous episode of Sydenham chorea and also in young women who have no history of a movement disorder. The movements can begin at any time, although the condition most frequently occurs 2 months after the drug is started. Symptoms resolve when the contraceptives are discontinued and usually recur if they are reinstituted.

Tardive dyskinesia presents as chorea and occurs in children, but is less frequent than in adults.[2] This may be due to a more limited use of psychotropic drugs in the pediatric age group or may be a function of the underlying conditions for which these drugs are used. Tongue and mouth movements are typical. There is chorea of the face; tongue lifting, rolling, and thrusting; masticatory movements; and forced jaw opening and deviation. If medication is stopped soon after symptoms begin, remission is possible.

Somewhat more common is the *withdrawal emergent syndrome*. Severe, continuous chorea involving the limbs and face begins immediately following the reduction or sudden discontinuation of large doses of psychotropic agents. This resolves without treatment over a period of several weeks to months.

Familial paroxysmal choreoathetosis refers to a group of conditions which includes a number of inherited disorders of movement. In the kinesigenic form, symptoms begin in late childhood or adolescence and attacks are triggered by sudden voluntary movements. The patient experiences paresthesias in the affected limb and then develops choreoathetoid movements and dystonic posturing. Symptoms are relieved by phenytoin and tend to diminish during adulthood.

The nonkinesigenic form begins in early childhood, and the attacks are not triggered by sudden movements. The dyskinesia is similar, but paresthesias are not a prominent feature. There is no therapeutic response to anticonvulsants.

Table 21-1 lists a number of other disorders associated with chorea.

ATHETOSIS

Athetoid cerebral palsy is the most common disorder in childhood associated with athetosis. This dyskinesia may also be seen in Wilson disease. It is often difficult to clearly differentiate chorea and athetosis in a specific patient.

TREMOR

Essential tremor is the most common form of tremor in both children and adults and can begin at any age. It is absent at rest, accentuated by attempting to hold the hands elevated, and often associated with an intention tremor. This is sometimes so prominent that a diagnosis of cerebellar ataxia is made. The

TABLE 21-1
Chorea in Childhood

Vascular	Drug induced
Sydenham chorea	Tardive dyskinesia
Systemic lupus erythematosus	Emergent dyskinesia
Anaphylactoid purpura	Miscellaneous
Posthemiplegic	Postanoxia
Metabolic	Postencephalitic
Lesch–Nyhan syndrome	Hereditary nonprogressive chorea
Wilson disease	Familial paroxysmal choreoathetosis
Degenerative	Kinesigenic
Huntington disease	Nonkinesigenic
Ataxia–telangiectsia	
Endocrine	
Oral contraceptives	
Thyrotoxicosis	

head is less commonly involved in children than in adults. An autosomal dominant mode of transmission is found in many families. If the tremor interferes with daily activities or is a major source of embarrassment, it can be ameliorated by the use of propranalol. This is given in doses of 10–40 mg every 6–8 hr. Propranalol is contraindicated if the patient has asthma or heart block. Ethanol ingestion also markedly reduces the tremor, but this is obviously not a useful therapeutic strategy.

Spasmus nutans is a condition restricted to early childhood. The patient presents with a horizontal nodding tremor of the head. This is usually associated with nystagmus, sometimes monocular, and occasionally with a head tilt. The etiology is not understood. There have been several reports of this syndrome associated with tumors in the region of the chiasm of the optic nerve. No specific treatment is available, but the condition resolves spontaneously in 1–2 years.

TICS

Simple tics are frequent in childhood and most commonly involve the eyes, face, neck, and shoulder. They can be partially suppressed voluntarily, but this typically produces a feeling of tension which is relieved by making the movement. The average age of onset is approximately 7 years. Boys are affected significantly more frequently than girls.

Tics become worse under stress. Because of this, a psychological etiology has been widely accepted, although this has never been rigorously proven, and the majority of tics resolve spontaneously within 3 months, with or without behavioral treatment. Haloperidol in doses of 0.5–2.0 mg/day will rapidly relieve most tics, although its use is seldom indicated.

Chronic motor tic disorder refers to a condition in which one or more motor tics continue for longer than 1 year.

Tic disorders lie along a spectrum of severity.[1] *Tourette syndrome* is the most severe and complex form. The diagnostic features are a changing repertory of motor and vocal tics, which begins in childhood and waxes and wanes spontaneously. The onset is usually with a single motor tic, indistinguishable from simple tics. As the condition progresses, however, it becomes apparent that new tics are added, some tics disappear, and several tics are present simultaneously. At some point, vocal tics then appear. These range in severity from inarticulate sounds such as coughing, sniffing, and throat clearing to loud and bizarre shrieks and cries.

Although these symptoms are the core features, a number of other unusual manifestations may be added. Among the most frequent are

- Complex stereotyped mannerisms
- Compulsive behavior
  - Touching
  - Smelling objects
  - Chewing on objects
  - Arranging objects
- Obsessive thinking
- Echolalia: echoing back the words of others
- Palilalia: repeating one's own words
- Coprolalia: involuntary utterance of obscene or blasphemous words

Between one-half and 70% of patients with Tourette syndrome have other individuals in their family with a tic disorder. They may meet the diagnostic criteria for Tourette syndrome, chronic motor tic disorder, or simple tics. These genetic data provide evidence that all of the tic disorders are interrelated and differ only in their severity and chronicity. Although early studies suggested an increased incidence among Ashkenazi Jews, this has not been confirmed. There does seem to be a low incidence among blacks.

Neurochemical studies suggest that the disorder is due to hypersensitivity of dopamine receptors in the central nervous system.[3] The observation that psychostimulant drugs (methylphenidate, dextroamphetamine, and pemoline) occasionally precipitate the symptoms of Tourette syndrome is consistent with this hypothesis.

Haloperidol, a potent dopamine receptor blocker, is the standard drug for treatment. This is begun at a dose of 0.25–0.5 mg/day and increased by 0.5 mg/day, every 5–7 days, until a therapeutic effect is obtained or side effects supervene. If a response is not obtained at a dose of 5–6 mg/day, it is unlikely that higher doses will be of any use. Substantial relief of the symptoms occurs in 80–85% of patients, but one-half will have side effects characteristic of neuroleptic drugs. Treatment often involves a compromise between therapeutic and side effects. Pimozide, a new dopamine receptor blocker, is also quite effective and appears to produce less sedation. Clonidine is useful for the treatment of some patients.

A spontaneous remission, partial or complete, occurs in middle or late adolescence in 30–40% of patients. There are no prognostic tools available, however, which can predict this outcome.

DYSTONIA

Dystonia musculorum deformans begins in midchildhood with the insidious and episodic appearance of uncontrolled movements of a limb, most commonly the foot. The spasms typically occur only during attempts to carry out specific movements, and the patient has some voluntary ability to inhibit them. For this reason, a psychiatric diagnosis is often considered. As the disease progresses, the spasms become more frequent and are less subject to voluntary control. Examination of the affected limb shows sustained contraction of both agonist and antagonist muscles; the spasm may be so severe that pain is produced. The examiner is able, at that stage, to passively correct the abnormal posture. Still later in the course, the deformity becomes fixed.

As the limb initially affected becomes progressively involved, the same process begins in other limbs; each may be at a different stage, but progression is inexorable. Some patients also develop dystonic spasms of the axial musculature, producing torticollis, tortipelvis, and scoliosis. The disease is restricted to the motor system, and there are neither sensory signs nor deterioration of cognitive function.

The most rapidly progressive form is seen in Ashkenazi Jews and is probably transmitted as an autosomal recessive trait. It begins in childhood, the limbs are more severely involved than the trunk and neck, and serious disability occurs by midadolescence. An autosomal dominant form affects all ethnic groups. These patients are more mildly involved, show prominent dystonia of axial muscles (torsion dystonia), and may have periods of stability or even remission. Sporadic cases can follow any pattern.

Drug treatment is unsatisfactory. Empirical trials of every drug known to have an effect on the basal ganglia, neurotransmitter metabolism, and muscle tone have been carried out. Occasional patients respond to a specific drug, but not frequently enough to allow development of any principles of therapy. Diazepam in high doses may be useful, but sedation is often a troublesome problem and reduction of the dose can produce withdrawal symptoms. Anticholinergic compounds, also in large doses, are used by some investigators. Stereotactic placement of lesions in the thalamus appears to produce improvement in one-third of patients, but recurrences are common. Bilateral lesions are often complicated by the development of pseudobulbar speech.

AKINESIA AND RIGIDITY

Disorders predominantly associated with akinesia or rigidity are rare in childhood. *Juvenile Parkinson disease* is usually sporadic, presents with features identical to those found in adults, and responds to the same therapeutic strategies. *Juvenile Huntington disease* differs from the adult form in that the majority of patients present with akinesia and rigidity. There may be some superimposed chorea, but this is not prominent. Behavior problems, progressive dementia, and seizures accompany the motor signs. There is no useful treatment. This disorder is transmitted as an autosomal dominant trait, and clinical diagnosis depends on a thorough family history. New techniques of DNA analysis have been used to detect the presence of the gene. Further refinement of this methodology will allow development of a biological marker for confirming the diagnosis and determining the carrier state.

The *neuroleptic malignant syndrome* is a potentially life-threatening complication associated with the use of antipsychotic tranquilizers.[4,5] The cardinal features are fever, a movement disorder, and a change in mental status. The most common dyskinesia is rigidity, which may be so severe that it is associated with rhabdomyolysis. The creatinine phosphokinase level in serum is usually elevated. Movements resembling tardive dyskinesia have also been reported. In addition to fever, other autonomic signs, such as tachycardia, diaphoresis, and labile blood pressure, are present. Depression in the state of consciousness is common, and the patient may become comatose. The neuroleptic drug should be discontinued. Treatment with dantrolene sodium or bromocriptine may produce rapid resolution of the symptoms.

MOVEMENT DISORDERS AS PART OF GENERALIZED NEUROLOGICAL DISEASES

The majority of the disorders discussed in this chapter, with the exception of Huntington disease, are restricted almost entirely to the motor system. Diseases associated with diffuse neuronal involvement, such as some cases of ceroid lipofuscinosis, may have a dyskinesia as part of the clinical picture. This information can be found in the appropriate chapters.

MOVEMENT DISORDERS AS PART OF GENERALIZED METABOLIC DISEASES

The prototype of disorders in this category is *Wilson disease*. There is deficient production of ceruloplasmin, a serum protein that binds copper. As a result, serum copper levels are low, urinary copper excretion is increased, and copper is deposited in many tissues of the body. This is responsible for the characteristic features of the disorder.

One-half of patients initially present with neurological signs and symptoms. Most typically, there is the rapid onset and progression of tremor. This is either fine and rhythmical or large-amplitude and "flapping." Pseudobulbar signs, ataxia, dysarthria, and rigidity develop; dementia and seizures are rare.

The remainder of the patients present with hepatic cirrhosis and portal hypertension. Wilson disease should be considered in any child with unexplained liver disease. Although neurological and hepatic manifestations are the best known, Wilson disease is also associated with thrombocytopenia, leukopenia, hemolytic anemia, proximal renal tubular resorption defects, metabolic bone disease, osteoporosis, and arthritis.

Diagnosis is aided by the finding of a Kayser–Fleischer ring, an area of discoloration at the limbus of the cornea. Slit-lamp microscopy confirms that it is in Descemet's membrane. Definitive diagnosis requires demonstration of a low ceruloplasmin level, low serum copper levels, and increased urinary excretion of copper. Liver biopsy confirms an increased hepatic copper content.

Treatment has two components. Copper intake is decreased by dietary modification. Administration of penicillamine causes the mobilization and excretion of tissue copper. If therapy is begun early, the long-term prognosis is good, although treatment must be lifelong. There may even be regression of preexisting neurological deficits. Genetic counseling must be a part of management, as the disorder is transmitted by an autosomal recessive gene.

REFERENCES

1. Golden, G. S., 1982, Movement disorders in children: Tourette syndrome, *Dev. Behav. Pediatr.* **3**:209–216.
2. Gualtieri, C. T., Barnhill, J., McGimsey, J., and Schell, D., 1980, Tardive dyskinesia and other movement disorders in children treated with psychotropic drugs, *J. Am. Acad. Child Psychiatry,* **19**:419–510.
3. Singer, H. S., Butler, I. J., Tune, L. E., Seifert, W. E., and Coyle, J. T., 1982, Dopamine dysfunction in Tourette syndrome, *Ann. Neurol.* **12**:361–366.
4. Klein, S. K., Levinsohn, M. W., and Blumer, J. L., 1985, Accidental chlorpromazine ingestion as a cause of the neuroleptic malignant syndrome in children, *J. Pediatr.* **107**:970–973.
5. Guze, B. H., and Baxter, L. R., 1985, Neuroleptic malignant syndrome, *N. Engl. J. Med.* **313**:163–166.

ADDITIONAL READING

Barbeau, A. (ed.), 1981, *Disorders of Movement,* J.B. Lippincott, Philadelphia.
Marsden, C. D., 1982, The mysterious motor function of the basal ganglia: The Robert Wartenberg Lecture, *Neurology* **32**:514–539.

22

Sleep Disorders

Sleep is a universal phenomenon in higher animals, and although the need for it is clearly recognized, its physiological purpose and the factors producing it are not understood. There is a well-defined evolution of sleep patterns in the individual, and disorders of sleep have age-specific characteristics. A rational clinical approach to complaints of disordered sleep requires understanding of the developmental aspects of normal sleep.

Adult sleep is characterized by the regular alteration of two different physiological patterns, rapid-eye-movement (REM) sleep and non-rapid-eye-movement (NREM) sleep. The electoencephalogram shows four basic stages. Stage 1, a low-voltage fast pattern, occurs in both REM and NREM sleep. The addition of sleep spindles and vertex sharp waves (K complexes) to this background distinguishes stage 2 sleep. Stages 3 and 4 show high-voltage, slow-wave activity. Stages 2, 3, and 4 are associated only with NREM sleep.

During REM sleep, there are rapid conjugate eye movements, loss of tone in the chin muscles, small myoclonic jerks of the fingers, an irregular pulse, and irregular respirations with brief periods of apnea. NREM sleep is characterized by lack of rapid eye movements, maintenance of muscle tone, a slow, regular pulse, and slow, regular respirations. The adult, upon falling asleep, shows a gradual transition from stage 1 NREM sleep, through stages 2 and 3 to stage 4. There then are shifts back and forth through the various levels. The first REM period occurs quite regularly 90 min after the onset of sleep. These then recur at somewhat shorter intervals, and there are four to six REM periods during the average night, with a return to NREM sleep in between. Approximately 20% of sleep time is in the REM phase.

The premature or full-term neonate shows, in addition to REM and NREM sleep, a third pattern, indeterminate sleep.[1] This is the major characteristic at 34 weeks of gestational age and has largely disappeared by postnatal age 3 months. The full-term infant spends approximately 50% of sleep time in REM sleep. Other features differentiating the infant from the adult include REM at the onset of sleep and a briefer interval between REM cycles. Organization of sleep patterns with a long period of sleep at night, for which parents are most grateful, occurs by 3 months of age. There are typically two naps during the day, with the remainder of the time spent awake. The age at which the naps are given up is quite variable.

Total sleep time is also highly variable, although the average neonate sleeps nearly 17 hr each day. This is reduced to 14 hr by age 6 months, 13 by 1 year, and 10.5 by 6 years. There is a slight decrease by the beginning of adolescence, and the usual adult pattern of 7–8 hr of sleep each night is attained by age 13–14 years.

APPROACH TO THE PATIENT

A simple way of approaching the analysis of sleep problems is to divide them into conditions that produce insomnia, hypersomnia, or disordered sleep. The latter category is used to refer to those disorders that regularly interrupt sleep or always occur in association with sleep, even if awakening does not occur. Nocturnal seizures and vascular headaches beginning during sleep are discussed in the appropriate chapters.

INSOMNIA

Insomnia is one of the most frequent complaints in adult medicine. This is variously characterized as the inability to fall asleep, frequent nighttime awakenings, early-morning awakening, or the feeling of inadequate rest after a night's sleep. Children occasionally voice this complaint, but it is more frequently called to the physician's attention by the child's parents. The condition is usually self-limited and responds to assurances that it will improve.

The parents should understand that anxiety at bedtime is a normal developmental phenomenon. It is perfectly acceptable for the child to use brief rituals, a night-light, a treasured object (or several), or thumb sucking to aid in falling asleep.

If the complaint of insomnia is persistent, and the child also has daytime somnolence, further investigation is warranted. Serious emotional problems associated with major life stress, anxiety, or depression may be the underlying cause. If so, referral for evaluation and treatment would be appropriate. Exploration of the social environment and sleeping arrangements is also often productive. Simple suggestions may allow these to be modified. More serious causes of disturbed sleep with daytime hypersomnia are discussed later in this chapter.

It is rarely appropriate to use sedative medication for complaints of insomnia in a child. Most drugs disturb the normal structure of the night's sleep, lose their effectiveness within 2 weeks, and are associated with rebound insomnia when they are discontinued. If the child disturbs the parents at night, behavioral approaches should be used to keep him in his room and playing quietly until he again falls asleep.

Children with central nervous system anomalies or damage often have poorly organized sleep, excessive irritability, and a rather abrasive cry. If this continues to be a problem and is disruptive to the family, sedation is sometimes needed. Chloral hydrate, in doses of 50–100 mg/kg body weight, can be given 45–60 min before the child is put to bed.

HYPERSOMNIA

Hypersomnia occurring at night is an unusual condition, typically beginning in adolescence. There are excessively long periods of sleep, and awakening is difficult. Some patients will be confused and drowsy for as long as 1–2 hours after being aroused. Sleep studies have shown no abnormalities. Psychological problems such as depression are often associated with this disorder.

Narcolepsy rarely begins before adolescence. Boys are affected more frequently than girls, and an autosomal dominant mode of transmission has been reported in some families. The narcoleptic triad consists of uncontrollable attacks of sleep during the day, hypnagogic hallucinations, and cataplexy. Hypnagogic hallucinations occur when the patient is falling asleep, are quite vivid, and may be associated with sleep paralysis. This is transient inability to move; there is no respiratory embarrassment. Many normal individuals have similar episodes occasionally, but they are more frequent in the narcoleptic. Cataplexy refers to sudden loss of muscle tone with inability to move one or more muscle groups. It may be so severe that postural tone is lost and the patient falls. Emotional stimuli and laughing will precipitate cataplexy in some individuals.

The sleep attacks are associated with REM at the onset, a pattern never seen in normal sleep. It is now known that the narcoleptic has large numbers of "microsleep" episodes during the day characterized by brief bursts of theta activity of a REM pattern. These may not be easily recognized clinically, but can interfere with the ability to learn and to be productive at work.

The most effective treatment is the use of dextroamphetamine or methylphenidate. These must often be given in large doses, which can be titrated against the clinical effect, and continuous administration is required. Tricyclic antidepressants are less useful for the sleep attacks, but may be more effective in treating the other symptoms.

The *sleep apnea–hypersomnia syndrome* occurs in childhood and adolescence and is a potentially important cause of morbidity. Several different complaints bring the child to medical attention. These include persistent daytime somnolence, declining school performance, and loud snoring at night. Investigation documents that the patient is having apneic spells during sleep, lasting as long as 1 min and sometimes occurring hundreds of times each night. Each episode is terminated by spontaneous partial or full arousal, interfering with sleep and producing drowsiness during the day. During the apneic spell, hypoxia, hypercapnea, and acidosis occur. Systemic and pulmonary hypertension and cor pulmonale result if the condition is not properly diagnosed and treatment instituted.

Sleep apnea in adults can be categorized into central (primary) or obstructive types. In older children and adolescents, it is almost always obstructive.[2] The combination of partial anatomical obstruction of the upper airway and relaxation of the muscles of the tongue and throat during sleep produces the symptoms. Causes of obstruction include hypertrophied tonsils and adenoids, anatomical malformations of the face, micrognathia, and cleft palate repair. If the problem cannot be corrected surgically, a permanent tracheostomy must be placed. This is left plugged during the day and opened before the child goes to sleep.

The *pickwickian syndrome* consists of daytime somnolence in the presence of massive obesity. There is respiratory compromise with hypercarbia and carbon dioxide narcosis. Treatment is most difficult and is dependent on major, sustained weight loss. Untreated, there is a risk of pulmonary hypertension developing secondary to the sustained hypercarbia.

DISTURBED SLEEP

Nightmares are extremely common, especially in preschool children. They are dreams with frightening content; the child believes that they are real, and it may take a good deal of effort to calm him and get him back to sleep. The child should be encouraged to return to his own bed and given whatever special object he wants to help him get back to sleep. If he is allowed into the parents' bed, a pattern of behavior may develop that is very difficult to change. Psychological consultation is rarely required unless the nightmares are so frequent that they are severely disruptive or the child has other signs of psychological disturbance.

Night terrors (pavor nocturnus) are unrelated to nightmares. These occur during arousal from stage 3 or 4 sleep. The child suddenly sits upright in bed, stares and appears frightened, and may scream or cry inconsolably. Attacks last approximately 10 min, and the child then returns to undisturbed sleep. In the morning, there is no recall of dream content or of the episode. This condition occurs predominantly in preschool children, is benign and self-limited, and is not a sign of psychological problems. Treatment is rarely required, but if the attacks occur daily and are extremely disruptive, a brief trial of diazepam, 0.5–2 mg at bedtime, is usually rapidly effective.

Sleepwalking (somnambulism) and *sleeptalking* (somniloquy) begin during school age and adolescence. The child sits up in bed or gets up and walks. The eyes are open and staring, but the activities are not purposeful. It is difficult to awaken the patient or to communicate with him. Sleeptalking may occur with or without sleepwalking. These phenomena appear during stage 4 sleep. There is no effective treatment. It is important to understand that the sleepwalking child does not have any critical judgment, and that serious injuries may occur during these episodes. The environment must be arranged so that the child cannot easily injure himself.

Nocturnal enuresis is usually included among the sleep disorders, as it almost always occurs during NREM sleep. There is controversy as to whether or not it is restricted to stage 3 and 4 sleep. Enuretic children demonstrate increased intravesical pressures during slow-wave sleep, when compared to controls. The condition is more common in males, and a family history is often present. Bed wetting during sleep is seen in up to 15% of 5-year-olds.

If the child has primary enuresis, that is, has never been dry at night for a significant period of time, an underlying psychological cause is almost never found. Wetting during the day as well as at night, or secondary enuresis, especially after age 5 years, is compatible with either organic or psychological factors. A urinary tract infection should be ruled out, but there is little or no need for x-ray studies of the kidneys and bladder in most instances. New information concerning this disorder is forthcoming from urodynamic studies, which are now being applied to children.

Many approaches to treatment are available, suggesting that none is consistently effective. These have included various behavioral techniques, pad and buzzer systems, and administration of imipramine. Before any claim for therapeutic success can be made, it is important to remember that enuresis, especially in boys, cannot be considered abnormal prior to age 4 or 5 years, the spontaneous "cure" rate is 10% per year, and 3–5% of children will remain enuretic into late adolescence and, occasionally, adulthood.

SUDDEN INFANT DEATH SYNDROME

Although there is no proof that sudden infant death syndrome (SIDS) is a sleep disorder, it is discussed at this point because of its regular occurrence during sleep. SIDS probably causes at least 5000 deaths each year. The typical child is between 2 and 4 months of age. There is an association with preterm delivery, low socioeconomic status, winter months, and being male. Siblings have an increased risk. The child seems well when put to bed, but sometime later is found dead. A number of autopsy findings have been reported, but none consistent enough to be diagnostic or to fully explain the cause of death. Many, such as petechiae on the pericardium, mild pulmonary edema, and pulmonary vascular congestion, can be associated with death from anoxia or attempts to respire in the face of upper airway obstruction.

The relationship of SIDS to sleep has been suggested by two observations. The first is "near-miss SIDS," a situation in which an adult finds the child moribund during sleep and achieves successful resuscitation. The second is increasing awareness of the existence of significant apneic episodes during sleep in all infants, but especially those born preterm. At this time it seems reasonable to hypothesize that SIDS may be due to a maturational abnormality in the control of respiration during sleep.[3] The data contain enough conflicts, however, to prevent any more definitive statement.

Ondine's curse, or congenital central alveolar hypoventilation, is a rare condition in which there is failure of the automatic control of ventilation during sleep.[4] The child becomes anoxic and hypercarbic because of failure to respire adequately; no upper airway obstruction is present. There is some evidence that central receptors do not respond to increasing levels of carbon dioxide. Cor pulmonale is a frequent cause of death. There have been only a few case reports, and no long-term follow-up studies are available.

REFERENCES

1. Coons, S., and Guilleminault, C., 1982, Development of sleep–wake patterns and non-rapid eye movement sleep stages in the first six months of life in normal infants, *Pediatrics* **69:**793–798.
2. Brouilette, R. T., Fernbach, S. K., and Hunt, C. E., 1982, Obstructive sleep apnea in infants and children, *J. Pediatr.* **100:**31–40.
3. Lacey, D. J., 1983, Sleep EEG abnormalities in children with near-miss sudden infant death syndrome, in siblings, and in infants with recurrent apnea, *J. Pediatr.* **102:**854–859.
4. Fleming, P. J., Cade, D., Bryan, M. H., and Bryan, A. C., 1980, Congenital central hypoventilation and sleep state, *Pediatrics* **66:**425–428.

ADDITIONAL READING

Anders, T. F., Carskaden, M. A., and Dement, W. C., 1980, Sleep and sleepiness in children and adolescents, *Pediatr. Clin., North Am.* **27:**29–43.

23

Disorders of Higher Cognitive Function

Mental retardation, a global disorder of higher cognitive function, has been discussed in Chapter 9. This section will concentrate on those conditions in which the cognitive deficit is more circumscribed and overall intelligence is preserved. This is, to some extent, an artificial construct, as the meaning of a full-scale IQ score in the face of specific cognitive disabilities is not clear.

The attainment of higher-order intellectual skills follows a reasonably consistent time schedule, as does any developmental phenomenon. There are several theoretical frameworks that allow understanding of this progression. The work of Piaget is a useful approach and can be referred to for details.

When general intelligence seems to develop normally, but performance in school does not meet expectations, a learning disability should be suspected. The concept of learning disability has gone through a number of changes over the last 50 years. It was clearly recognized early on that children with documented brain damage, acquired either perinatally or postnatally, had difficulties in memory, learning, and behavior. In the absence of obvious brain damage, however, there was a great tendency to blame school failure on psychological problems. The concept of a "block" for learning, based on psychodynamic hypotheses, was one outcome of this reasoning. A good deal of time was spent on therapy to assist children to overcome this block and motivate them to achieve in school.

During the 1950s it became apparent that many children with no obvious evidence of brain damage had cognitive and behavioral abnormalities identical to those found in patients with documented abnormalities of the CNS. This concept was then formalized in 1966 by an NIH task force, which introduced the term "minimal brain dysfunction" (MBD).[1] Several alternative definitions were offered, all of which shared three features:

1. General intelligence is normal or near normal.

2. There are varying combinations of impairment in perception, conceptualization, language, memory, motor function, and control of attention.
3. There is no other cause to account for the school failure.

The introduction of this concept was extremely important, as it clearly focused on abnormalities in brain function. Problems occurred, however, when the term MBD was used as a specific diagnosis, rather than a conceptual framework. School systems, physicians, and psychologists lost sight of the major differences between children, and this tended to stifle the development of individualized diagnoses and specific plans for remedial education. It is best to avoid the term MBD and to focus on the child's specific strengths and weaknesses, skills and deficits.

Faced with these varying approaches, many school systems developed operational criteria that did allow for specificity in diagnosis, but made no assumptions concerning the underlying mechanisms. Learning disabilities were generally accepted as existing when full-scale IQ was normal and academic performance in one or more areas was at least two standard deviations below the expected grade level on standardized tests. It was also necessary to rule out emotional and social factors that could interfere with schoolwork.

These definitions provided specific criteria that allowed for the classification of children and determination of who would be eligible for special services. There were two problems with this approach, however. First is the assumption that full-scale IQ and academic achievement are always closely correlated. This is, in general, true but does not allow for developmental variations, individual differences in cognitive style, individual strengths and weaknesses, and differences in motivation. The second problem is the use of exclusionary criteria. These might make it difficult to classify a child from a disrupted home of low socioeconomic status as being learning disabled. Despite these issues, a discrepancy between IQ and academic achievement is widely used as the defining criterion.

Research into the underlying causes of learning disabilities is currently following two very different tracks, neuropsychological testing and neurophysiological studies. Neuropsychology as a clinical science rapidly developed following World War II, when the Veterans Administration hospitals provided a large population of patients with static residua of head injuries. The basic approach is to develop tests that probe specific cognitive tasks and correlate the abnormalities defined with the known CNS pathology. The assumption is then made that the impaired function is normally served by the area of brain that had been damaged.

This lesion–deficit approach has been applied to children, but with varying degrees of success. One problem is that the disorders that affect children are generally not discrete, circumscribed abnormalities, but are the result of abnormal development or diffuse processes such as meningitis and head trauma. The second confounding factor is that of plasticity, the ability of the immature brain to regain lost functions. The extent to which this is a result of either anatomical repair or functional reorganization is not clear, although the second factor is probably the most important.

Neurophysiological techniques are primarily based on computer-assisted analysis of bioelectrical brain activity, especially that evoked by sensory stimuli or recorded during the performance of specific cognitive tasks. This provides quantitative data or maps of brain activity that allow comparison of clinical subjects and controls. Newer techniques such as nuclear magnetic resonance imaging and positron emission tomography are now being applied to these problems. Attempts to correlate these physiological studies with deficits on neuropsychological testing may allow the development of a new approach to functional localization in children.

APPROACH TO THE PATIENT

When a child presents with unexpected school failure, the first task is to differentiate a school problem from a learning disability. Poor performance can be due to many factors other than a learning disability, some of the most important of which are

1. Underlying chronic illness
2. Defect in vision or hearing
3. Unrecognized mental retardation
4. Major emotional problems
5. Serious sociocultural deprivation
5. Inadequate school experience

It should be remembered, however, that although these factors may complicate the diagnostic process, they can coexist with a learning disability. Careful testing to define the cognitive deficit is most important.

The history is directed toward uncovering features that are known to be associated with developmental or acquired abnormalities of the CNS. This is no different than the routine neurological history, although special emphasis should be placed on developmental patterns and progress, especially in the areas of language and fine motor function. Abnormalities in these abilities are frequently forerunners of other cognitive problems.

The physical examination is used to rule out underlying medical conditions. Any acute or chronic illness can interfere with sustained peak performance. The general neurological examination can define any focal or lateralizing abnormalities.

Soft signs play a prominent role in the literature on cognitive dysfunction. These can be defined as deficits in motor or sensory performance which are abnormal only in the context of the child's age. They would be normal if found in younger children. Other authors include as soft signs those findings which have localizing significance but are not associated with any functional disability. An example would be the presence of a Babinski sign without other evidence of a hemiparesis.

Many published reports attempt to correlate the presence of soft signs with cognitive disabilities. Each investigator, however, uses his own test battery, norms are often based on a small number of subjects, and correlations between studies are poor. The meaning of these abnormalities is not clear. A child with severe learning disabilities can have a completely normal motor examination. Children with large numbers of soft signs and extremely poor coordination, on the other hand, may excel academically. It is important to remember, however, that an incompetent motor system can be a source of major problems in the classroom setting and in the schoolyard, independent of any learning disability.

LEARNING DISABILITIES

Dyslexia, the inability to learn to read at or near grade level, is the most common learning disability. This may be an isolated condition or associated with problems in spelling and writing. Dyslexia is a familial disorder in some cases and affects boys considerably more often than girls.

A moment's reflection will give a picture of the enormous complexity of the tasks involved in reading, starting with the perception and decoding of written symbols and ending with apprehension of the complex thoughts that the author was trying to convey. Reading disability could conceivably result from abnormal function at any point along this pathway.

A number of specific syndromes or subgroups of dyslexia have been defined by neuropsychological testing.[2] Although these are not universally accepted, and other workers have developed different frameworks, they serve as a useful example of an attempt to differentiate dyslexic children on the basis of specific processing deficits. These syndromes are

1. Language disorder syndrome. These children have difficulty naming objects and have one or more additional language deficits. Verbal IQ is significantly lower than performance IQ.
2. Visual–spatial perceptual syndrome. Language is not impaired, but there is a deficit in visual–spatial perception and memory. Performance IQ is depressed.
3. Articulation and graphomotor discoordination syndrome. There are major problems with fine motor coordination. The children often have articulation problems due to oromotor apraxia, the inability to consistently produce proper sounds even though all of the component movements can be made individually.
4. Sequencing deficit syndrome. These children have difficulty maintaining the sequence of words, sentences, and digits.

In each of these cases the presenting problem is difficulty learning to read. Because the causes are so different, it is reasonable to assume that associated features, treatment, and prognosis vary greatly and must be defined for the specific patient. Any single system of remediation that purports to be useful for all children with dyslexia is suspect.

There is a good deal of disagreement concerning the prognosis of dyslexia. It seems to be most favorable if there are no other associated cognitive deficits and if the patient has normal intelligence. Some children never become competent readers despite intensive remedial efforts. It is important that the remainder of their education not be allowed to pass them by, and arrangements should be made to use alternate materials, such as recorded books and other audiovisual aids.

Dysgraphia, inefficient and illegible writing, can be either an isolated problem or associated with other learning disabilities. In many, but not all, cases there is other evidence of impairment of fine motor coordination. The child cannot write both rapidly and legibly, and so the school must make special allowances. Spelling may or may not be disrupted, although it is usually inadequate if dyslexia is also present. If spelling skills are intact, early training in the use of a typewriter or word processor is most helpful.

Dyscalculia, difficulty in arithmetic, is one of the less common of the learning disabilities. There is a complex sequence of operations needed to carry out even simple calculations, analogous to the complexities of reading. Dysfunction at any point in this chain will disrupt performance. If the child can learn the correct use of the major arithmetical operations and convert word problems into a proper sequence of steps, the use of a small calculator will provide immense benefit.

Dyspraxia is a severe deficit in motor performance. Defining characteristics include normal strength, tone, coordination, and sensory function, but the inability to skillfully carry out complex voluntary motor acts. This has also been referred to as a motor planning deficit. A number of subgroups can be defined, depending on whether the difficulty is in using real objects, pretending to use objects, or imitating the examiner's movements. Apraxia of gait may be an associated problem or may exist independently.

Constructional apraxia refers to the inability to reproduce patterns and designs made with blocks or pencil and paper. As with other disorders of higher cognitive function, there can be any combination of deficits.

Disorders of memory, as isolated deficits, are unusual in children. They are most commonly found following severe head injury. There may be memory deficits associated with other cognitive disorders, but in those cases they are only part of a complex series of disabilities.

Attention Deficit Disorder

A constellation of behavioral abnormalities including a short attention span, distractability, motor restlessness, and hyperactivity is frequently observed in children with learning disabilities. This syndrome was first clearly described following the epidemic of encephalitis lethargica that was prevalent in the years 1916–1926. During the 1930s studies showed that similar symptoms were more commonly present in those mentally retarded individuals who had suffered a definable encephalopathic event than those with familial or genetically derived mental retardation. Based on these data, the concept was put forth that brain damage was the cause of the behavioral abnormalities. It soon became obvious, however, that most children with this disorder had neither mental retardation nor evidence of brain damage. It is now generally accepted that hyperactive children do not form a homogeneous group.[3] Similar symptoms can be caused by a number of other behavioral and psychological problems, the most prominent being conduct disorder.

Early definitions of this syndrome of hyperactivity or hyperkinesis focused on the level of motor activity. With the publication of the *Diagnostic and Statistical Manual of Mental Disorders,* 3rd ed. (DSM-III),[4] the name and perspective have both changed, and the term attention deficit disorder (ADD) was introduced. The primary symptoms are now considered to be an abnormally short attention span and distractability; motor hyperactivity is frequently associated, but this symptom is not required (Table 23-1). Unfortunately, the diagnostic criteria are qualitative and somewhat subjective rather than quantitative.

There are a number of rating scales, which are useful for structuring observations about the child and assessing changes in a given child's behavior following the introduction of therapy (Table 23-2).[5] These scales can be administered by the physician, teacher, or parent. A score of 15 or higher has been used to separate the 10% of children with the highest activity level. This cutting criterion varies slightly when the children are selected by sex and ethnicity.[6] Rating scales such as these are not diagnostic instruments, but serve as adjuncts to the clinical diagnosis.

TABLE 23-1
Diagnostic Features of Attention Deficit Disorder[a]

Inattentiveness (at least three of the following)	Hyperactivity (at least two of the following)
Does not finish things started	Runs about or climbs on things
Does not seem to listen	Cannot sit still or fidgets excessively
Distractable	Difficulty staying seated
Cannot sustain attention	Moves excessively during sleep
Does not stick to play activity	Continuously active
Impulsivity (at least two of the following)	
Acts before thinking	
Shifts from one activity to another	
Difficulty organizing work	
Needs a lot of supervision	
Calls out in class	
Cannot await turn	

[a]Modified from American Psychiatric Association.[4]

TABLE 23-2
Conners Behavior Rating Scale[a]

Scale items
1. Restless or overactive
2. Excitable, impulsive
3. Disturbs other children
4. Fails to finish things he starts, short attention span
5. Constantly fidgeting
6. Inattentive, easily distracted
7. Demands must be met immediately, easily frustrated
8. Cries often and easily
9. Mood changes quickly and drastically
10. Temper outbursts, explosive and unpredictable behavior

Each item is scored as[b]
0 Not at all
1 Just a little
2 Pretty much
3 Very much

[a]Modified from Goyette et al.[5]
[b]Highest possible score is 30.

ADD must always be defined developmentally, in terms of an inadequate attention span for the child's age. There are no absolute diagnostic criteria. Boys are affected 7–10 times more frequently than girls. Neurological examination is usually normal. There is not a one-to-one correlation between ADD and learning disabilities. Some children can show all of the characteristic features of ADD and still learn at the expected rate; many children with severe learning disabilities have a perfectly adequate attention span.

The treatment of ADD is even more controversial than the diagnostic criteria. Therapy is generally based on the use of psychostimulant drugs, most commonly methylphenidate. There is little argument that the children, during treatment, have less motor activity, are less intrusive, and seem to sustain attention for longer periods of time. They are more easily tolerated by adults in the environment and by their peers.

The controversy centers around the effects on cognitive function. Laboratory studies show improvement in short-term learning tasks requiring sustained performance. The evidence for overall academic improvement, and increased ability to handle complex and more abstract types of learning, is less convincing.[7] It is often disappointing to parents and teachers to find that there is no improvement in academic performance following successful therapy for the hyperactivity.

The concept that hyperactive children have an idiosyncratic reaction to stimulant drugs and that they can be used as a diagnostic test to separate organic from psychologically based hyperactivity has not been supported. It appears that normal children show changes in activity level, behavior, and performance similar to those of the patient group.[8]

The optimum dose of methylphenidate is 0.3–0.6 mg/kg per day. One problem in setting a drug level is that the dose producing the best improvement of cognitive testing is less than that which is most effective in reducing the motor activity.[9] Whether or not drug holidays should be instituted during weekends or periods of school vacation depends to a large extent on the parent's perception of the child's behavior at home. Treating a child with medication on the basis of the inability of others to cope is not a scientifically based approach, however, and the physician must carefully weigh all of the factors involved before deciding on the advisability of drug holidays.

Children under 5 years of age often respond poorly to stimulants. They become restless and irritable or appear oversedated and are described by their parents as acting like "zombies." Some children show an increase, rather than decrease, in activity level. Loss of appetite with weight loss and temporary growth failure also occurs. During a drug holiday, catchup growth takes place.

There are few serious medical complications with the use of psychostimulants. Excessive postexercise tachycardia, persisting as long as 1 year following discontinuation of medication, has been reported, but the clinical significance of this finding is not clear.[10]

The development or worsening of simple tics or Tourette syndrome occurs on occasion. If tics begin after therapy has been initiated, the medication should be discontinued. The child with both ADD and a tic disorder presents a difficult clinical dilemma. If ADD is the major problem, a cautious trial of methylphenidate might be attempted. If there is an exacerbation of the tics, the medication should be discontinued and behavioral strategies employed to manage the ADD if at all possible. Further use of psychostimulants should be approached with great caution, and only if the ADD is clearly so severe that the increased number and severity of tics and the possible need for the concurrent administration of haloperidol is acceptable.

Children with ADD do respond to behavior modification techniques.[11] This form of treatment is a problem for many school districts, however, because of the large amount of skilled staff time and one-on-one teaching that is required.

Language Disorders

Language disorders in children are complex, but in recent years a good deal of research has increased our understanding and provided useful clinical classifications. The majority of severe language disorders appear to be developmental in nature, although it is not known whether the underlying problem is structural or functional.

Acquired language disorders are less common. Children under 4 years of age who suffer an acute insult to the left cerebral hemisphere can be rendered aphasic. Recovery of language is rapid and in most cases is complete. Between 4 and 8 years of age, the same general pattern is seen, although recovery is slower and careful testing often shows some deficit in complex language skills.

Children older than 8 years of age have the patterns of recovery and types of residual aphasia similar to those of adult patients.

The classification of Rapin and Allen[12] appears to have a good deal of validity and utility when applied to patients and will be briefly summarized.

Verbal auditory agnosia refers to the inability to decode the phonological aspects of speech, the first step necessary for the understanding of language. These children do not understand spoken language but generally comprehend the meaning of nonspeech sounds in the environment, can communicate with gestures, will use toys appropriately, and may learn to read. In other words, internal symbolic language is intact. Peripheral hearing is normal, but the children function as if they were deaf.

This syndrome may be present from birth. An acquired form is associated with temporal lobe epileptogenic activity, frequently bilateral. Seizures may also occur. If speech was already present, it is lost, and the patient becomes mute or nearly so.

There are no reliable prognostic tools, but some patients will make a good recovery. Seizures resolve and the EEG becomes normal. The role of anticonvulsants in this improvement has been the source of controversy. As the course of the disorder is prolonged and the prognosis unpredictable, it is most important that the child's educational and communication needs be met. A total communication approach (manual language and oral speech), as with a deaf child, is most appropriate and effective.

The *semantic–pragmatic syndrome* is associated with difficulty in understanding the more complex aspects of language and the appropriate use of language for communication. The child understands words and speaks using properly formed sentences, but verbal productions are often inappropriate and not quite on target. Some of these children are echolalic and have behavior problems.

In the *mixed phonological–syntactic syndrome* understanding of language is good but there is a deficit in spoken language. The vocabulary is small, syntax immature, and articulation poor with numerous errors and poor intelligibility. An oromotor apraxia may be present, and some children have generally impaired motor function. As with many of the language disorders, reading problems are frequently associated. An even greater discrepancy between intact comprehension and severely disturbed expression is seen in the *phonological programming deficit syndrome*.

INFANTILE AUTISM

The term infantile autism was introduced by Kanner, in 1943, to describe children who showed severely decreased or absent interaction with others, a failure to use language to communicate, and a compulsive desire to keep the environment unchanged. He originally stated that they were quite skillful in fine motor tasks and had good cognitive function.

Although psychodynamic hypotheses were originally used to explain the etiology of infantile autism, and treatment strategies were based on these theories, it is now clear that autistic behavior is found in many different conditions. Most, if not all, of these children have underlying abnormalities of the CNS. This is seen in the association of this syndrome with such conditions as tuberous sclerosis and phenylketonuria. A substantial percentage of autistic children will have seizures by the time they are adolescents.

The DSM-III outlines the currently used diagnostic criteria (Table 23-3).[4]

The behavioral abnormalities are so striking that they are usually the first feature to bring the patient to attention. The child does not interact with other people, even the parents, in meaningful fashion. This behavior may be present from early infancy when the baby does not show the usual anticipatory reaction to being picked up and does not "cuddle" the way other children do. This autistic aloofness remains a constant feature to some degree.

Many children have stereotyped mannerisms, such as hand flapping, or develop excessive attachment to an object and manifest severe panic if this is removed. They become extremely upset at what seem to be minimal changes in the environment or routine. When the children are older, some personal interactions may develop, but they always have a peculiar quality. A minority of autistic children will ever become fully independent and self-supporting.

Children with infantile autism have, in addition to the classic behavioral abnormalities, major cognitive and language deficits.[13] The cognitive deficit is usually global, and only 15% of autistic children have an overall IQ in the normal range. There is a direct correlation between IQ and the ultimate prognosis. A small group of these children have splinter skills which are out of proportion with their overall cognitive level. They may be able to take complex mechanical objects apart and put them back together, memorize many songs, or mentally multiply long numbers. These are usually isolated skills, however, with little or no functional value and no importance in determining prognosis.

The language disorder is complex, but two major subgroups can be defined.[12] In the *fluent autistic syndrome* the children have reasonably normal articulation and comprehension. They are echolalic, however, and the pragmatic aspects of language (use of language as a tool for communication) are severely impaired.

Children with the *nonfluent severe autistic syndrome* are mute or have severely disturbed articulation. Comprehension is also impaired, and other cognitive def-

---

TABLE 23-3
Diagnostic Features of Infantile Autism[a]

Onset before age 30 months
Pervasive lack of responsiveness to other people
Deficits in language development
Abnormal language and speech
Bizarre response to environment
Absence of features of schizophrenia

[a]Modified from American Psychiatric Association.[4]

icits are present. The autistic child who is not attempting to use language for communication by age 5 years has an extremely poor prognosis.

CONTROVERSIAL THERAPIES

Disorders of higher cognitive function are chronic, handicapping, and usually not associated with easily demonstrable pathology of the CNS. The standard approaches to therapy are educational and behavioral, and progress is slow and difficult to measure. Medication plays an extremely limited role in the management of these children, except for the use of methylphenidate in selected cases of ADD. These factors obviously produce frustration on the part of the child, parents, and school, and they will often go on a search for a quicker and more dramatic approach to treatment.

In response to this situation, a number of controversial nutritional and physical therapies have been developed and are in widespread use. These all, on critical analysis, share certain defining characteristics:[14]

1. The theoretical basis underlying the therapy is not consistent with current biological knowledge.
2. They are said to be of benefit for a broad range of problems.
3. It is stated that there is no possibility of serious side effects.
4. The treatment is popularized without support for its use from properly designed studies or publication in peer-reviewed journals.
5. When controlled studies are carried out and do not support the concept, the rebuttal is that the experiments were inadequately designed or that there is a conspiracy to suppress the treatment method.
6. A cult aspect develops, and the therapy finds support among proselytizing lay groups.

The best known and most popular of the controversial therapies is the *Feingold diet*. The hypothesis is that learning disabilities and hyperactivity are due to a genetically determined, nonimmunological response to artificial coloring agents and other food additives. Feingold stated that 40–50% of these children improved when placed on an additive-free diet, and that dietary infractions caused a severe, immediate behavioral relapse.

A number of controlled studies, using either a diet–placebo crossover design or a challenge for children who were said to be reactors, have been carried out. No consistent or reliable effects were found.

Although attempts to remove unnecessary chemical agents from foods are to be commended, there are several potential adverse side effects of this diet. These include the expense and difficulty of managing the diet and the need to change the eating patterns of the entire family. In addition, the child, who is already stigmatized by his peers, is further marked as being different. He is limited in his participation in many social functions with other children because of the dietary restrictions.

Orthomolecular therapy (megavitamins) derives originally from work on the biochemical basis of schizophrenia in adults. Megavitamins have been claimed to be useful in the treatment of infantile autism, juvenile schizophrenia, Down syndrome, mental retardation, and learning disabilities, but these claims have not been supported in well-designed, controlled studies.

Orthomolecular therapy relies on massive doses of a large number of nutritional supplements, mainly vitamins. Each of these agents has the potential for toxicity. It is of note that nutritional therapies do not have to meet the same standards for safety and efficacy as are imposed on drugs. This has contributed to the popularization of these treatment methods.

Orthomolecular mineral therapy has even less of a theoretical basis than megavitamins. It has become much more popular since the introduction of hair mineral analysis. There are major problems with this technique, however, involving standard setting, determination of norms, intralaboratory correlations, and methods of sample collection. In addition, the relationship of the concentration of minerals in the hair to the body economy of these substances is poorly understood.

Some preliminary studies suggested differences in the concentration of a number of minerals, when comparing control subjects and learning-disabled children. These have not been replicated.

There is little or no information on the metabolic balance of many of these substances when ingested in large amounts over a prolonged period of time. It is known that a positive balance of many minerals can damage organ systems, but that this may take a long period of time.

Patterning is the best known of the physical therapies. The theory on which this is based is that the damaged CNS can be made to develop along normal pathways by the passive imposition of a carefully defined series of patterns of movement of the head and limbs.

Here again, the few controlled studies available have not provided support for this concept. Problems arise from the major time commitment necessary to carry out the program. If it is not effective, the blame is placed on the parents for failure to comply adequately or on the physician for delaying the referral for therapy.

Vestibular stimulation has been used for the treatment of many different developmental disabilities. Well-designed studies have not been carried out. A new approach, based on the concept that vestibular function is abnormal in children with learning disabilities, is the use of motion-sickness drugs. This has received extremely wide publicity through the public media, but no scientific support.

Optometric training is the prescription of exercises that are said to improve ocular tracking, eye muscle balance, and binocular fixation. This technique has been applied predominantly to children with reading problems.

There is no neurophysiological basis to support the claim that beginning reading, basically a skill involving the decoding of linguistic symbols, depends on the accuracy and efficiency of eye movements. It is possible that the deficits in motility, if they exist, could interfere with rapid reading in older individuals, but that is a different problem than that of dyslexia.

The relationship of *sugar metabolism* to behavior has become a popular preoccupation. As with most of the approaches discussed in this section, this has not been supported by well-designed studies. Foods are very complex chemically, and recent work has shown that *a priori* assumptions concerning which foods contain free carbohydrate and rapidly affect blood sugar levels are overly simplistic.

A host of new controversial therapies are introduced each year. Most do not catch the popular imagination, however. The physician would be well advised to keep up with the lay literature, which seems to be very open to publishing information about any new treatment approach. It is important to always insist on proper scientific proof before accepting any of these novel methods. The patient's long-term interests are not served by an unnecessary and unproductive expenditure of time and money.

REFERENCES

1. Clements, S. D., 1966, *Minimal Brain Dysfunction in Children,* US Department of Health, Education, and Welfare, Washington, DC.
2. Mattis, S., French, J. H., and Rapin, I., 1975, Dyslexia in young children: Three independent neuropsychological syndromes, *Dev. Med. Child. Neurol.* **17:**150–163.
3. Levine, M. D., Busch, B., and Aufseeser, C., 1982, The dimension of inattention among children with school problems, *Pediatrics* **70:**387–395.
4. American Psychiatric Association, 1980, *Diagnostic and Statistical Manual of Mental Disorders,* 3rd ed., American Psychiatric Association, Washington, DC.
5. Goyette, C. H., Conners, C. K., and Ulrich, R. F., 1978, Normative data on revised Conners Parent and Teacher Rating Scales, *J. Abnorm. Child Psychol.* **6:**221–236.
6. Adams, R. M., Macy, D. J., Kocsis, J. J., and Sullivan, A. R., 1984, Attention deficit disorder with hyperactivity: Normative data for Conners Behavior Rating Scale, *Texas Med.* **80:**58–61.
7. Barkley, R. A., and Cunningham, C. E., 1978, Do stimulant drugs improve the academic performance of hyperkinetic children? *Clin. Pediatr.* **17:**85–92.
8. Rapaport, J. L., Buchsbaum, M. S., Zahn, T. P., Weingartner, H., Ludlow, C., and Mikkelsen, E. J., 1978, Dextroamphetamine: Cognitive and behavioral effects in normal prepubertal boys, *Science* **199:**560–563.
9. Brown, R. T., and Sleator, E. K., 1979, Methylphenidate in hyperkinetic children: Differences in dose effects on impulsive behavior, *Pediatrics* **64:**408–411.
10. Ballard, J. E., Boileau, R. A., Sleator, E. K., Massey, B. H., and Sprague, R. L., 1976, Cardiovascular responses of hyperactive children to methylphenidate, *JAMA* **236:**2870–2874.
11. O'Leary, S. G., and Pelham, W. E., 1978, Behavior therapy and withdrawal of stimulant medication in hyperactive children, *Pediatrics* **61:**211–217.
12. Rapin, I., and Allen, D. A., 1982, Developmental language disorders: Nosologic considerations, in: *Neuropsychology of Language, Reading, and Spelling* (U. Kirk, ed.), Academic Press, New York.
13. Morgan, S. B., 1984, Helping parents understand the diagnosis of autism, *Dev. Behav. Pediatr.* **5:**78–85.
14. Golden, G. S., 1980, Nonstandard therapies in the developmental disabilities, *Am. J. Dis. Child.* **134:**487–491.

ADDITIONAL READING

Feagans, L., 1983, A current view of learning disabilities, *J. Pediatr.* **102:**487–493.
Golden, G. S., 1982, Neurobiological correlates of learning disabilities, *Ann. Neurol.* **12:**409–418.
Rapin, I., 1982, *Children with Brain Dysfunction,* Raven Press, New York.

III

Specific Symptoms

24

Increased Intracranial Pressure

Increased intracranial pressure is a life-threatening condition and almost always signals the presence of serious neurological disease. Rapid and efficient evaluation of any child presenting with signs or symptoms of intracranial hypertension is mandatory, and treatment must be prompt and effective.

The cranial vault is a closed cavity, and the compliance of the intracranial contents is low. Small changes in the volume of blood or cerebrospinal fluid (CSF), the presence of cerebral edema, or the development of a mass lesion all can rapidly produce large increases in pressure. Secondary effects, such as herniation of intracranial contents and impairment of cerebral vascular perfusion, will damage tissue, cause further swelling, and initiate a cycle that can quickly lead to death.

The bulk of CSF is produced by the choroid plexuses of the lateral, third, and fourth ventricles by an active metabolic process (Chapter 10). The rate of production is approximately 0.3 ml/min and is independent of intracranial pressure. This means that CSF production continues virtually unchanged, despite large increases in intracranial pressure. CSF flows from the lateral ventricles through the third and fourth ventricles. It exits into the cisterna magna through the midline foramen of Magendie and the paired lateral foramina of Luschka. The fluid then circulates through the basal cisterns and the subarachnoid spaces of the brain and spinal cord and is reabsorbed through the arachnoid villi of the superior sagittal sinus. This system has the capacity to absorb three to four times the normal rate of production of CSF and still maintain pressure at a steady state. If spinal fluid pathways are blocked, secondary routes of absorption through tears in the ependymal lining of the ventricles can provide some compensation and allow the pressure to stabilize.

Theoretically, increased pressure could result from excess CSF production, a block in CSF flow, or failure of absorption through the arachnoid granulations. The first mechanism is rarely involved but possibly occurs with choroid plexus papillomas. This would only produce increased intracranial pressure if the excess production exceeded the absorptive capacity. Failure of absorption basically represents a block in flow at the most distal site, and so most hydrocephalus can be simply thought of as being the result of a mechanical problem with CSF flow.

An increased intracranial vascular volume, as an isolated factor, rarely causes increased intracranial pressure. During states when pressure is elevated, however, increase in flow, such as produced by hypercapnea, can compound the problem. Reduction of blood flow, induced by hyperventilation, can be used therapeutically.

A mass lesion, such as a hematoma or neoplasm, causes an increase in pressure by two mechanisms. The first is by adding volume to a system of low compliance. In addition, there may be direct impingement on CSF pathways or distortion of brain with secondary impairment of CSF flow.

Cerebral edema can also be produced by several mechanisms. Vasogenic edema occurs when there is breakdown of the blood–brain barrier and entry of osmotically active substances and water into the extracellular space of the brain. This can be focal or diffuse.

Cytotoxic edema results from swelling of neurons or glia and is found following diffuse metabolic insults such as anoxia or hypoglycemia. An unusual form of edema occurs as blebs within myelin sheaths following poisoning with organic tin compounds and as a feature of Canavan spongy degeneration of the CNS. Edema and increased intracranial pressure can also be produced by impairment of cerebral venous drainage or major changes in serum osmolality.

There are two mechanisms by which increased intracranial pressure causes irreversible CNS damage or death. The first is by impairing cerebral vascular perfusion. As the intracranial pressure approaches or becomes higher than the mean arterial pressure, there will be inadequate cerebral blood flow. This produces ischemic damage, which then superimposes cytotoxic edema on the existing pathological process.

The second mechanism is that of herniation. Intracranial contents shift from areas of greater swelling to lesser, and toward the basal cisterns, posterior fossa, and foramen magnum. Herniation of the mesial temporal lobe (the uncus) through the tentorial notch, or herniation of the cerebellar tonsils through the foramen magnum, produces brain stem compression, hemorrhage into the brain stem, and death. Less common, but no less serious, are herniation of posterior fossa contents up through the tentorial notch or of the cingulate gyrus under the falx cerebri.

In the young infant, the dynamic relationships discussed are modified because of the open fontanelles and suture lines. Acutely increased pressure can still be lethal, but accommodation to less severe degrees can be made by progressive enlargement of the head. During the first few years of life, if the increase in pressure is not too great and the time course is prolonged, some compensation through head growth is still possible. This is rarely an effective mechanism after age 5 years.

APPROACH TO THE PATIENT

Increased intracranial pressure should be suspected in any patient who presents with the recent onset of severe headaches or a change in the frequency or pattern of previous headaches. Cephalgia that awakens the person at night or is present on arising in the morning is most commonly vascular (migrainous) in origin, but also can be a sign of intracranial hypertension. The same is true of headaches that are increased in intensity by a Valsalva maneuver, bending over, or sudden changes in position. Other important warning signs are progressive somnolence, transient episodes of loss of vision (visual obscurations), sudden vomiting without nausea, and changes in personality or cognitive abilities.

Examination of the infant should always include measurement of the head circumference and palpation of the fontanelle and suture lines. Dilated veins over the scalp also may be apparent. In the older child, papilledema, the classic sign of increased intracranial pressure, should be present if the problem has existed for at least several days (Figure 24-1). The earliest funduscopic sign is loss of the normal venous pulsations. This is followed by blurring and elevation of the optic disc and, as the pressure increases, hemorrhages into the retina. Even though this part of the examination is extremely important, it is almost always inadvisable to dilate the pupils in an attempt to visualize the fundus more clearly. This will mask the pupillary changes that are one of the earliest and most important signs of uncal herniation.

Extraocular movements must be carefully evaluated. Sixth-nerve palsies,

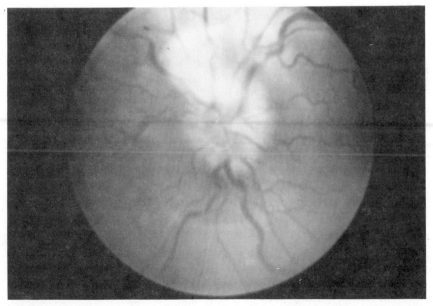

FIGURE 24-1. Papilledema. The optic disc is swollen and elevated, the disc margins are blurred, and the veins are engorged.

with inability of either eye to be moved laterally, are a common sign of increased intracranial pressure, although without localizing value. A third-nerve palsy, manifested either as pupillary dilatation or by the eye assuming a lateral and downward position with impaired medial movement, is a warning sign of uncal herniation and a call for immediate emergency management.

The presence of decorticate or decerebrate posturing also is a sign of impending herniation. The remainder of the neurological examination is directed toward defining the localization of the intracranial lesion.

CT scan of the head has had a major impact on the diagnosis and management of increased intracranial pressure. This is the preferred initial diagnostic procedure and should be performed on an emergency basis, both with and without the administration of a contrast agent. It will provide evidence for the existence of a mass lesion, obstruction of cerebrospinal fluid flow with hydrocephalus, or cerebral edema.

If, after the CT scan has been obtained, it appears that only cerebral edema is present, the evaluation must then pursue the most likely diagnostic possibilities based on the history of the illness. A major problem arises if intracranial infection is suspected but there is also unequivocal evidence of increased intracranial pressure. Lumbar puncture is associated with a risk of herniation, but is necessary in order to make a specific diagnosis and to identify the pathogen. It is sometimes appropriate to delay the procedure briefly while rapid reduction of pressure is attempted.

TREATMENT OF INCREASED INTRACRANIAL PRESSURE

There are three approaches to the treatment of increased intracranial pressure: surgical, physiological, and medical. A surgical approach is obviously required if a mass lesion or hydrocephalus is present. Many centers now use intracranial pressure monitoring for any patient with increased intracranial pressure and impaired consciousness.[1] The measurement can be intraventricular, subarachnoid, or subdural, but is useful only if the apparatus is properly placed, not occluded, and regularly calibrated. This technique is important as it allows continuous monitoring of intracranial pressure and comparison with simultaneously measured mean arterial pressure. It also allows detection of sustained high pressure accompanied by plateau waves and assists in the rational use of therapeutic agents.

Physiological approaches are an important part of management. The patient's head is elevated to decrease hydrostatic pressure and facilitate venous drainage. Maintenance of adequate ventilation is important, as hypercapnia increases cerebral blood flow and intracranial pressure. Fluid should be restricted to minimal maintenance levels but not to such an extreme that cardiac output and arterial perfusion pressure are impaired. Fever, which increases the metabolic needs of all tissues including those of the brain, should be treated with a cooling blanket if necessary.

Hyperventilation can be used to lower the P_{CO_2} to 20–22 mm Hg. This produces vasoconstriction of intracranial vessels and reduces cerebral blood flow. At this level of hypocarbia, the circulation will not be impaired to the extent that ischemia results. Lower levels may be hazardous if sustained.

The most useful medical therapy relies on osmotic agents.[2] Mannitol, as a 20% solution, has almost entirely replaced other substances such as urea, as there is less of a rebound of pressure when it is discontinued. This is given in small, repeated doses (0.25 mg/kg) when intracranial pressure is being monitored. A less satisfactory approach is using a large bolus of 1 mg/kg every 4 hr based only on the clinical assessment of the patient.

Dexamethasone, in doses of 0.1–0.25 mg/kg, is used almost routinely if increased intracranial pressure is present, although critical evidence of efficacy is, in most cases, lacking. It clearly is effective for edema surrounding brain tumors, but is probably not of major use in cerebral edema due to trauma or anoxia.

Paralyzing the patient with a nondepolarizing neuromuscular blocking agent prevents random movements, decerebrate posturing, and coughing, all of which can cause major spikes in intracranial pressure. The disadvantage of this procedure is that the value of repeated neurological examinations is lost, and a coma scale cannot be used to follow the patient's course.

Coma induced by short-acting barbiturates reduces the cerebral metabolic rate and may protect the brain during periods when cerebral blood flow is compromised. It may also reduce intracranial pressure directly, although the mechanism is not fully understood. This technique is under study, and is not currently part of routine clinical practice.[3]

Many other therapeutic modalities have been tried, although their usefulness is often limited and they are associated with major potential problems. Hypothermia is difficult to achieve and is associated with a rebound in pressure when it is discontinued. Limited surgical decompressions can lead to infarction of brain where it herniates through the bony defect. Large decompressions are often associated with major brain herniation (fungus cerebri) and hydrocephalus. As a last resort in the patient with trauma and necrosis of the temporal lobes, surgery with removal of damaged tissue, an internal decompression, is sometimes carried out. This can only be performed unilaterally or major permanent deficits in memory will occur. Removal of the anterior temporal lobe of the dominant hemisphere should be limited to avoid impairment of language function. Edematous brain will usually fill the space rapidly, however, making surgical closure difficult.

SPECIFIC DISORDERS

The most common causes of increased intracranial pressure in children are the same as those found in adults and include head trauma, asphyxia, vascular disorders, infections, and neoplasms. These are discussed in the appropriate

TABLE 24-1
Conditions Associated with Pseudotumor Cerebri

Physiological states	Oral contraceptives
Menarche	Tetracyclines
Obesity	Vitamin A overdose or deficiency
Pregnancy	Other conditions
Systemic diseases	Cerebral venous thrombosis
Adrenal insufficiency	Guillain–Barré syndrome
Cushing syndrome	Head trauma
Hypoparathyroidism	Infections
Polycythemia	Superior vena cava obstruction
Systemic lupus erythematosus	
Toxic states	
Corticosteroid administration or withdrawal	

chapters. Two conditions that are difficult to classify and are most common in the pediatric age group are Reye syndrome (discussed in Chapter 13) and pseudotumor cerebri.

Pseudotumor cerebri is a term used to refer to chronically increased intracranial pressure resulting from cerebral edema and unassociated with either focal neurological signs or impairment in the state of consciousness. The presenting complaint is headache, and neurological examination reveals papilledema and little else. Abducens palsies are sometimes found, but have no specific localizing value. CT of the head is normal or shows some evidence of white-matter edema and a small ventricular system.

A large number of associated conditions have been reported (Table 24-1), making a single pathophysiological mechanism unlikely.[4] The diagnostic approach is guided by the history and evidence on examination of other signs of systemic illness.

Although pseudotumor cerebri has also been referred to by the term "benign increased intracranial pressure," it can lead to optic atrophy and irreversible visual loss. One of the most important warning signs is the occurrence of transient visual obscurations, but these are not always present. If the headaches are incapacitating or visual field examination shows progressive enlargement of the blind spot, a sign that visual loss is imminent, treatment should be considered. Dexamethasone in therapeutic doses is used, but this is associated with the usual risks of long-term administration of corticosteroids. Oral glycerol, 1 mg/kg orally every 6–8 hr, will often be effective. This probably acts as an osmotically active agent, although direct metabolic effects have been postulated. A major problem with glycerol is its high caloric content. This may contribute to obesity, which, in itself, has been associated with pseudotumor cerebri.

REFERENCES

1. Mickell, J. J., Reigel, D. H., Cook, D. R., Binda, R. E., and Safer, P., 1977, Intracranial pressure: Monitoring and normalization therapy in children, *Pediatrics* **59**:606–613.

2. McDonald, J. T., and Uden, D. L., 1982, Intravenous glycerol and mannitol therapy in children with intracranial hypertension, *Neurology* **32:**437–440.
3. Miller, J. D., 1979, Barbiturates and raised intracranial pressure, *Ann. Neurol.* **6:**189–193.
4. Weisberg, L. A., and Chutorian, A. M., 1977, Pseudotumor cerebri of childhood, *Am. J. Dis. Child.* **131:**1243–1248.

ADDITIONAL READING

Batzdorf, U., 1976, The management of cerebral edema in pediatric practice, *Pediatrics* **58:**78–87.
Goldstein, G. W., 1979, Pathogenesis of brain edema and hemorrhage: Role of the brain capillary, *Pediatrics* **64:**357–360.

25

Ataxia

Ataxia refers to the inability to carry out age-appropriate voluntary skilled movements because of lack of coordination. In the clinical setting, this term implies that the pathophysiological process involves the cerebellum or cerebellar connections in the brain stem. Assumptions concerning the portion of the cerebellar system involved can be made from specific abnormalities on examination.

Stabilization of the head and trunk involves the midline cerebellar vermis. Dysfunction of this region produces titubation, a tremulousness of the head and trunk when the patient is sitting; this disappears in the recumbent position. Gait is abnormal with a wide base, staggering, and frequent falls. Young children do not always compensate with widening of the base, and the increased number of falls may be the major clue. With pathology isolated to the vermis, there is no ataxia or intention tremor of the limbs. Speech is impaired; there is a scanning quality with slowing and loss of normal rhythm. Nystagmus, especially on vertical gaze, is almost always present.

Each cerebellar hemisphere controls coordination of the ipsilateral limbs. The hallmark of pathological involvement is intention tremor. Horizontal nystagmus, most pronounced on looking to the side of the lesion, is frequently present. Factors determining whether or not gait is involved depend on the severity of the limb ataxia, whether or not there is distortion of the brain stem by a mass, and direct involvement of the vermis.

Lesions affecting primarily the brain stem are associated with cerebellar signs. Connections to and from the cerebellum pass through this structure, and the pontine nuclei, superior olive, and red nucleus are part of this system. Involvement of the vestibular nuclei and their connections also cause abnormalities in coordination and gait and produce severe nystagmus. Vertigo and nausea are typical of acute lesions of the vestibular system.

APPROACH TO THE PATIENT

The first task when evaluating the child with incoordination is to verify that the problem is ataxia. Generalized weakness can produce a staggering gait, instability of the head and trunk when sitting, and what can be mistaken for an intention tremor. Weakness is documented by demonstrating abnormalities on manual or functional muscle testing. There is one important caution, however. The child with severe cerebellar involvement may appear to be weak and hypotonic.

Sensory abnormalities, especially involving joint position sense, also produce incoordination. A useful diagnostic clue for proprioceptive abnormalities is that performance is better if the child is allowed to watch the affected limb during performance of the test, and skills deteriorate with the eyes closed. With cerebellar lesions, performance is equally poor with and without visual guidance.

Involuntary movements such as chorea, tics, and myoclonus can interject themselves into attempts at skilled movements and simulate ataxia. These movements, except for intention myoclonus, are usually also present at rest, however. The interrelationships between ataxia and myoclonus are complex, as a number of disorders produce both.

Ataxia, especially of gait, is occasionally seen in the presence of hydrocephalus or lesions involving the frontal lobes. This is due to compression or stretching of fibers belonging to the circuit loop beginning and ending in the frontal regions and involving the cerebellar and brain stem nuclei as well as the cerebellar cortex.

Differentiation of vestibular and cerebellar lesions is often difficult, and if the brain stem is the primary site of the pathological process, both systems are often involved. Vestibular lesions should be strongly suspected in the presence of spontaneous or positional vertigo, a tendency to always fall to one side, nystagmus out of proportion to the degree of ataxia, or severe incoordination without involvement of speech.

The examination of the ataxic patient will help define the structures involved, using the principles outlined earlier. One of the most important issues is differentiating pure cerebellar disease from conditions involving the brain stem or supratentorial structures.

A most useful tool in the differential diagnosis of disorders causing ataxia is the history. Specific diseases are suggested if the pattern can be defined as congenital, of acute onset, intermittent, or progressive. Table 25-1 lists some of the more important causes found in children.

CONGENITAL ATAXIA

The diagnosis of *ataxic cerebral palsy* should always be viewed with suspicion, as a number of anatomical and biochemical abnormalities are associated with ataxia that is present from early infancy. Less than 10% of motor disorders due to static perinatal encephalopathies present with ataxia as the most prominent sign. Computerized tomography often reveals agenesis or dysgenesis of the cerebellum, Arnold–Chiari malformation, or a Dandy–Walker malformation. Degenerative disorders, such as metachromatic leukodystrophy, may begin so

TABLE 25-1
Causes of Ataxia

Congenital ataxia	Hyperammonemia
Ataxic cerebral palsy	Hartnup disease
Cerebellar dysgenesis	Maple syrup urine disease
Arnold–Chiari malformation	Progressive ataxia
Dandy-Walker malformation	Brain tumor
Ataxia of sudden onset	Spinocerebellar degeneration
Acute cerebellar ataxia	Ataxia–telangiectasia
Infantile polymyoclonus	Abetalipoproteinemia
Toxins	Neuronal ceroid lipofuscinosis
Trauma	Metachromatic leukodystrophy
Arteriovenous malformation	Refsum disease
Meningitis	Subacute necrotizing encephalomyelitis
Encephalitis	Ramsay Hunt syndrome
Intermittent ataxia	
Basilar artery migraine	

early in life that the ataxia appears to be congenital. Other clinical signs and the progressive nature of the disorder soon become apparent.

ATAXIA OF SUDDEN ONSET

Acute cerebellar ataxia is the most common syndrome presenting with severe ataxia of sudden onset in childhood. A young child, previously well, has a minor viral illness. Two to three weeks later there is the sudden onset of severe ataxia. This always involves trunk and gait to a marked degree and frequently also produces limb ataxia. Nystagmus is present, as is cerebellar speech. Cerebrospinal fluid is normal, or a lymphocytic pleocytosis may be present. Recovery is generally rapid but may take several months. It is usually complete, although some children are left with permanent cerebellar dysfunction. A number of different viral agents, including mumps, varicella, and Epstein–Barr virus, have been associated with this condition.

Toxins must always be considered as a cause of the acute onset of ataxia in a child. Any CNS depressant can cause these findings. Ethanol, sedatives, tranquilizers, and anticonvulsants are the most common. Progressive obtundation is an important diagnostic clue.

Infantile polymyoclonus illustrates the complex relationships between ataxia and myoclonus and highlights the diagnostic difficulties. In this condition a young child develops the acute onset of what appears to be ataxia associated with multiple, continuous myoclonic jerks of the limbs and trunk. Opsoclonus, chaotic, large-amplitude, conjugate eye movements, is frequently present. The child often undergoes a personality change with marked irritability. Some cases are associated with neuroblastoma, most commonly in the chest. Removal of the tumor leads to resolution of the symptoms, and recurrence of the neoplasm is heralded by a return of the clinical signs. There are many other etiologies, including viral illnesses, and most cases are not associated with neuroblastoma. Treatment with corticosteroids or ACTH is effective,[1] although many of the children are left with learning disabilities and abnormalities in coordination.

Arteriovenous malformations of the cerebellum or brain stem can present with ataxia. Acute hemorrhage into these structures is a life-threatening event. The diagnosis of *trauma* can be made from the history and the presence of soft tissue signs.

INTERMITTENT ATAXIA

Conditions causing intermittent ataxia normally are only considered when a second attack has occurred. They should be suspected, however, if a specific diagnosis cannot be made during the initial episode. This will allow early definition of the underlying problem. *Basilar artery migraine* in the young child frequently presents with ataxia but without severe headache, although as the child grows, headache becomes more prominent.[2] During adolescence, the neurological signs tend to be lost, and a more typical pattern of migraine supervenes. The diagnosis should be suspected when there is the acute onset of ataxia, often associated with other signs of brain stem involvement, which rapidly clears and leaves the child with no residua. Commonly associated features are visual abnormalities, extraocular palsies, and alternating hemipareses.

Metabolic disorders associated with intermittent ataxia include Hartnup disease, a form of maple syrup urine disease, and a number of variants of hyperammonemia. Evaluation of the child should include blood ammonia determinations and urinary and serum amino acid studies obtained during the attacks. If no cause for the ataxia can be found, repeated ingestions of *CNS depressants* should be considered. In older children, this can result from substance abuse, and in younger children, accidental ingestion or administration by a caretaker is possible.

PROGRESSIVE ATAXIA

The most common cause of progressive ataxia in childhood is a *brain tumor*. Ataxia is frequently the first symptom, as the majority of CNS neoplasms in children involve the cerebellum and brain stem. Early diagnosis is important because of the danger of complications resulting from increased intracranial pressure. In addition, some tumors, such as medulloblastoma, can seed the subarachnoid space. Although there is no proof that early diagnosis and treatment will prevent this, delay is certainly unwarranted.

Friedreich ataxia is the most common spinocerebellar degeneration occurring in childhood. It typically presents in adolescence, but early signs may be present in the school years. Progressive gait ataxia is followed by involvement of the head and trunk, limbs, and speech. Muscle weakness is present, as is the unusual combination of areflexia and bilateral Babinski signs. Position sense loss is espccially marked in the legs. Other associated features include retinitis pigmentosa, oculomotor palsies, and sensorineural deafness. Cardiomyopathy occurs and is often the cause of death.

Skeletal deformities, especially pes cavus and kyphoscoliosis, are almost always present and are frequently found in family members who have no evidence of clinical involvement of the CNS. There appear to be different genetic patterns in individual families, and classic cases are transmitted by both autosomal dominant and recessive modes. There are no specific laboratory aids to diagnosis, although a good deal of current research is directed toward defining abnormalities of the pyruvate dehydrogenase enzyme complex.

Other *spinocerebellar degenerations* should be considered when progressive ataxia is associated with abnormalities of any other major neurological system. These include optic atrophy or retinal degeneration, sensorineural deafness, oculomotor palsies, neuropathy or myopathy, and spinal cord dysfunction. In many cases, the disorder appears to be unique to a particular family and only fits the description of similar conditions approximately.

Ataxia–telangiectasia presents in the preschool years with progressive ataxia involving the axial musculature initially and then the limbs and speech.[3] Choreoathetoid movements develop at about the same time and are also progressive. Oculomotor apraxia is present. Bulbar telangiectasiae are a striking feature of this condition and can appear at any age. Telangiectasiae develop in other areas, including the eyelids, face, arms, and legs.

Thymic abnormalities are associated with deficient cellular immunity. In addition, there are decreased levels of IgA and IgE and may be increased levels of IgG and IgM. Recurrent infections are frequent and need vigorous and intensive treatment. No other specific tests or therapeutic modalities are available. The disease is transmitted as an autosomal recessive condition.

A number of *metabolic disorders* must be considered in any child with progressive ataxia. These include abetalipoproteinemia, ceroid lipofuscinosis, neuronal storage disorders with definable lysosomal enzyme abnormalities, metachromatic leukodystrophy, and Refsum disease. These are rather rare conditions and are all associated with other evidence of degeneration of the CNS. This will become apparent as the patient is followed.

Subacute necrotizing encephalomyelopathy (Chapter 16) occasionally presents with acute or intermittent ataxia. As with the other metabolic disorders, the course aids definition of the correct diagnosis.

REFERENCES

1. Tal, Y., Jaffe, M., Sharf, B., and Amir, N., 1983, Steroid-dependent state in a child with opsoclonus, *J. Pediatr.* **103**:420–421.
2. Lapkin, M. L., and Golden, G. S., 1978, Basilar artery migraine, *Am. J. Dis. Child.* **132**:278–281.
3. Teplitz, R. L., 1978, Ataxia telangiectasia, *Arch. Neurol.* **35**:553–554.

26

Headache

Headache is one of the most common neurological complaints of childhood. Only seizures and problems with behavior and learning are referred more frequently to the pediatric neurologist. This symptom always raises the specter of serious, and perhaps life-threatening, neurological disease. An understanding of the mechanisms of cephalalgia, and a thorough history and neurological examination, allow the physician to quickly clarify the issues and prescribe appropriate therapy.

Pain in the head and face can emanate from every intracranial and extracranial structure with the exception of the brain itself. Infections of the scalp or destructive lesions of the skull, such as osteomyelitis and eosinophilic granuloma, produce localized pain and tenderness over the affected area. The paranasal sinuses and mastoids, if infected, also cause localized pain and are tender to percussion. Signs of infection, such as swelling and erythema, and systemic signs, such as fever, are present. In the case of infection or a mass within the orbit, exophthalmos and limitation of extraocular movement are typically present.

Pain from intracranial sources derives mainly from pressure or traction on the dura, its reflections, and the large arteries and veins. Intracranial inflammatory processes also affect the same structures.

The pain of vascular (migraine) headaches appears to originate from involvement of the arteries of the scalp.[1] Vascular headaches have three phases. Vasoconstriction occurs initially and is not associated with symptoms unless intracranial vessels are involved, in which case an aura can be produced. This mechanism is also an important factor in the production of the neurological signs that are a part of complicated migraine. Vasodilation, predominantly of extracranial vessels, produces the headache with its pulsatile characteristics. Vasoactive substances are then released, producing the third phase of inflammation, edema, and tenderness. At this stage, the process can no longer be reversed by medication but can only be treated symptomatically with analgesics.

The pathogenetic factors that initiate this chain of events are not completely known. The initial vasoconstriction may be triggered by the autonomic nervous system, although this does not explain the localized nature of the headache. At the same time, there is an outpouring of serotonin from platelets, a marked rise in serum serotonin, and increased platelet aggregability. Later in the headache, there is a great increase in urinary 5-HIAA. Local anoxia and acidosis in the region of the involved arteries are associated with an uptake in serotonin and release of vasoactive substances, which produce vasodilation, pain, and tenderness.

An alternate hypothesis, based on animal studies, implicates prostaglandin E_1. Intracarotid injection of this substance produces vasodilation and increased flow in external vessels and reduced intracranial flow due to a steal phenomenon.[2]

The mechanisms involved in muscle contraction headaches are less clear. Muscles of the scalp and neck enter a state of tonic contraction, which is not under the patient's voluntary control. There may be additional factors of vasoconstriction and local muscle ischemia, but the triggering events producing this are not known.

APPROACH TO THE PATIENT

Almost 35% of all children will have complained of headache by age 7 years.[3] Of these, 2.5% will have had repeated severe headaches, and 1.4% can be diagnosed as having migraine. By age 17 years, 54% of children have a history of headache. Fifteen percent of patients in this group have had severe headaches; 5.3%, migraine. Despite the common nature of this symptom, the complaint should always be taken seriously. The tendency to ascribe all headaches to life stresses should be resisted.

The most important diagnostic tool is the history. The key historical elements needed for formulating a differential diagnosis will be outlined in the following sections. Certain general points are important, however. Headaches that awaken the patient from sleep are almost always organic in nature and suggest migraine or increased intracranial pressure. In the latter case, the pain improves when the patient gets out of bed whereas migraine worsens with attempted activity. If the patient has had severe headaches for a substantial period of time, and no new signs or symptoms have developed, the condition is not likely to be due to serious organic disease.

A complete general physical examination will help eliminate systemic illness and disease localized to structures of the head and neck. The neurological examination is directed toward two major areas: ruling out increased intracranial pressure and searching for focal neurological signs. Papilledema is a reliable sign in any patient over 2 or 3 years of age. Younger children will have evidence of a bulging fontanelle or splitting of the sutures and excessively rapid head growth.

Neurodiagnostic studies are rarely required or useful. As headaches are quite common in childhood, it is impractical and extremely costly to order CT scans, skull x-ray studies, and electroencephalograms for every patient with this complaint. The most important indications for a full diagnostic evaluation are abnormal findings on neurological examination[4] or evidence of increased intracranial pressure. Historical features raising concern that a headache may be due to an intracranial lesion are the recent onset of severe cephalalgia, a major change in the pattern of the symptoms, and a progressive increase in severity. Neuroradiological studies are also appropriate if other signs of serious neurological disease, such as seizures, develop.

SYMPTOMATIC HEADACHES

One of the most frequent causes of headache in children is acute systemic illness, especially if associated with fever. Certain infections, such as influenza and rickettsial diseases, have headache as a regular component. If the headache persists, or if it is accompanied by somnolence or nuchal rigidity, a lumbar puncture is required to rule out intracranial infection. Other systemic disorders associated with headache include intoxications, hypertension, hypoxia, and carbon monoxide poisoning. Posttraumatic headaches can last for many months.

Disease of the paranasal sinuses and mastoids is not as common a cause of chronic headache in children as is generally believed. The history should be consistent with involvement of these structures, and examination should show localized tenderness. Purulent rhinitis or otitis media should also be present. If there are no clinical features of sinusitis or mastoiditis, and only minor roentgenographic findings are present, the diagnosis cannot be supported.

Ocular disorders also are not a common cause of chronic headaches, despite the frequent use of the diagnosis of eyestrain. Hyperopic children may have symptoms after reading for long periods of time, but myopes and children with strabismus will not have this difficulty.

MUSCLE CONTRACTION HEADACHES

Although stress appears to be related to many headaches, the term muscle contraction headaches is preferable to tension headaches, as it speaks to the pathophysiology. The typical headache comes on gradually as the day progresses, never awakens the patient from sleep, and is not present on awakening in the morning. It is diffuse, localized to the frontal or occipital regions, or most prominent at the vertex. The quality of the pain is that of pressure or a tight band, and it is rarely lancinating, burning, or pulsatile. There is no aura, associated neurological signs, or nausea and vomiting.

The general physical and neurological examinations should be normal, both during the attack and in the interictal period. With a typical history and normal examination, no laboratory tests or neurodiagnostic studies are necessary.

Treatment is based almost entirely on the use of simple analgesics. Aspirin, 20 mg/kg per dose every 4 hr, to a maximum of 625 mg/dose every 4 hr, is effective, but repeated doses should be used with caution in children under 2 years of age, patients with a history of ulcer disease, and those in whom gastric discomfort occurs. A different analgesic should be used in patients with influenza or varicella, because of concerns about Reye syndrome. Acetaminophen is equally useful in doses one and one-half those recommended for aspirin. Some patients require proprietary compounds containing salicylates or acetaminophen and a short-acting barbiturate. Stronger analgesics are never indicated, as headaches are often a lifelong problem, and the abuse potential of the other drugs is too great.

If the patient does not respond well and the diagnosis is not in question, but the symptoms are incapacitating, a brief trial of imipramine, 2.5 mg/kg per day, is sometimes useful, although this is not an approved indication for this drug in children. Many adults respond well to a course of amitriptyline, but this drug is also not approved for use in children under 12 years of age. Biofeedback and other relaxation techniques can be used for older children, but there are few controlled studies supporting their efficacy.

Counseling of the parents and child is an essential part of treatment. This should be a joint session so that each person has received the same information. It is important that the validity of the child's complaints be accepted and assurance given that the headaches are not due to serious neurological disease. Reasons for not obtaining sophisticated neurodiagnostic tests should be discussed. A permanent cure should not be promised, as headaches are, in most patients, a recurring condition throughout their life. Therapy is presented as a method of ameliorating symptoms, not providing a cure for an underlying condition. The family can be assured that there is a very high probability of a spontaneous remission at some point, and that this may last for a considerable period of time. Finally, the child should be encouraged to continue to function to the greatest extent possible, and procedures to minimize secondary gain should be instituted.

The role of psychological counseling in the treatment of headaches is not clear. An occasional patient is seen in whom the etiology of the complaints is clearly the life situation or family interactions. This obviously requires intervention. Behavioral treatment is also important when the family's response to the symptoms or the child's use of the symptoms is a major problem.

VASCULAR HEADACHES

The term vascular headaches refers to migraine and its variants. The major conditions seen in children are the following:

- Classic migraine
- Common migraine

- Complicated migraine
  - Hemiplegic
  - Basilar artery
  - Ophthalmoplegic
  - Acute confusional reaction
  - Alice-in-Wonderland syndrome

Classic migraine is not common in the preadolescent child, although it can occasionally be seen as early as 5 years of age. The major diagnostic features, not all of which are manifested by every patient, are

- Prodromal personality change
- Visual phenomena
- Pulsatile headache
- Nausea and vomiting
- Family history of migraine

The most common personality change is irritability, but other patients become hypomanic. This may be present for a day or more before the headache actually begins. The visual phenomena, if present, are highly variable and sometimes quite spectacular.[5] They include dark or scintillating scotomata, displays that rival the aurora borealis, and dense visual field deficits. This is followed by the subacute and then crescendo onset of pulsatile cephalalgia restricted to one side of the head and often including the eye. The patients have photophobia and phonophobia and take to their beds. Nausea and vomiting occur as the pain is increasing. Sleep provides some relief, although the patient has residual tenderness to palpation along the course of the superficial temporal arteries on the affected side.

Common migraine is the variant most frequently seen in prepubertal children. This shares many of the features of classic migraine, but lacks the visual phenomena and clearly unilateral distribution of the headache. A family history of migraine provides useful additional information and should be carefully sought. Migraine should be considered in any child with recurrent headaches and a family history of migraine.

Complicated migraine refers to the association of neurological signs and symptoms with the attack of headache. The best known is hemiplegic migraine.[6] During the prodromal or early phase of the headache, the child rapidly develops a dense hemiplegia, visual field defect, and, if the left hemisphere is involved, aphasia. The headache becomes increasingly severe, and the patient presents as if there had been a major intracranial hemorrhage with associated structural brain damage. Within a day or 2, the headache is gone and the neurological signs resolve.

A family history of hemiplegic migraine is sometimes obtained, and if this is present, a permanent neurological deficit is rare. Sporadic hemiplegic migraine occasionally leaves the patient with a completed stroke. If this occurs, full evaluation to search for underlying vascular disease is mandatory. The pro-phylactic use of propranalol decreases the frequency of attacks.

Basilar artery migraine presents with the signs and symptoms typically found in older patients with vertebrobasilar insufficiency. Vertigo, vague dizziness, and ataxia are the most frequent complaints.[7] These may be associated with ophthal-moplegia, alternating hemipareses, drop attacks, tinnitus, visual disturbances including blindness, and loss of consciousness. The episodes are highly stereo-typed but resolve spontaneously and do not leave the patient with a fixed deficit.

Younger children often present with the neurological signs but without prominent complaints of headache. Adolescents usually have severe headache localized to the occipital region. As the children grow older, the basilar artery symptoms disappear, and more typical migraine appears, although vertigo fre-quently remains part of the patient's symptom complex. A family history of migraine, especially on the maternal side, is commonly found.

If headache is associated with ophthalmoplegia as an isolated sign, the patient requires a full evaluation. Although this may be a migraine variant, *ophthalmoplegic migraine,* many of these patients actually have an aneurysm of the circle of Willis.

The child with an *acute confusional reaction* presents with headache and what appears to be a toxic delirium.[8] There is confusion, disorientation, lethargy, and irritability. Evaluation is directed toward ruling out intoxication, seizures, trauma, intracranial hemorrhage, and encephalitis. The presence of the severe headache, headaches between attacks of confusion, and a family history of migraine are useful diagnostic clues. An attack of acute confusional reaction may be precipitated by head trauma, adding further difficulty to the differential diagnosis.

The *Alice-in-Wonderland syndrome* occurs in the setting of a clear sensorium and causes the patient extreme anxiety. The children have perceptions of strange changes in the size and shape of their body or parts of their body, visual distortions, abnormalities in time sense, and, occasionally, hallucinations.[9] These may occur initially without prominent headache, although there are usually headaches between attacks. The differential diagnosis includes psychiatric dis-orders, intoxications, and seizures.

The initial treatment of migraine in children, especially common migraine, relies on the same analgesics used for muscle contraction headaches. They are surprisingly effective, especially in young children. As the child becomes older, and especially if an aura is present, ergotamine-containing compounds are use-ful. A number of compounds, often containing mixtures of ergotamine tartrate, a barbiturate, caffeine, and atropine alkaloids, are available. The physician should become familiar with one for oral administration and one that can be used by suppository. The patient must understand that there is a maximum number of pills that can be taken each week, and although they need to be taken early in an attack, they cannot be used for every minor headache.

Although ergotamine-containing drugs do not usually cause problems in patients with complicated migraine, there is fear that their vasoconstrictor properties will accentuate the symptoms. In these patients, children who do not obtain relief from other medications, and those who awaken at night with headaches, prophylactic medication can be used. Propranolol is begun at a level of 20–40 mg/day in divided doses and increased as needed. The maximum dose is equivalent to 160–240 mg/day in an adult, adjusted for the child's size.[10] A trial of 6–10 weeks is necessary to determine whether the medication is effective.

Many other drugs have been used to treat migraine. Methysergide is extremely effective prophylactically in adults, but is not recommended for children because of potentially severe side effects such as retroperitoneal fibrosis. Some patients respond to cyproheptadine, anticonvulsants, amitriptyline, imipramine, prostaglandin inhibitors, nonsteroidal antiinflammatory agents, and drugs that interfere with platelet aggregability. Experience with them in children is limited. Strong analgesics should rarely, if ever, be used. The same principles of counseling as outlined for muscle contraction headaches are important.

Cluster headaches are uncommon in children. Males are affected considerably more frequently than females. Attacks come in cycles with several brief episodes of excruciating pain each day for a number of weeks. Remission then occurs and can last months or years. The pain is extremely intense and initially localized to the eye on one side. It is steady in character. Tearing of the eye, a stuffy nose, and sweating occur on the affected side.

Treatment is similar to that of migraine, relying on ergotamine-containing drugs; simple analgesics are not effective. Refractory cases will respond to treatment with corticosteroids. Lithium carbonate also appears to be effective in protecting against attacks.

REFERENCES

1. Brown, J. K., 1977, Migraine and migraine equivalents in children, *Dev. Med. Child. Neurol.* **19**:683–695.
2. Welch, K. M. A., Spira, P. J., Knowles, L., and Lance, J. W., 1974, Effects of prostaglandins on the internal and external carotid blood flow in the monkey, *Neurology* **24**:705–710.
3. Bille, B., 1962, Migraine in school children, *Acta Paediatr.* **51**(Suppl. 136):1–151.
4. Larson, E. B., Omenn, G. S., and Lewis, H., 1980, Diagnostic evaluation of headache, *JAMA* **243**:359–362.
5. Hachinski, V. C., Porchawka, J., and Steele, J. C., 1973, Visual symptoms in the migraine syndrome, *Neurology* **23**:570–579.
6. Lai, C-W., Ziegler, D. K., Lansky, L. L., and Torres, F., 1982, Hemiplegic migraine in childhood: Diagnostic and therapeutic aspects, *J. Pediatr.* **101**:696–699.
7. Lapkin, M. L., and Golden, G. S., 1978, Basilar artery migraine, *Am. J. Dis. Child.* **132**:278–281.
8. Ehyai, A., and Fenichel, G., 1978, The natural history of acute confusional migraine, *Arch. Neurol.* **35**:368–369.
9. Golden, G. S., 1979, The Alice in Wonderland syndrome in juvenile migraine, *Pediatrics* **63**:517–519.
10. Rosen, J. A., 1983, Observations on the efficacy of propranalol for the prophylaxis of migraine, *Ann. Neurol.* **13**:92–93.

ADDITIONAL READING

Congdon, P. J., and Forsythe, W. I., 1979, Migraine in childhood: A study of 300 children, *Dev. Med. Child. Neurol.* **21:**209–216.

Golden, G. S., 1982, The child with headaches, *Dev. Behav. Pediatr.* **3:**114–117.

Lance, J. W., 1981, Headache, *Ann. Neurol.* **10:**1–10.

27

Coma

The child in coma represents an acute pediatric emergency. The physician is faced with the tasks of initiating emergency management, defining the cause of the alteration in consciousness, and instituting specific therapeutic procedures, all of which must be carried out simultaneously. Important entities associated with coma are discussed in other chapters. The focus here is on the initial diagnosis and management.

Consciousness is defined as the state of awareness of oneself and the environment and the ability to respond to internal and external stimuli.[1] Although the cerebral cortex is involved in processing stimuli and then organizing and effecting the patient's response, the brain stem ascending reticular activating system is responsible for maintaining alertness. Coma, in the strictest sense, always implies brain stem dysfunction. Extensive diffuse damage to the cortex will make it impossible for the patient to respond, however.

APPROACH TO THE PATIENT

When confronted with a child with a depressed state of consciousness, the following procedures must be rapidly carried out:

- Assessment of vital signs
- Evaluation of associated diseases or injuries
- Assessment of level of consciousness
- Neurological examination

The assessment of vital signs is no different than that mandated by any emergency situation. Airway, pulse, and blood pressure are tended to in that order, and corrective action is taken as necessary. Search for an underlying disease or ingestion of a toxin is aided by a rapid and directed history. A rapid, but complete physical examination, with special attention to thoracic and abdominal injuries and fractures of the long bones, is performed next. Any patient found comatose following trauma or under unknown circumstances should be assumed to have an associated spinal cord injury, and proper procedures used during transport. A small amount of extra care can prevent a tragic outcome.

At this point attention is turned to assessment of the level of consciousness. The term coma, in an absolute sense, refers to lack of any spontaneous actions on the part of the patient and lack of response to any external stimuli. It is best to avoid the use of other terms (e.g., lethargy, somnolence, stupor, light coma), which are subject to a good deal of individual definition. A structured, semiquantitative approach using a scoring method such as the Glasgow Coma Scale is much more reliable.[2]

This provides criteria that allow a score to be assigned. Scoring is simple and interrater reliability is good (Table 27-1). Changes in the score over time are used as an index of changes in the level of consciousness. There have been many clinical studies correlating the outcome of coma from various causes with the coma score.

There are problems with the use of the Glasgow Coma Scale in young children, especially in the area of assessing verbal responses. An analogous scale for use in infants and toddlers has been developed (Table 27-2).[3]

The neurological examination provides several types of information:

Level of central nervous system lesion
Structural or metabolic etiology
Presence of focal pathology

TABLE 27-1
Glasgow Coma Scale[a]

Response	Score
Eye opening	
Spontaneous	4
To speech	3
To pain	2
None	1
Verbal	
Oriented	5
Confused	4
Inappropriate words	3
Sounds	2
None	1
Motor	
Obeys commands	6
Localizes painful stimulus	5
Withdraws from pain	4
Flexion	3
Extension	2
None	1

[a]From Teasdale and Jennett.[2]

TABLE 27-2
Children's Coma Score[a]

Response	Score
Ocular	
Pursuit	4
EOM[b] intact, reactive pupils	3
EOM impaired or fixed pupils	2
EOM paralyzed, fixed pupils	1
Verbal	
Cries	3
Spontaneous respirations	2
Apneic	1
Motor	
Flexes and extends	4
Withdraws from painful stimuli	3
Hypertonic	2
Flaccid	1

[a]From Raimondi and Hirschauer.[3]
[b]EOM, extraocular muscles.

A structured approach to the neurological examination, based on a limited number of procedures, allows determination of the level of the lesion in the CNS. These are the respiratory pattern, pupil size and reactivity, ocular movements, and motor function.[1] This also provides a tool for following the patient's course. A summary of this schema is presented in Table 27-3.

This approach also provides an important clue to the presence of toxic or metabolic causes of the coma. These should be suspected whenever lower brain stem functions are abnormal but higher-level functions remain intact. A typical example is the maintenance of normal pupil size and reactivity in the face of apnea and absent caloric responses. These findings imply that the coma results from either a toxic etiology or, rarely, a discrete lesion of the medulla. A complete neurological examination determines whether or not there is any clear evidence of a focal lesion of the brain or of spinal cord involvement.

If the cause of the coma is unknown, blood should be taken for determination of glucose, electrolytes, blood urea nitrogen, calcium and phosphorus, ammonia, serum transaminase levels, and toxicological studies. This is easily accomplished when an intravenous needle is inserted as part of the emergency management. Glucose (1–2 ml/kg of a 50% solution) should then be infused as empirical treatment for hypoglycemia.

CT scan of the head, both with and without contrast enhancement, should be performed early in the evaluation of any patient with impaired consciousness due to head trauma or unknown causes. This assists in defining the etiology and can provide rapid assessment of the need for neurosurgical intervention. While the patient is in the radiology suite, anterior–posterior and lateral views of the cervical spine should be obtained. There are few indications for radionuclide

TABLE 27-3
Examination of the Unconscious Patient[a]

Transtentorial herniation	
Early diencephalic stage	
Respirations	Sighs and yawns or Cheyne–Stokes
Pupils	Small, symmetrical, react
Calorics	Full deviation
Motor	Removes noxious stimulus
	Bilateral Babinski signs
Late diencepalic stage	
Respirations	Cheyne–Stokes
Pupils	Small, symmetrical, react
Calorics	Full deviation
Motor	Decorticate posturing
Midbrain–upper pons stage	
Respirations	Regular hyperventilation
Pupils	Midposition, fixed, irregular
Calorics	Impaired, often dysconjugate
Motor	Decerebrate posturing
Lower pons–upper medulla stage	
Respirations	Shallow regular or ataxic
Pupils	Midposition, fixed
Calorics	No response
Motor	No response
Uncal herniation	
Early third-nerve stage	
Respirations	Eupneic
Pupils	Unilateral dilated, sluggish
Calorics	Present or dysconjugate
Motor	Removes noxious stimulus
Late third-nerve stage	
Respirations	Regular hyperventilation
Pupils	Unilateral dilated, unreactive
Calorics	Involved eye does not move
Motor	Decerebrate or decorticate

[a]Modified from Plum and Posner.[1]

brain scans, cerebral arteriography, and other neurodiagnostic procedures at this point.

The electroencephalogram (EEG) of the comatose patient is always abnormal. A normal record suggests that the patient is not really comatose but may be displaying psychogenic coma, although in the locked-in syndrome, the EEG also may appear virtually normal. Electrical status epilepticus can present with a depressed state of consciousness and a paucity of neurological signs. The EEG should be diagnostic. Focal lesions such as brain abscess, tumors, and hematomas are more accurately diagnosed by the CT scan.

Lumbar puncture has limited usefulness and is performed only if there is reason to suspect an infection of the CNS or a specific need to document the presence of subarachnoid blood. If signs of increased intracranial pressure are present, lumbar puncture must be approached with the greatest caution. The administration of a rapidly acting osmotic agent, such as mannitol, prior to the spinal tap and removal of the smallest amount of fluid required to provide the needed diagnostic information will lessen the risk of herniation, but not remove it entirely.

ETIOLOGY OF COMA

The major causes of coma in childhood are head trauma and intracranial infection. An unrecognized seizure should also be suspected, even if there is no prior history of a seizure disorder. Accidental ingestion of a medication or toxic substance is an important consideration in the toddler, as is use of illicit drugs and intoxicants in the older school-age child and adolescent.

Impaired consciousness also results from a number of progressive disorders of the CNS. The diagnostic pattern is one of gradual deterioration of the patient, rather than sudden onset of neurological signs. Neoplasms, slow virus infections, and degenerative diseases are the major considerations.

The possibility of systemic disease should be carefully evaluated. Reye syndrome is one of the most frequent causes of acute encephalopathy in childhood. Diseases impairing renal or hepatic function can present either acutely or subacutely. Unusual metabolic disorders should be considered if the child has had repeated episodes of coma or there is a family history of a metabolic disorder. These include abnormalities in ammonia and short-chain fatty acid metabolism, diabetes, and hypoglycemia.

Structural lesions, such as a brain tumor or an intracerebral hematoma due to an aneurysm of arteriovenous malformation, are usually associated with focal neurological signs on examination. Increased intracranial pressure is a frequent concomitant of these lesions.

PSYCHOGENIC COMA

This state is uncommon in children, but occurs more frequently in adolescents. The major feature is the appearance of coma with an otherwise normal neurological examination. Pupillary reactions and caloric responses are intact, respirations are normal, and there is no evidence of spasticity. Lack of response to painful stimuli is a less useful sign. If diagnostic uncertainty remains, an EEG that shows a normal awake record provides useful confirmatory evidence that the patient is not comatose.

PERSISTENT VEGETATIVE STATE

Following head trauma, anoxia, or other diffuse insults to the CNS, the patient may enter a state in which the eyes are open and wake–sleep cycles are present, but there is neither speech nor any other evidence of meaningful contact with other persons. There are varying degrees of spasticity, and other neurological findings are sometimes present. The patient is not dependent on life-support systems. Although this condition can occur transiently during recovery from coma, its persistence for longer than 3 months is an ominous sign.[4]

LOCKED-IN SYNDROME

Destruction of the base of the pons, most frequently due to thrombosis of the basilar artery, produces a state in which the patient is awake and alert but cannot speak and has spastic quadriplegia. The only means of communication is the establishment of a coded series of eye blinks. Wake–sleep cycles are present, and the EEG is reasonably normal.

IRREVERSIBLE COMA

Irreversible coma, or brain death, refers to a state in which the brain has been damaged to such an extent that there is permanent and irreversible loss of cerebral cortical and brain stem function. The major features are the following:

- No spontaneous movement or breathing
- No response, either voluntary or reflex, to external stimuli
- Absence of all brain stem reflexes
- Isoelectric EEG

The criteria are not valid if there is marked hypothermia or toxic levels of CNS depressant drugs. Most clinicians feel more secure in making the diagnosis if the same findings are present on a second examination 12–24 hr after the first. If there is some urgency in establishing the presence of irreversible coma (e.g., the need for organ transplantation), special procedures can document the absence of cerebral blood flow. These include carotid angiography and radionuclide brain scanning. The absence of blood flow through the intracranial vessels is definitive evidence of brain death.

Although the criteria for irreversible coma were initially established in adults, they appear to be valid for older children. They have not yet, however, been critically evaluated in large series of neonates and infants. Such techniques as Doppler ultrasonography can be used to demonstrate abnormalities in, and the loss of, intracerebral blood flow.[5]

REFERENCES

1. Plum, F., and Posner, J. B., 1980, *The Diagnosis of Stupor and Coma,* FA Davis, Philadelphia.
2. Teasdale, G., and Jennett, B., 1974, Assessment of coma and impaired consciousness: A practical scale, *Lancet* **2:**81–84.

3. Raimondi, A. J., and Hirschauer, J., 1984, Head injury in the infant and toddler: Coma scoring and outcome scale, *Child's Brain* **11:**12–35.
4. Gillies, J. D., and Seshia, S. S., 1980, Vegetative state following coma in childhood: Evolution and outcome, *Dev. Med. Child. Neurol.* **22:**642–648.
5. McMenamin, J. B., and Volpe, J. J., 1983, Doppler ultrasonography in the determination of neonatal brain death, *Ann. Neurol.* **14:**302–307.

ADDITIONAL READING

Johnston, R. B., and Mellits, E. D., 1980, Pediatric coma: Prognosis and outcome. *Dev. Med. Child. Neurol.* **22:**3–12.
Seshia, S. S., Seshia, M. M. K., and Sachdeva, R. K., 1977, Coma in childhood, *Dev. Med. Child. Neurol.* **19:**614–628.

IV

Neurological Complications

Neonatal Neurology

The major physiological task of the newborn infant is to successfully make the transition from the intrauterine to the extrauterine environment. During this period of time there are many pitfalls, including the occurrence of hypoxia and hypotension, both of which can damage the CNS, and trauma, which can affect the peripheral nervous system as well as the CNS. This chapter will concentrate on the consequences of these pathogenetic factors and certain metabolic disorders that derive from the neonate's immature homeostatic mechanisms.

The fetus, *in utero*, is obviously dependent on transplacental transport for continuous supplies of oxygen and glucose, and for removal of metabolic products. Little blood circulates through the lungs; right ventricular output is shunted through the ductus arteriosus to the descending aorta. Left ventricular output supplies the upper portion of the body, including the brain. The fetus is exposed to a relatively low P_{O_2}, although metabolism is still mainly aerobic.

During the course of labor, and in the immediate postnatal period, the integrity of the fetus depends on the following:

- Maintenance of placental circulation
- Maintenance of fetal circulation
- Continuous supply of oxygen
- Continuous supply of glucose
- Transition to neonatal circulation
- Expansion of lungs
- Development of sustained respirations
- Closure of the ductus arteriosus

A failure at any point in this chain of events puts the child's brain at great risk.

Neonatal neurology has become increasingly important as there have been major improvements in the critical care of the newborn infant. Children who would have died only a few years ago now survive, and many do well. Others are seriously impaired neurologically. A cost–benefit analysis is nearly impossible, as techniques of care change more rapidly than follow-up data can be obtained. Ethical issues also become involved, and now the courts and the federal government are taking an active interest in the problems of the seriously ill neonate.

APPROACH TO THE PATIENT

The health and physiological status of the fetus can be measured in a number of ways. Ultrasonography provides an accurate estimate of fetal size and can demonstrate major anomalies such as anencephaly, myelomeningocele, and hydrocephalus. Chromosomal abnormalities can be defined using fetal cells obtained by amniocentesis or chorionic villus biopsy. Assay of α-fetoprotein in the amniotic fluid assists in the diagnosis of the 80–85% of neural tube defects that are not skin-covered. Newer techniques, such as fetal blood sampling and fetal skin biopsy, are opening the way for the intrauterine diagnosis of a large number of metabolic and genetic diseases.

An assessment of the maturity of the fetus is important if elective cesarean section or induction of labor is planned, or if a decision needs to be made concerning the advisability of attempts to stop premature labor. Premature birth, respiratory distress, and subependymal and intraventricular hemorrhage are closely correlated. In addition to a determination of fetal size with ultrasonography, maturation of the lungs can be determined by measuring the ratio of lecithin to sphingomyelin in the amniotic fluid. A ratio of 2:1 or more is found at 35 weeks of gestation and predicts a decreased risk of respiratory distress syndrome.

There are a number of methods of monitoring of the fetus's status that can be used during the course of labor. These detect abnormalities that indicate that the fetus may be in physiological difficulty. Although the correlation of these findings with neurological damage is not absolute, they are a warning that the child must be followed closely.

The passage of meconium into the amniotic fluid has long been recognized as a sign of fetal distress and is associated with increased perinatal mortality. Meconium aspiration adds another set of problems, as it interferes with proper expansion of the lungs and impairs respiration.

Monitoring of the fetal heart rate is another method of obtaining a warning of fetal distress. Early (type I) decelerations of the heart rate begin with the onset of uterine contractions; the heart rate returns to its baseline value as the contraction stops. These are not associated with fetal distress. Late (type II) decelerations are delayed beyond the onset of uterine contractions and continue after the contraction is finished. Type II decelerations are a sign of perinatal asphyxia.

The most direct evidence for an impaired physiological status of the fetus can be obtained through fetal blood monitoring. The specimen is taken from the scalp. Values suggesting asphyxia are a pH of 7.20 or less, or a base deficit greater than 10 meq/liter.

Postnatally, the child's status can be monitored with periodic neurological examinations. This is discussed in Chapters 3 and 4.

HYPOXIC–ISCHEMIC ENCEPHALOPATHY

Hypoxia refers to a decreased content of oxygen in the blood; ischemia is reduced blood flow. These can occur separately, but in most cases of perinatal asphyxia, there is some component of each. The brain tolerates hypoxia longer than ischemia. As long as the circulation remains intact, some oxygen can be extracted even though the content is greatly diminished, and the products of anaerobic metabolism, carbon dioxide and lactic acid, are removed.

The most important pathological change following an episode of perinatal asphyxia is neuronal injury. This involves all regions of the brain, although some areas appear to be more sensitive than others. Especially at risk are the cerebral cortex, hippocampus, inferior colliculus, and cerebellum. Involvement of the basal ganglia produces status marmoratus, a marbled appearance resulting from neuronal loss with gliosis and areas of hypermyelination. There may also be necrosis of large areas of brain. The outcome can range from a single porencephalic cyst to hydranencephaly.[1]

Attempts have been made to use clinical signs to assess the degree of asphyxia.[2] There are three stages, each indicating a progressively greater degree of damage. These are the following:

- Stage I: Hyperalertness, hyperreflexia, dilated pupils, and tachycardia
- Stage II: Lethargy, hyperreflexia, miosis, bradycardia, seizures, hypotonia, weak suck, weak Moro reflex
- Stage III: Stupor, flaccidity, small to midposition pupils that react slowly, hyporeflexia, hypothermia, absent suck, absent Moro reflex

These stages correlate fairly well with the risk of death or a poor neurological outcome.[3]

Children with severe encephalopathy show changing signs as they are followed in the nursery.[1] The most typical progression is as follows:

- Birth to 12 hr: Stupor, periodic respirations, normal pupillary and oculomotor responses, hypotonia, seizures
- 12–24 hr: Apparent increase in alertness, seizures, apnea, tremulousness, weakness
- 24–72 hr: Stupor, respiratory arrest, oculomotor abnormalities, deterioration

- After 72 hr: Improving level of consciousness, hypotonia, weakness. Abnormalities in sucking, swallowing, tongue movements, and the gag reflex are also present.

There have been many attempts to find features of the history, neurological examination, and laboratory evaluation that correlate with the long-term outcome. Most obstetrical antepartum and intrapartum variables have little predictive value. A more severe stage of encephalopathy and the presence of intractable seizures appear to be associated with neurological damage.[3-5]

The CT scan is quite useful in formulating a prognosis for the full-term infant.[6] A group of 62 patients with hypoxic–ischemic encephalopathy were followed to at least 18 months of age. Serious motor or intellectual handicaps were found in 11 of the 15 children with intraventricular or parenchymal hemorrhage documented by CT scan. Eighteen of twenty infants with large areas of hypodensity in gray and white matter were abnormal on follow-up evaluation.

The CT scan is less useful in identifying ischemic lesions in the brain of the asphyxiated premature infant with a birth weight of less than 1500 g.[7] A correlation between intraventricular hemorrhage and hydrocephalus was present, but no feature of the scan was predictive of the child's neurological status at age 18 months. Only 4 of 56 scans were normal, despite the fact that 60% of the children were normal and an additional 16% had only slightly depressed scores on the Bayley scales. The most common finding was dilation of the ventricles and widening of the subarachnoid space.

The principles of acute management are simple, although implementation can be quite complex. Metabolic derangements are corrected and homeostasis is supported. Attention must be paid to assuring adequate oxygen and glucose supplies, maintaining systemic blood pressure and vascular perfusion of the brain, and promoting the removal of excess lactic acid and carbon dioxide. Seizures are treated with phenobarbital; an initial loading dose of 20 mg/kg is given, and then a maintenance dose of 5–7 mg/kg per day as needed, with close monitoring of serum anticonvulsant levels. There is little or no firm evidence that administration of corticosteroids, methods used to control cerebral edema in older patients, or barbiturate-induced coma are useful.

The prognosis following hypoxic–ischemic encephalopathy, as noted, depends on the severity of the insult and the localization of the damage. The most serious outcome is spastic quadriparesis with severe mental retardation and seizures. The child typically is hypotonic through the first 3–9 months of life and then shows gradually increasing spasticity. Early warning signs include a tendency to hold the head retroflexed and the assumption of an opisthotonic posture when agitated. Pathological reflexes, such as an obligatory tonic neck reflex, are found on examination. There are feeding difficulties due to depressed or uncoordinated sucking, tongue protrusion with any stimulus about the mouth, and inadequate swallowing. These are a result of pseudobulbar paralysis.

Mental retardation, in severely involved children, is at the severe or profound level. These children are usually nonambulatory and remain completely dependent. Defects in vision and hearing are a result of diffuse cortical destruction or damage to the end organs. Seizures are difficult to control. Many of the children have a mixed pattern of seizures and an EEG that evolves into the slow spike-and-wave pattern characteristic of the Lennox–Gastaut syndrome.

Long-term management is also complex. Traditional approaches are used for the therapy of the neuromuscular problem and the seizure disorder. These children also are subject to repeated serious respiratory infections because of gastroesophageal reflux and aspiration of food. Other problems include decubitus ulcers, poor bone mineralization with fractures, joint dislocations, urinary tract infections, and fecal impactions. The use of anticonvulsants, particularly phenytoin, in this group of children has been associated with rickets. This can be treated with vitamin D supplementation.

Parental counseling is most important, as severely handicapped children are a source of chronic family stress. At some point, many families are willing to consider alternate living arrangements for the severely handicapped child. These include foster home placement, community-based facilities, or institutional settings. The periods of transition during which placement is generally considered are when the prognosis first becomes certain, at school entry, at the onset of adolescence, and when the patient becomes an adult. This option also must be reevaluated any time the child's problems result in major disruption within the family and when the parents reach the age when they are no longer physically able to provide care.

SUBEPENDYMAL–INTRAVENTRICULAR HEMORRHAGE

This entity, as noted in Chapter 15, is primarily seen in the premature infant, and its frequency of occurrence is inversely related to the child's birth weight. The traditional teaching has always been that intraventricular hemorrhage is associated with the respiratory distress syndrome and presents with catastrophic deterioration in the child's clinical course and an almost invariably fatal outcome. The increased availability of CT scans and ultrasonography has revealed, however, that the incidence of this lesion is much higher than originally thought, and that survival is possible (Figure 28-1). Now, with the routine use of ultrasonography in many nurseries, it is clear that some degree of intracranial bleeding is extremely common in the small premature infant, and that clinical signs are often minimal.

The incidence of hemorrhage is 31% in children with a gestational age of 34 weeks or less; it is 48% in the group with gestational age of 29 weeks or less. All of the hemorrhages occur in the first 72 hr of life, with at least 25% found to be present at 6 hr.[8]

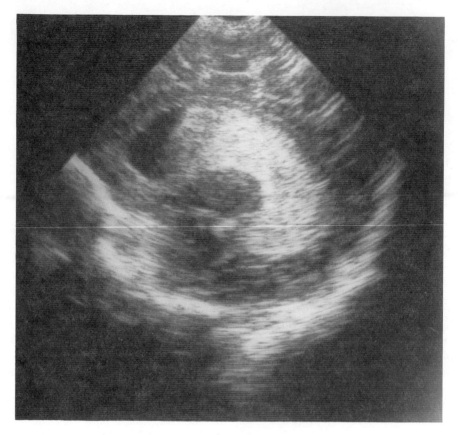

FIGURE 28-1. Sagittal sonogram demonstrating a large intraventricular hemorrhage in a premature infant.

Two different clinical syndromes have been identified.[1] The catastrophic syndrome is the pattern traditionally associated with this entity. The major characteristics are

- Rapid evolution
- Stupor progressing to coma
- Respiratory disturbance progressing to apnea
- Generalized tonic seizures
- Decerebrate (extensor) posturing
- Pupils unreactive to light
- No response to vestibular stimulation
- Flaccid quadriparesis
- Increased intracranial pressure
- Falling hematocrit
- Hypotension, bradycardia, acidosis

The saltatory syndrome has only been recognized in recent years.[1] The features are often overlooked; subependymal or intraventricular hemorrhage should be considered whenever there is any change in the infant's course. The typical manifestations of the saltatory syndrome are

- Stuttering evolution over hours or days
- Stupor and altered motility
- Hypotonia
- Abnormal eye position or movements
- Respiratory disturbances
- Falling hematocrit

A less common lesion is an intracerebellar hematoma. This occurs most commonly in children under 32 weeks of gestation. Because of the rapidly fatal outcome, a clearly defined clinical syndrome has not yet emerged. Flaccid quadriparesis, abnormalities of eye position and movement, and episodes of tonic extension of the limbs have been reported. Cerebellar hematomas can be visualized with ultrasonography.[9]

CT scans and ultrasonography now allow the hemorrhages to be classified by their location and extent. This is important, as the survival rate and severity of residua correlate with these features. The basic schema is as follows:[10]

- Grade I: Hemorrhage confined to the subependymal germinal layer
- Grade II: Intraventricular hemorrhage without ventricular dilation
- Grade III: Intraventricular hemorrhage with ventricular dilation
- Grade IV: Intraventricular hemorrhage with extension into the parenchyma of the brain

The abnormalities found on long-term follow-up are the result of either parenchymal damage or ventricular dilation. Injury to the brain may be diffuse, in which case it is probably due to hypoxic–ischemic encephalopathy coexisting with the hemorrhage. The neurological deficits are the same as for any child with asphyxia and include spastic quadriparesis, mental retardation, and seizures.

In other patients, brain destruction is largely restricted to the subependymal white matter. The descending (corticospinal) tracts originating in the motor cortex are organized so that the fibers subserving leg function are closest to the lateral ventricles. These suffer the brunt of the damage, and the resultant deficit is spastic diplegia. Intelligence is generally well preserved, and seizures are uncommon.

The grade of hemorrhage[11] and presence of ventriculomegaly[12] are the most powerful predictors of neurological outcome. Birth weight and grade of hemorrhage both correlate with the need for special education. These factors and paternal social class are related to overall intellectual performance.[13]

The presence and severity of progressive ventricular dilation also correlate well with the grade of hemorrhage. This often occurs without the usual clinical signs of increased intracranial pressure and without excessive increase in head circumference. It is clear that some of these patients have hydrocephalus, with obstruction at the level of the aqueduct of Sylvius or the subarachnoid space. In other patients, however, the ventricular enlargement is secondary to loss of brain parenchyma.

Uncertainty about the underlying pathophysiology in any specific case makes the evaluation of treatment methods difficult and prognostic statements hazardous. Nonsurgical methods such as repeated lumbar puncture, administration of osmotic agents, and drugs that decrease CSF production have been tried. Many children will eventually require placement of a ventriculoperitoneal shunt.

A systematic approach to management has been developed.[1] This relies on information obtained from serial ultrasonography or CT scans. If ventricular dilation is not progressive, therapy is not required. With a slow increase in ventricular size, nonsurgical methods are tried. If they fail, a ventriculostomy is temporarily placed, and if there is continued progression after 5–7 days of drainage, a shunt is performed. With stabilization of the situation at any point in the treatment program, no further procedures are carried out.

In the case of a rapidly progressive increase in ventricular size, a ventriculostomy is used as the first approach, and this is followed by shunting if dilation continues.

Factors that predict sustained benefit from repeated lumbar punctures include the demonstration of communication between the lateral ventricles and lumbar subarachnoid space by documenting decreased ventricular size and decreased ventricular pressure when cerebrospinal fluid is removed. The second predictive factor is the ability to remove relatively large volumes of cerebrospinal fluid with each procedure.[14]

Supratentorial intracerebral hemorrhage in the full-term neonate is most commonly associated with hypoxic–ischemic injury.[15] Contributory factors include polycythemia and birth trauma, although no precipitating cause can be found in approximately one-half of patients. The majority of children in whom a cause was found will be left with moderate to severe neurological handicaps. Normal development was most common in the group with no definable etiology.

PERINATAL TRAUMA

Head trauma in the neonate can be conceptualized using the same format as with the older individual. The major problems are injury to the skull, the presence of intracranial hematomas, and damage to the brain itself. Linear *skull fractures* are unusual and have no significance in themselves. Growing fracture (leptomeningeal cyst) is uncommon in children in the newborn period. Depressed skull fractures are much more common and almost always are a complication of forceps delivery.[16] In most cases, the involved area is depressed as if it were a ping-pong ball. Criteria for therapy are not clear, but if simple suction devices cannot correct the situation, neurosurgical intervention must be considered.

Isolated *cerebral contusion* or *laceration* rarely occurs; these are usually associated with extracerebral hematomas. *Acute subdural hematomas* are the most common. The children are pale, lethargic, and have a poor suck and cry. Reflex responses, such as the Moro, are weak or absent. A bulging fontanelle and other signs of increased intracranial pressure may be present. Convulsions sometimes occur and are often difficult to control.

Management is largely supportive. Seizures should be treated vigorously. If the hematoma is acting as a space-occupying mass lesion, subdural taps will reduce the pressure. The child's hematocrit must be followed closely, as blood loss can be considerable.

The outcome of symptomatic head injury in the neonate is not good. Less than one-third of the children are normal on long-term follow-up. Almost one-half die or are left severely handicapped.[16]

Spinal cord injury in the neonatal period has been discussed in Chapter 14.

The most common type of injury to the peripheral nervous system involves the brachial plexus. The classic finding is *Erb palsy.* The trauma results from forcible distraction of the head and shoulder and involves the upper plexus, most commonly the C_{5-7} segments. The arm is held abducted and internally rotated at the shoulder, extended and pronated at the elbow, and flexed at the wrist and fingers (Figure 28-2). If the C_4 root is also involved, the ipsilateral leaf of the diaphragm will be paralyzed. Sensory deficits are difficult to document.

Prognosis depends on whether the brachial plexus has suffered a stretch injury or nerve roots have been avulsed from the spinal cord. This determination cannot be made initially, but avulsion should be suspected if there is no return of function in the first few months. Although myelography is not performed routinely, this will demonstrate a leak of the contrast medium through the nerve root sleeve if the root is torn.

Treatment is directed toward prevention of contractures and protecting the shoulder from dislocation. Eighty to ninety percent of children will make a complete recovery by age 1 year.

Klumpke paralysis involves the lower plexus and is manifested as a flail hand. Horner syndrome (ptosis, miosis, enophthalmos, and anhydrosis) is also present in many cases, as there is damage to the C_8-T_1 roots. Prognosis for recovery is poor in Klumpke paralysis, as it is in injuries involving the total plexus.

Facial paralysis must be differentiated from the asymmetrical crying-face syndrome. The prognosis is good. Injury to other peripheral or cranial nerves is uncommon.

DISORDERS SPECIFIC TO THE NEONATAL PERIOD

A number of disorders related to the transition from intrauterine to independent extrauterine existence are not the result of trauma or inadequate

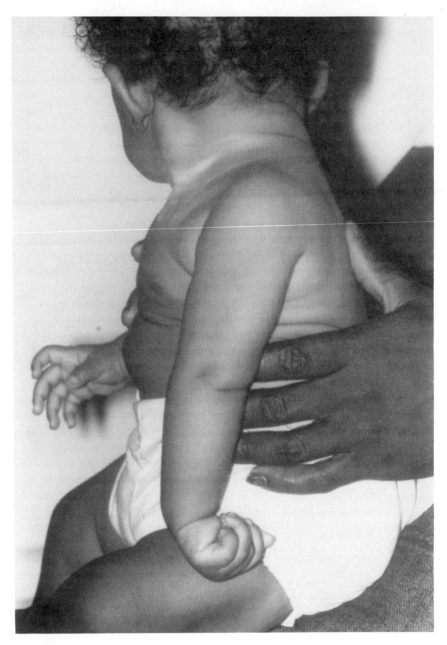

FIGURE 28-2. Infant with Erb palsy of the left arm, demonstrating the characteristic posture of the arm and hand.

adjustments of the cardiorespiratory system. They are related to other problems with the child becoming responsible for his own homeostasis and also result from immaturity of specific organ systems. Many of these conditions have CNS manifestations.

The definition of *hypoglycemia* in the neonate is the subject of some dispute.

The generally accepted lower limits of normal are a blood glucose of 20 mg/dl in the premature infant and 30 mg/dl in the child born at term. As the clinical manifestations of hypoglycemia are often subtle, Volpe[1] recommends setting the critical level at 30 mg/dl for the premature and 40 mg/dl for the infant at term.

Infants seem to be able to tolerate a lower glucose level than that which will support the function of the mature brain because of their ability to utilize amino acids, lipids, and ketone bodies as metabolic substrates for energy metabolism. If glucose levels fall to the point where cerebral function cannot be adequately maintained, the damage is diffuse and involves neurons primarily.

Four major types of hypoglycemia are seen in neonates.[17] Early transitional–adaptive hypoglycemia is found most commonly in infants of diabetic mothers, premature infants who have suffered perinatal asphyxia or intrauterine malnutrition, and children with erythroblastosis. The incidence is increased by delaying feedings. Hypoglycemia is early, mild, and easily treated. There are few specific clinical signs.

Secondary hypoglycemia occurs in babies with acquired damage to, or congenital anomalies of, the CNS and in children with other types of serious illness. It becomes manifest on the first day of life with symptoms such as lethargy, jitteriness, irritability, and seizures. The hypoglycemia is mild and easily treated.

Classical transient neonatal hypoglycemia is most common in children who are small for gestational age or those delivered by a mother with toxemia. Onset is on the first day of life for one-half of the children, and it almost always occurs before 72 hr. These infants are generally symptomatic. The abnormality in blood sugar level is severe and prolonged, and response to treatment is slow.

Severe recurrent or persistent hypoglycemia is rare. This finding should always trigger a thorough search for an underlying primary metabolic disorder (Table 28-1).

Treatment of neonatal hypoglycemia is dependent on supplying adequate amounts of glucose intravenously. If the blood sugar level cannot be maintained, corticosteroids are also used. It is important to slowly decrease the rate of glucose administration, when discontinuing therapy, to prevent rebound hypoglycemia.

TABLE 28-1
Causes of Recurrent or Persistent Hypoglycemia[a]

Defects in carbohydrate metabolism	Hyperinsulism
Glycogen storage disease, type 1	Beckwith–Wiedemann syndrome
Glycogen synthase deficiency	Islet cell adenoma
Fructose intolerance	Nesidioblastosis
Galactosemia	Beta-cell hyperplasia
Fructose-1,6-diphosphatase deficiency	Defects in amino acid metabolism
Endocrine abnormalities	Maple syrup urine disease
Hypopituitarism	Propionic acidemia
Lack of cortisol	Methylmalonic acidemia
Adrenal hemorrhage	Tyrosinemia
Adrenogenital syndrome	

[a]From Cornblath and Schwartz.[17]

The outcome depends on the severity and duration of hypoglycemia. Children with neurological abnormalities and seizures are more likely to have residua than those who are asymptomatic. There is little information available as to whether subtle damage is caused by mild, asymptomatic hypoglycemia.

Hypocalcemia is present in the neonate if the serum calcium level is below 7 mg/dl. Children at highest risk are those who are premature, small for gestational age, or have suffered perinatal asphyxia, and infants of diabetic mothers. Clinical signs are irritability, jitteriness, tremors, and seizures. *Hypomagnesemia* frequently accompanies hypocalcemia, although it may occur as an isolated metabolic abnormality. It is usually necessary to provide supplemental magnesium when hypocalcemia is being treated, and this should be considered if calcium replacement alone does not relieve the infant's symptoms.

Hypocalcemia occurring after the first week of life can be caused by many factors. The classical syndrome follows ingestion of whole cow milk, which has a phosphorus load beyond that which can be excreted by the infant's kidneys. Other etiological factors include hypoparathyroidism, liver disease, and intestinal malabsorption.

Hypermagnesemia is seen in patients whose mothers were treated with magnesium sulfate for eclampsia.[18] Symptoms are lethargy, poor suck and cry, hyporeflexia, and weakness, sometimes progressing to complete paralysis.

Neonatal narcotics withdrawal is a problem occurring in infants whose mothers were addicted to heroin or methadone during pregnancy. The major symptoms are tremulousness and irritability, reduced sleep, constant hunger, and increased muscle tone and reflexes. In the case of methadone addiction, the symptoms come on later, the course of the illness is more prolonged, and seizures are more common.

Mildly affected children need no treatment. If symptoms are severe, or if seizures occur, a more active approach must be taken. Phenobarbital and chlorpromazine are the drugs most commonly used. Other methods of therapy include administration of paregoric or diazepam. Follow-up studies have shown no major neurological deficits when the children are compared to a control group matched for socioeconomic status. There is an increased risk of sudden infant death syndrome in children who have undergone methadone withdrawal in the neonatal period.

Congenital hypothyroidism (cretinism) can occur as a result of any one of a number of abnormalities of structure and function of the thyroid gland. Severe cases are easily recognized clinically by the signs of poor postnatal growth, lethargy, feeding problems, constipation, and prolonged physiological jaundice. There are typical physical features, which include a coarse, puffy face with a large tongue and dull expression; enlarged abdomen with an umbilical hernia; and hypothermia. Laboratory studies document the defect in production of thyroid hormone. Bone age is delayed, providing confirmatory evidence for the diagnosis.

Most neonatal screening programs test for T_4. As this may be low in children with decreased levels of thyroid-binding globulin, an elevated level of thyroid-stimulating hormone should also be present before the diagnosis is accepted. These screening programs have shown that hypothyroidism is not a rare condition, and that many mildly affected children do not have obvious clinical abnormalities.

The importance of the early diagnosis of congenital hypothyroidism cannot be overemphasized, as this is one of the few preventable causes of mental retardation. The best chance for normal development occurs if treatment is begun in the first month of life. Unfortunately, those children who have severe clinical manifestations early in infancy may not reach their full intellectual potential even with prompt, early treatment.

Bilirubin encephalopathy (kernicterus) is becoming a rare condition. This disorder is characterized by the deposition of bilirubin in the basal ganglia and other subcortical nuclei of the infant's brain. Acute symptoms include lethargy, poor feeding, hypotonia, and loss of the Moro reflex in association with a significantly elevated serum indirect bilirubin level. There are episodes of opisthotonic posturing. Death often occurs during the acute illness. If the child survives, there is hypotonia for a number of months and then evolution into the classic triad of athetoid cerebral palsy, paralysis of upward gaze, and sensorineural deafness.

There is a clear relationship between the bilirubin level at which damage occurs and the child's birth weight and gestational age. The risk is diminished after the child is several days old, but is increased by sepsis, anoxia, acidosis, and any drug that displaces bilirubin from protein-binding sites. Unconjugated bilirubin crosses the blood–brain barrier and causes the damage, and the risk is dependent on the concentration of this compound, rather than the total bilirubin level.

No specific treatment exists once neurological damage has taken place. Efforts must be made to prevent the serum bilirubin concentration from rising to toxic levels, taking into account all of the factors discussed previously.

Neonatal hyperviscosity syndrome is being recognized with increased frequency. The diagnosis should be suspected if the venous hematocrit is over 65%. These children have an increased incidence of tachypnea, cyanosis, and hypoglycemia. On follow-up evaluation, motor and other neurological abnormalities are found more frequently than in a control group. Hyperviscosity, rather than the associated hypoglycemia, seems to be the major factor involved.[19]

NEONATAL SEIZURES

Seizures occurring in the newborn infant are discussed in Chapter 16. It should be emphasized that the clinical signs may be obvious or can be quite subtle. The types of abnormalities seen include[1]

- Tonic deviation of the eyes
- Eyelid blinking or fluttering
- Sucking, drooling, lip smacking

- Stereotyped "rowing," "swimming," or "pedaling" movements
- Apneic spells[20]

Any serious insult to the CNS can cause seizures, although hypoxic–ischemic encephalopathy is the most common. The ultimate prognosis depends almost entirely on the underlying cause of the seizures.

The initial treatment calls for large doses of anticonvulsants, so that an adequate blood level can be rapidly achieved. Either phenobarbital or phenytoin can be given at a dose of 20 mg/kg initially. Blood levels are then monitored, and additional medication administered as required. The appropriate duration of treatment is not clear, and there is a good deal of variability in the protocols used by different clinicians. Factors taken into consideration include the cause of the seizures, ease with which control was achieved, and the presence or absence of neurological abnormalities on follow-up evaluation.

The diagnosis of a seizure disorder may be inappropriately applied to the *jittery newborn and infant*. The presence of a tremor in this age group is often associated with an exaggerated startle response, hypertonicity, and increased general movement.[21] This can be caused by many different factors which affect the CNS. Treatment should be directed toward the etiological problem, not the tremor itself. Coarse tremor is more significant than fine tremor, and some of these children are found to have choreiform movements when they are older.

REFERENCES

1. Volpe, J. J., 1981, *Neurology of the Newborn*, W. B. Saunders, Philadelphia.
2. Sarnat, H. B., and Sarnat, M. S., 1978, Neonatal encephalopathy following fetal distress, *Arch. Neurol.* **33**:696–705.
3. Finer, N. N., Robertson, C. M., Richards, R. T., Pinnell, R. N., and Peters, K. L., 1981, Hypoxic–ischemic encephalopathy in term neonates: Perinatal factors and outcome, *J. Pediatr.* **98**:112–117.
4. Finer, N. N., Robertson, C. M., Peters, K. L., and Coward, J. H., 1983, Factors affecting outcome in hypoxic–ischemic encephalopathy in term infants, *Am. J. Dis. Child.* **137**:21–25.
5. Coen, R. W., McCutchen, C. B., Wermer, D., Snyder, J., and Gluck, F. E., 1932, Continuous monitoring of the electroencephalogram following perinatal asphyxia, *J. Pediatr.* **100**:628–630.
6. Fitzhardinge, P. M., Flodmark, O., Fitz, C. R., and Ashby, S., 1981, The prognostic value of computed tomography as an adjunct to assessment of the term infant with postasphyxial encephalopathy, *J. Pediatr.* **99**:777–781.
7. Fitzhardinge, P. M., Flodmark, O., Fitz, C. R., and Ashby, S., 1982, The prognostic value of computed tomography of the brain in asphyxiated premature infants, *J. Pediatr.* **100**:476–481.
8. Dolfin, T., Skidmore, M. B., Fong, K. W., Hoskins, E. M., and Shennand, A. T., 1983, Incidence, severity, and timing of subependymal and intraventricular hemorrhages in preterm infants born in a perinatal unit as detected by serial real-time ultrasound, *Pediatrics* **71**:541–546.
9. Perlman, J. M., Nelson, J. S., McAlister, W. H., and Volpe, J. J., 1983, Intracerebellar hemorrhage in a premature newborn: Diagnosis by real-time ultrasound and correlation of autopsy findings, *Pediatrics* **71**:159–162.
10. Papile, L-A, Burstein, J., Burstein, R., and Koffler, H., 1978, Incidence and evolution of subependymal and intraventricular hemorrhage: A study of infants with birth weights less than 1500 gm, *J. Pediatr.* **92**:529–534.

11. Tekolste, K. A., Bennett, F. C., and Mack, L. A., 1985, Follow-up of infants receiving cranial ultrasound for intracranial hemorrhage, *Am. J. Dis. Child.* **139:**299–303.
12. Graziani, L. J., Pesto, M., Stanley, C., Steben, J., Desai, H., Desai, S., Foy, P. M., Branca, P., and Goldberg, B. B., 1985, Cranial ultrasound and clinical studies in preterm infants, *J. Pediatr.* **106:**269–276.
13. Williamson, W. D., Desmond, M. M., Wilson, G. S., Murphy, M. A., Rozelle, J., Garcia-Prats, J. A., 1983, Survival of low-birth-weight infants with neonatal intraventricular hemorrhage, *Am. J. Dis. Child.* **137:**1181–1184.
14. Kreusser, K. L., Tarby, T. J., Kovnar, E., Taylor, D. A., Hill, A., and Volpe, J. J., 1985, Serial lumbar puncture for at least temporary amelioration of neonatal posthemorrhagic hydrocephalus, *Pediatrics* **75:**719–724.
15. Bergman, I., Bauer, R. E., Barmada, M. A., Latchaw, R. E., Taylor, H.G., David, R., Painter, M. J., 1985, Intracerebral hemorrhage in the full-term neonatal infant, *Pediatrics* **75:**488–496.
16. Natelson, S. E., and Sayers, M. P., 1973, The fate of children sustaining severe head trauma at birth, *Pediatrics* **51:**169–174.
17. Cornblath, M., and Schwartz, P., 1976, *Disorders of Carbohydrate Metabolism in Infancy,* W.B. Saunders, Philadelphia.
18. Rasch, D. K., Huber, P. A., Richardson, C. J., L'Hommedieu, C. S., Nelson, T. E., and Reddi, R., 1982, Neurobehavioral effects of neonatal hypermagnesemia, *J. Pediatr.* **100:**272–276.
19. Black, V. D., Lubchenco, L. O., Luckey, D. W., Koops, B. L., McGuinness, G. A., Powell, D. P., and Tomlinson, A. L., 1982, Developmental and neurologic sequelae of neonatal hyperviscosity syndrome, *Pediatrics* **69:**426–431.
20. Watanabe, K., Hara, K., Miyazaki, S., Hakamada, S., and Kuroyanagi, M., 1982, Apneic seizures in the newborn, *Am. J. Dis. Child.* **136:**980–984.
21. Rosman, N. P., Donnally, J. H. and Braun, M. A., 1984, The jittery newborn and infant: A review, *Dev. Behav. Pediatr.* **5:**263–273.

ADDITIONAL READING

Hill, A., and Volpe, J. J., 1981, Seizures, hypoxic–ischemic brain injury and intraventricular hemorrhage in the newborn, *Ann. Neurol.* **10:**109–121.

Neurological Complications of Pediatric Disease

The acute onset of a neurological problem, such as coma or seizures, is dramatic when it occurs and demands immediate evaluation and emergency treatment. In this context, it is easy to overlook the possibility that the nervous system abnormality does not represent a primary neurological disorder but is secondary to systemic disease or failure of one or more organ systems. Ascertainment of an underlying condition obviously has important implications for treatment.

Systemic diseases and abnormalities in the function of the CNS and systemic diseases can be related in three ways:

1. The disease simultaneously involves multiple organ systems, including the CNS (e.g., systemic lupus erythematosus).
2. Metabolic changes produced by the disease secondarily involve the CNS (e.g., hepatic encephalopathy).
3. The nervous system is affected as a toxic reaction to drugs being used to treat the systemic disease (e.g., vincristine neuropathy).

This chapter will also cover conditions produced by toxins and by physical agents excluding trauma.

APPROACH TO THE PATIENT

A simple guideline is important if the clinician wishes to avoid diagnostic errors. Any child who presents with abnormalities involving the function of the nervous system should be considered to have an underlying systemic disease until proven otherwise. This is an extremely useful approach to neurological differential diagnosis.

The approach to a specific patient obviously depends on the mode of clinical presentation and the important features revealed by the history, physical examination, and neurological examination. The selective use of laboratory procedures also requires a critical analysis of the information obtained at the bedside. Uncritical ordering of screening procedures, test batteries, baseline studies, and laboratory profiles frequently provides the clinician with one or more false positive results. This can quickly lead even the experienced diagnostician down expensive and time-consuming blind alleys.

DISORDERS OF WATER AND ELECTROLYTE METABOLISM

The brain has reasonably good capacity to maintain its internal milieu despite rather marked changes in serum electrolyte concentrations. The blood–brain barrier, a property of the tight junctions between capillary endothelial cells, does not allow passive egress and ingress of these solutes, and active metabolic processes are used to regulate their concentrations. Water, on the other hand, diffuses in and out of the CNS rapidly. For this reason, the brain is sensitive to changes in osmotic pressure. Significantly decreased serum osmolality can produce cerebral edema; in a hyperosmolar state, dehydration and shrinkage of cerebral tissue occurs.

Nervous system function depends on the maintenance of an electrochemical gradient across nerve cell membranes. Major alterations in electrolyte concentration alter this gradient, produce changes in mentation and consciousness, and can also cause seizures. Slow changes in water and electrolyte concentrations are better tolerated than rapid shifts, whether the change is away from or toward the normal level.

Isotonic dehydration does not affect the CNS directly. Impaired function results if the dehydration is so severe that vascular collapse occurs, or if the illness is associated with a severe metabolic acidosis.

Hyponatremia results from dehydration in which the loss of sodium exceeds that of water, from dilution by ill-advised attempts to rehydrate the patient with an excessively hypotonic solution, or from water intoxication without dehydration. Excessive sodium loss also occurs as part of adrenocortical insufficiency, either primary or as part of the adrenogenital syndrome. Children with cystic fibrosis suffer excessive sodium loss in perspiration when exposed to a warm environment. The syndrome of inappropriate secretion of antidiuretic hormone (ADH) following head injury or CNS infections is a controversial issue. In most cases, the hyponatremia is actually due to the administration of hypotonic solutions or excessive amounts of fluid.

The neurological signs of hyponatremia are drowsiness, irritability, and seizures. Mild degrees of hyponatremia (above 120 meq/liter) are tolerated well, but if serum sodium levels fall rapidly, the symptoms are exaggerated and the patient may become comatose and have evidence of cerebral edema. Overly rapid correction of hyponatremia by the administration of hypertonic saline solution has been associated with central pontine myelinolysis.

Treatment of severe hyponatremic dehydration starts with rapid restoration of the vascular volume. Excessively hypotonic solutions should not be used for fluid replacement. Attempts to quickly correct the sodium deficit are unwarranted. If the patient is having seizures, however, cautious administration of hypertonic saline may be necessary, as the convulsions will probably not respond to the usual anticonvulsants. In the case of hyponatremia due to water intoxication, the use of hypertonic saline is also indicated if convulsions are present.

Hypernatremia in children is usually associated with severe dehydration and a disproportionate loss of water. The patient presents with a depressed state of consciousness and seizures which respond poorly to therapy with anticonvulsants. Treatment requires prompt restoration of the circulating blood volume, but cautious reduction of the sodium concentration. Overly rapid correction is associated with an increase in seizures, cerebral edema, and multiple areas of petechial hemorrhage within the brain.

Salt poisoning also produces severe hypernatremia. Most cases have been due to the inadvertent use of salt instead of sugar when making up infant formulas, or the treatment of dehydrated children with home-mixed fluids containing excessive amounts of sodium. The principles of treatment are the same, although there is usually no deficit in blood volume.

Diabetes insipidus results from a reduction or loss of ADH (vasopressin) production. This most commonly caused by suprasellar or hypothalamic tumors and can also be seen following severe head trauma. The child presents with polyuria, polydipsia, and poor growth. Hypernatremia is a result of excessive water loss. Treatment focuses on the replacement of ADH or use of desmopressin acetate, a synthetic analog.

Chronic hypernatremia is also present in *nephrogenic diabetes insipidus.* This abnormality in the renal conservation of water is inherited as an X-linked recessive condition. The boys have polyuria and polydipsia, grow poorly, and are frequently mentally retarded.

Severe *hypokalemia* produces flaccid paralysis of the muscles. This may easily be mistaken for Guillain–Barré syndrome. The most common etiology of symptomatic hypokalemia is the chronic use of diuretics. A rare, but interesting, cause is the ingestion of large amounts of licorice over a long period of time. A substance in the licorice, glycyrrhizinic acid, has aldosteronelike activity. *Hyperkalemia* rarely presents with neuromuscular or CNS manifestations, because of the cardiotoxic effects of high serum concentrations of potassium.

Hypocalcemia presenting beyond the neonatal period is rare, except when associated with rickets, either nutritional or metabolic, or with a malabsorption syndrome. It has also been reported to occur following the use of pediatric enemas containing a high concentration of sodium dihydrogen phosphate. Absorption of the phosphate is the causative factor. The most common clinical abnormality accompanying hypocalcemia is carpopedal spasm. Laryngeal stridor and paresthesias are sometimes present. Seizures also occur. Treatment is based on the administration of calcium. This must be done cautiously, because of the risk of cardiac toxicity.

Hypercalcemia is rare, except as a result of vitamin D intoxication. Infantile hypercalcemia associated with supravalvular aortic stenosis, mental retardation, and characteristic facial appearance has been reported. Calcium levels return to normal later in childhood. Symptoms of hypercalcemia include drowsiness, irritability, and weakness. Sustained high levels can produce disorientation and coma.

VITAMIN DEFICIENCIES AND EXCESSES

The complex relationships between general malnutrition, brain growth, and cognitive function have been discussed in Chapter 1. Clinical vitamin deficiencies are rare in this country, although they are seen in immigrants from less developed nations. A new cause of *protein–calorie* and *vitamin malnutrition* has recently been reported, however. This is the use of unusual diets by certain groups. Examples of diets that put the growing child at great risk are macrobiotic diets, unsupplemented pure vegan diets, and the use of artificial infant formulas made entirely from unmodified vegetable sources.[1,2]

Vitamin A deficiency is associated with corneal ulcerations and loss of night vision. It has been reported to produce pseudotumor cerebri, although increased intracranial pressure is much more typically a result of hypervitaminosis A. This usually requires large doses over a prolonged period of time, but patients can be seen with increased intracranial pressure following the ingestion of only modest doses. Pseudotumor cerebri also occurs during treatment of acne with isotretinoin, a vitamin A analog. Other manifestations of vitamin A toxicity include pain and swelling of the extremities, skin changes, and hepatomegaly.

Thiamine (vitamin B_1) deficiency is rare in children. In areas of the world where infantile beriberi occurs, the patients, in addition to poor growth, vomiting, diarrhea, skin rash, and myocardial abnormalities, present with peripheral neuropathy, lethargy, and mental changes. With severe deficiency, Wernicke syndrome (oculomotor palsies, ataxia, and coma) can occur.

Riboflavin (vitamin B_2) deficiency rarely occurs as an isolated problem, but is usually associated with deficiencies of the other B-group vitamins. It apparently does not cause any specific neurological disorder.

Deficiency of *niacin* is associated with general symptoms such as irritability and cognitive dysfunction. The major neurological abnormality is a mixed motor and sensory neuropathy.

Pyridoxine (vitamin B_6) deficiency in infants is associated with seizures. This was clearly demonstrated when infants were fed a proprietary formula that was inadvertently deficient in pyridoxine. Irritability and seizures began within 1–6 months after use of this product was begun.

Peripheral neuropathy can occur as a result of pyridoxine deficiency caused by administration of isoniazid for the treatment of tuberculosis. This is less common in children than in adults and can be prevented by pyridoxine supplementation.

Pyridoxine dependency is a rare metabolic disorder; the children have seizures which are refractory to standard therapy but can be treated by the administration of pharmacological doses of pyridoxine.[3] The increased need for this substance is permanent. Transient pyridoxine dependency in infants is seen following maternal ingestion of large doses of pyridoxine during pregnancy. Neonatal seizures occur and can be prevented by temporarily providing supplemental pyridoxine.

Vitamin B$_{12}$ deficiency is rare, although it is seen in children taking vegan diets. It has also been reported in nursing infants of mothers with vitamin B$_{12}$–deficient diets or pernicious anemia. The major clinical abnormality is macrocytic anemia. Neurological signs are unusual in children, but when they occur include ataxia, spastic paraparesis, peripheral neuropathy, and coma.

Several types of juvenile pernicious anemia, with or without associated neurological abnormalities, occur. Classical juvenile pernicious anemia, as in the adult form, is due to an absence of gastric intrinsic factor. A congenital deficiency of transcobalamin II presents in early infancy. Vitamin B$_{12}$ deficiency is also seen with gastrointestinal diseases that interfere with the function of the terminal ileum.

The major manifestation of *folic acid* deficiency is anemia. This disorder can occur with diets restricted to goat's milk or powdered milk. Specific involvement of the CNS has not been documented. There is now some evidence that supplementing the maternal diet with folic acid reduces the incidence of neural tube defects.

Neurological deficits are also not a specific feature of *vitamin C* deficiency, although intracranial hemorrhage can occur in scurvy. Because of the pain caused by subperiosteal hemorrhages, the children are reluctant to move and are thought to be weak and hypotonic. The diagnostic clue is evidence of severe pain when the child's limbs are manipulated.

Vitamin D deficiency is uncommon, as most commercially available milk has vitamins D and A added. The child fed an unusual vegetable-based diet is at risk. The hypocalcemia associated with rickets can present as tetany and may be associated with seizures. Excessive intake of vitamin D produces hypercalcemia. These children are irritable and have weakness and hypotonia.

Vitamin E deficiency as a causative factor in some cases of neuroaxonal dystrophy has been suggested by the finding of a similar histological picture in children with cystic fibrosis and biliary atresia.[4] Suggestions of the usefulness of vitamin E in the treatment of neuronal ceroid lipofuscinosis have not been borne out.

Hemorrhagic disease of the newborn, a result of *vitamin K* deficiency, can cause bleeding into the CNS. Hypoprothrombinemia, due to vitamin K deficiency, is associated with hepatic dysfunction in older children. Bleeding into any organ, including the brain, can occur.

Muscular pain can result from *biotin* deficiency. A deficiency of *pantothenic acid* has been associated with a burning sensation of the feet.

ENDOCRINE DISORDERS

The most striking features of disease of the *pituitary gland* or the hypothalamopituitary axis in children are growth failure and diabetes insipidus. The only common cause of pituitary dysfunction in childhood is a suprasellar or hypothalamic tumor. Suspicion should be raised when a child's growth rate decelerates, and the growth chart shows a progressive decrease in the height percentile. This finding should always trigger a comprehensive evaluation.

The often-associated finding of bitemporal hemianopia is difficult to document in a child. Complaints of decreasing visual acuity are also uncommon, until optic atrophy has become severe.

Pituitary adenomas are rare tumors in childhood. They may present with gigantism. Neurological manifestations are largely restricted to a chiasmal syndrome with bitemporal hemianopia. Severe kyphosis with complaint of back pain is also common.

Isosexual precocious puberty in boys is associated with a suprasellar or hypothalamic tumor in approximately one-half of cases. A thorough evaluation is obviously required. Only 10% of girls with true precocious puberty will have demonstrable lesions. A CT scan is indicated, however, as the procedure is noninvasive and the yield will be reasonably high.

Hypothyroidism in early life is associated with cretinism. This disorder in the neonate is discussed in Chapter 28. Onset in later childhood causes slowing of growth, myxedema, and retardation of cognitive development. Proximal muscle weakness is commonly present. There is a good deal of variability in the findings, depending on the severity of the endocrine disorder and the age at which hypothyroidism occurs.

Early signs of *hyperthyroidism* in children are hyperactivity, behavioral changes, and tremor. Chorea occasionally occurs. Ocular palsies and exophthalmos may also be seen. A number of neuromuscular problems have been associated with thyrotoxicosis. These include myopathy, myasthenia gravis, and periodic paralysis. The differential diagnosis is obviously complex.

Thyrotoxic myopathy has the usual limb–girdle distribution, with major involvement of the legs. Exophthalmos may be present, but ptosis and extraocular palsies do not occur. Deep-tendon reflexes are brisk, and there is no response to either edrophonium or physostigmine. The myasthenic syndrome often includes ptosis and paralysis of eye muscles, and the weakness improves with administration of acetylcholine esterase inhibitors. Diagnosis of periodic paralysis rests on the history and course of the illness.

Hypoparathyroidism is associated with tetany and seizures, as is any condition causing hypocalcemia. Behavioral changes are also common. Pseudotumor cerebri occurs in some patients. Diagnostic clues to this condition include the presence of cataracts, dental abnormalities, and mucocutaneous candidiasis.

Hyperparathyroidism, and the associated hypercalcemia causes generalized weakness but no specific neurological signs in older children. When it occurs in infancy, however, mental retardation frequently occurs.

Adrenocortical insufficiency produces effects on CNS function only through changes in serum electrolyte concentration. Adrenoleukodystrophy is associated with adrenal insufficiency. Acute adrenal failure occurs as part of the Waterhouse–Friderichsen syndrome associated with meningococcemia.

Cushing disease is caused by excessive production of ACTH by the pituitary, which then stimulates excessive production of adrenal steroids. This disorder is extremely rare in childhood. *Cushing syndrome,* due to adrenal hyperplasia or an adrenal adenoma, is much more common. Neurological signs are nonspecific and include behavioral changes, weakness, and lethargy.

The *adrenogenital syndrome* (virilizing adrenal hyperplasia) presents with virilization in girls and pseudoprecocious puberty in boys. This is differentiated from true precocious puberty, as the testes are not enlarged in the adrenogenital syndrome. This differential point is important, so that an unnecessary search for a suprasellar tumor is not begun. Neurological signs and symptoms occur only as a result of the electrolyte abnormalities.

Coma, due to ketoacidosis, is the presenting event in up to 20% of children with *diabetes mellitus.* This is life-threatening and may be associated with cerebral edema.[5] Diabetic coma must be differentiated from other disorders producing coma and ketoacidosis, such as metabolic abnormalities of the short-chain fatty acids. In the patient with known diabetes, impairment of the sensorium always requires the differentiation of ketoacidosis and hypoglycemia. If there is any doubt, a blood specimen for glucose determination should be obtained and glucose administered immediately.

The major long-term neurological complication of diabetes is peripheral neuropathy. Changes in nerve conduction velocity are found early in the course of the disease. As many as 20% of patients are involved 10 years after the onset of the condition. After 20 years, one-half of patients will be symptomatic. Currently available data suggest that complications can be kept to a minimum if close control of the diabetes is maintained.[6]

Nonketotic hyperosmolar coma is not common in children. This condition occurs when there is an extremely high sustained blood glucose level, usually over 600 mg/dl. There is little or no ketosis. Focal signs may be present. Many of the children have preexisting neurological abnormalities. Permanent neurological damage has been reported to follow this condition, and there is a high mortality rate.[7]

METABOLIC ENCEPHALOPATHIES

Any disorder that seriously upsets systemic homeostasis will impair the function of the CNS. This is often the most subtle sign of failure of another organ system. The major acute metabolic encephalopathies of importance in pediatrics are those due to uremia, hepatic failure, and hypoglycemia. Respira-

abolic disorders and is not specific for uremia. It is elicited by _____ hold his arms outstretched with the wrists dorsiflexed. Sudden brief episodes of loss of tone cause the hands to drop and then assume the original position. If this is frequently repeated, it gives the appearance of a flapping tremor. Seizures are both myoclonic and focal. These commonly move from one muscle group to another.

The underlying metabolic basis of uremic encephalopathy is not fully understood. Serum urea nitrogen and creatinine levels are correlated with neurological symptoms to a good degree. Many patients who maintain reasonably low levels of these substances while on dialysis programs still remain symptomatic, however. Following renal transplantation, there is often a dramatic improvement in their condition. This suggests the presence of other toxic substances that are not easily dialyzable.[9]

Patients with renal failure have a number of other neurological problems. Hyponatremia and hypocalcemia are often present, and tetany sometimes occurs. A mixed sensorimotor neuropathy with paresthesias is common in patients with chronic uremia; this improves markedly following renal transplantation.[10]

Those with either acute or chronic renal failure are at risk for the development of hypertensive encephalopathy. The initial symptoms are headache, lethargy, and confusion. If treatment is not instituted rapidly, seizures and coma occur. Examination reveals severe hypertension, papilledema, retinal hemorrhages, and constriction of retinal arteries. Strokes, intracerebral bleeding, and cerebral edema with herniation can occur unless aggressive therapy to rapidly decrease the blood pressure is instituted.

The majority of patients with end-stage renal disease now have access to renal dialysis programs. An acute complication of this procedure is the dialysis disequilibrium syndrome. This is probably a result of the rapid removal of urea from the circulating blood and extracellular space. Egress of urea from cells is slow, and during the transition period, water moves into cells, producing intracellular cerebral edema. Lethargy, organic mental changes, and headache are the most common symptoms. Seizures may occur. In severe cases, signs of increased intracranial pressure, such as papilledema, are found. Treatment is conservative, as the symptoms improve when solute and water concentrations reequilibrate.

A rare complication of long-term hemodialysis is *dialysis dementia*. There is progressive dementia and seizures. This was originally reported in adults,[11] but has occurred in children. The cause of this condition is not known.

Patients who have renal transplantation require prolonged immunosuppressive therapy. This predisposes them to a new set of potential complications involving the CNS. These include infections with common and opportunistic organisms and the development of neoplasms. Cyclosporin, a new agent being used to reduce the risk of rejection, may be associated with a lower risk of these problems but can produce renal damage.

Hepatic encephalopathy is a serious complication of liver failure. It may occur in the context of acute liver disease or be superimposed on hepatic cirrhosis. There is rapidly progressive lethargy, confusion, and dysarthria. Examination reveals asterixis, ataxia, and intention tremor. Decorticate and decerebrate posturing may also occur. Some patients have evidence of spinal cord dysfunction, with spastic paraparesis. The EEG is severely abnormal and typically shows triphasic waves.

The two major precipitating factors in a patient with liver disease are excessive protein intake and gastrointestinal hemorrhage. Systemic illness, diuretics, and fluid and electrolyte imbalance can also accentuate symptoms. There is a correlation between the severity of symptoms and the ammonia level, although this is not absolute. Treatment is based on reducing protein intake and preventing the formation of ammonia by intestinal bacteria. This is accomplished by administering antibiotics, which markedly reduces the intestinal flora.

Patients with liver failure have a bleeding diathesis due to failure of production of prothrombin and a number of other clotting factors synthesized in the liver. The possibility of intracranial bleeding should be considered in any patient with hepatic disease who manifests signs and symptoms of CNS dysfunction. This should be ruled out before a diagnosis of hepatic encephalopathy is made.

Hypoglycemia is a rare disorder outside of the neonatal period. Although a large number of causes have been reported, most are uncommon. The major categories of conditions associated with hypoglycemia are [12]

- Hyperinsulinism
- Hepatic enzyme defects
- Endocrine deficiencies
  - Pituitary
  - Adrenal
- Ketotic hypoglycemia
- Drugs and toxins
- Miscellaneous
  - Reye syndrome
  - Malnutrition

Diagnosis can be a problem, as there is not a good correlation between symptoms and the measured blood sugar level during any given episode. Symptoms are more likely to occur if the rate of decrease in glucose level is rapid. There are two types of clinical manifestations, those resulting from adrenergic overactivity and those due to the hypoglycemia itself. The initial response to a falling bood sugar is the release of epinephrine by the adrenal glands. This produces tachycardia, anxiety, pallor, and diaphoresis.

If the hypoglycemia becomes severe, the patient is irritable and confused. A further decrease of blood sugar, or a sustained low level, can cause seizures and loss of consciousness. If this is not rapidly corrected, permanent damage, mainly to neurons, results. The child is left with mental retardation, behavior problems, and a seizure disorder.

The most comon type of hypoglycemia, a form restricted to childhood, is ketotic hypoglycemia. This first occurs in late infancy and the preschool years and resolves spontaneously by age 10 years. The usual triggering event is a prolonged fast, although the child is more susceptible during periods of illness. The diagnosis is suggested by the finding of ketonuria during an attack, and it can be documented if an episode is precipitated by a prolonged fast or a ketogenic diet. Treatment requires placing the child on several meals a day and avoiding prolonged periods without food intake, especially when the child is ill.

Children can develop hypoglycemia following ingestion of ethyl alcohol. The usual story is that the infant finds the remnants of cocktails in the house on Sunday morning and ingests them. Hypoglycemia comes on within an hour and can be quite severe and difficult to treat. Seizures and coma occur, and some of the reported cases have had a fatal outcome. The literature suggests that salicylates can also cause hypoglycemia in young patients. The relationship of this finding to the suggestive evidence that Reye syndrome can be precipitated by these compounds is not clear.

The complex issues concerning hypoglycemia, sugar ingestion, and behavior and learning abnormalities are discussed in Chapter 23. An important point is that the diagnosis of hypoglycemia is currently being made on the basis of inadequate documentation. If the child is, in fact, hypoglycemic, it is inappropriate to assume that this is "reactive hypoglycemia," and a detailed metabolic evaluation must be carried out. There is now some evidence that the entity of reactive hypoglycemia may not exist.

Acute *respiratory failure* in children is most commonly caused by infections of the upper respiratory tract or lungs, foreign body aspiration, and asthma. The earliest neurological signs are headache, restlessness, and impaired cognition. If hypoxia and hypercapnea remain severe, seizures can occur and the patient becomes comatose.

Respiratory insufficiency is a concomitant of a number of neurological diseases. These include those which involve the motor unit (anterior horn cell, peripheral nerve, myoneural junction, muscle), head and spinal cord injuries, and conditions associated with severe scoliosis.

CONGENITAL HEART DISEASE

Children with cyanotic congenital heart disease are at risk for a number of neurological problems. If the chronic hypoxia is severe, there is a delay in all developmental milestones, and many of these children will have permanent cognitive deficits.[13] There is some evidence that there is actually a progressive decline in intellectual level.[14]

The polycythemia that is commonly present predisposes the children, especially before age 2 years, to cerebral venous thromboses. Older patients are more likely to develop a cerebral abscess, and this should always be the first diagnostic consideration when a child with a cyanotic lesion presents with focal neurological signs, seizures, or increased intracranial pressure. Strokes due to emboli and bacterial endocarditis also occur.

There is less neurological risk if the child has an acyanotic lesion. The major problems are hypoxia due to congestive heart failure, hypertension with lesions such as coarctation of the aorta, and repeated episodes of pneumonia and other serious illnesses. If there are abnormalities of the mitral or aortic valves, emboli and bacterial endocarditis become important concerns. These also must be considered if acute neurological problems appear in a child who has had a valve replaced by a prosthesis or artificial valve.

Cognitive or behavioral changes following surgery for congenital heart disease suggest that an episode of cerebral hypoperfusion or anoxia occurred during the cardiac bypass portion of the procedure. Emboli from air, blood clots, and foreign material also can occur while the child is being maintained on the pump.

HEMATOLOGICAL DISEASES

The most common hematological diseases involving the nervous system are sickle cell anemia (Chapter 15) and leukemia (Chapter 19). A child with severe anemia from any cause tends to be irritable and lethargic. In general, however, cardiac failure occurs before CNS function is seriously impaired.

Intracranial hemorrhage is one of the most serious complications of any hemorrhagic diathesis. The typical symptoms of headache, alteration in state of consciousness, and meningeal signs occur. Whether or not there are focal findings on neurological examination depends on the localization and extent of the bleeding. Lumbar puncture is hazardous in such a setting, because of the risk of cerebral herniation and the possibility of causing even more subarachnoid bleeding. The CT scan is currently the most useful diagnostic procedure.

COLLAGEN VASCULAR DISEASES

Systemic lupus erythematosus (SLE) involves the CNS in up to one-half of cases. Behavioral abnormalities and seizures are the most common manifestations. Both of these features raise problems in differential diagnosis. If serious renal disease is present, this, rather than the cerebrovascular disease, may be the cause of seizures and organic mental symptoms. It is also difficult to separate the mental changes of the underlying disorder from those that can be induced by high-dosage corticosteroid therapy.

Less common neurological manifestations are chorea, strokes, transverse myelitis, and peripheral neuropathy. Rarely, a patient presents in coma with an acute encephalopathy and may rapidly die. In general, renal disease, not neurological involvement, is the life-limiting factor in SLE.

Polyarteritis nodosa is less common than SLE in childhood. Seizures frequently occur in this condition, but changes in mental status are unusual. Cerebrovascular accidents, peripheral neuropathy, and transverse myelitis have also been reported. Myositis with muscle pain and weakness is a prominent complaint in many of the children. As opposed to SLE, CNS damage is an important contributor to mortality in untreated polyarteritis nodosa.

There is a good deal of debate as to whether *Kawasaki disease* (mucocutaneous lymph node syndrome) and infantile polyarteritis nodosa are the same disorder. Kawasaki disease presents with high fever, stomatitis, inflammation of mucous membranes, a characteristic desquamating rash that includes the palms and soles, and lymphadenopathy. Involvement of the nervous system is usually limited to aseptic meningitis, but several patients with cerebral infarction have been reported.

Neurological abnormalities in *anaphylactoid purpura* (Henoch–Schönlein purpura) are uncommon, but there may be involvement of cerebral blood vessels with seizures, focal neurological deficits, and coma.[15] Polyradiculoneuropathies and mononeuropathies also occur. *Wegener granulomatosis* is associated with peripheral neuropathy. *Takayasu arteritis* produces visual loss in older individuals.

IMMUNOLOGICAL AND ALLERGIC DISORDERS

Immunological diseases present with repeated infections caused by common organisms, infections with unusual opportunistic organisms, persistent infections with agents that usually produce a self-limited illness, or any combination of these features. Patients taking immunosuppressive drugs for any reason are at risk for identical problems. CNS infections caused by fungi or protozoans may be found, and persistent infections with common viruses have also been reported.

Most allergic disorders are not associated with neurological signs and symptoms, but some of the drugs used to treat these conditions are potentially neurotoxic. Excessive doses of theophylline produce agitation and seizures which are sometimes refractory to treatment. Antihistamines have sedative properties, but can produce seizures and coma at toxic dose levels. Corticosteroids occasionally produce acute psychiatric symptoms or depression.

DRUG ABUSE

Most drugs of abuse have their primary effect on the CNS. The most commonly used drug in childhood and adolescence is *ethanol*. Acute intoxication is associated with loss of judgment, impaired coordination, and slurred speech. Larger doses can produce coma and death. Hypoglycemia following the ingestion of ethanol is a phenomenon seen mainly in preschool children.

The alcohol abstinence syndrome, precipitated by suddenly discontinuing intake of this drug after chronic use of large doses, is characterized by agitation, sleeplessness, and tachycardia. Fever and hallucinations occur in severe cases, and seizures are sometimes present. Most adolescents have not had sufficient exposure to alcohol to develop serious complications such as peripheral neuropathy, cerebellar degeneration, and Wernicke–Korsakoff syndrome. As there is a trend for alcohol abuse to begin at younger ages, the pediatrician will need to be aware of these conditions, however.

Small doses of *marijuana* produce effects similar to those of alcohol. The two drugs are synergistic in action. Chronic marijuana abuse has been associated with a syndrome of loss of motivation, loss of interest in age-appropriate activities, withdrawal from friends and social activities, and declining school performance.

Depressant drugs such as *barbiturates, glutethimide,* and *methaqualone* produce a picture of intoxication similar to that caused by alcohol and marijuana. After prolonged use, an abstinence syndrome follows attempts at discontinuing these drugs. The major features are anxiety, restlessness, and tremors. Seizures occur in many patients. There are also systemic abnormalities such as abdominal cramps, vomiting, and tachycardia. Detoxification must be approached cautiously, to prevent seizures.

Inhalants remain popular in some groups of adolescents in inner-city areas. The substances used are mainly hydrocarbons and halogenated hydrocarbons. Toxic effects vary with the specific substance, but include acute or chronic encephalopathy, polyneuropathy, hepatic toxicity, and renal disease. Large doses can produce coma, and death from suffocation has been reported when the material is inhaled from a plastic bag.

Phencyclidine (PCP) is the most popular of the potent hallucinogens at this time. The typical features of intoxication are an organic mental syndrome with hallucinosis and panic. Neurological signs following large doses include nystagmus, ataxia, dystonia, seizures, and coma. Systemic problems such as abnormalities in blood pressure regulation, hypothermia, and cardiac arrhythmias can be fatal.

Infants born to mothers who are chronic users of PCP have symptoms similar to those of the neonatal narcotic withdrawal syndrome. The drug also may be teratogenic.[16]

Lysergic acid diethylamide is less popular now than in past years. In addition to hallucinations, the patient shows signs of sympathetic nervous system overactivity, including tachycardia, dilated pupils, hyperthermia, and piloerection.

Stimulant drugs have retained their popularity. *Amphetamines* produce excitement, euphoria, and increased activity. When the effects of the drug wear off, however, the patient then develops depression, lethargy, and paranoia. Chronic use also is associated with a paranoid state. Intravenous administration of amphetamines has been associated with vasculitis and strokes.

There has been a startling increase in the use of *cocaine*. The patient cycles between euphoria when the drug is taken and profound depression when it is stopped or not available. Paranoia is very common in chronic users.

Although *opiates* are used for their euphoric effect, in large doses they are potent CNS and respiratory depressants. This effect is the cause of death in acute overdoses. As with any drug used intravenously under nonsterile conditions, sepsis and brain abscesses can occur. Sharing of needles is an important mechanism for the transmission of acquired immune deficiency syndrome. A number of uncommon neurological complications have been reported with opiate abuse. These include transverse myelitis and brachial neuritis. The etiology of these disorders is not known.

One of the important characteristics of opiate addiction is a severe abstinence syndrome when use of the drug is discontinued. Initially, the patient has restlessness, insomnia, and diarrhea. In severe cases, hypertension, tachycardia, and convulsions can occur.

PHYSICAL AGENTS

Neurological injury can result from environmental agents other than those causing direct mechanical trauma to the head, spine, and peripheral nerves. In some of these situations, damage to the CNS is the limiting factor in survival.

Drowning and *near drowning* produce complex physiological changes, which include hypoxia, acidosis, major shifts of fluid and electrolytes, and lung injury. The hypoxia is extremely severe during the period of submersion, and superimposed cardiac arrest places the brain at even higher risk. After adequate resuscitation, unrecognized hypoxia may be present secondary to shunting of blood through atelectatic areas of lung.

The major factor injuring the brain is hypoxia. This produces neuronal damage and death, and cerebral edema follows if the injury is extensive. The best clinical guideline for prognosis is the child's condition at the time of admission to the hospital. If this is good, recovery is usually complete. If the child is in a coma or has fixed dilated pupils, it is likely that there has been severe hypoxic encephalopathy with brain damage, and death usually occurs. The need for resuscitation in the emergency room is also a negative predictor.[17] Treatment is based on maintaining the child's cardiopulmonary status and preventing cerebral edema.

It is important to remember that drowning following a diving accident may be complicated by a spinal cord injury. It is obviously important to remove the individual from the water and begin resuscitation, but the cervical spine should be protected as carefully as possible during these maneuvers.

Cold-water drowning seems to protect the patient against neurological damage, even following prolonged periods of submersion. If the child is hypothermic, it is important to continue vigorous efforts at resuscitation for a considerable period of time. Hot-water drowning, as in a hot tub, has a devastating effect on the brain, even after relatively brief periods of immersion.

Burns are associated with damage to the nervous system for a number of reasons. During the fire, the inhalation of toxic gases such as carbon monoxide and hydrogen cyanide has a direct toxic effect on the brain. In addition, anoxia occurs as part of smoke inhalation. Vascular collapse from massive fluid loss in the severely burned patient can further compound the cerebral injury. Pulmonary damage caused by inhalation of flame or hot gases also contributes to anoxia. The result of all these factors is severe neuronal damage.

Burn encephalopathy is an entity that occurs after treatment has begun and the patient is stabilized. The major symptoms are seizures and an organic mental syndrome.[18] It is important to rule out fluid and electrolyte imbalance and sepsis with meningitis as a cause of the symptoms. Some cases of burn encephalopathy may have been due to the systemic absorption of hexachlorophene which was used to wash the patients. This procedure is no longer in common use, but encephalopathy still occurs. Its etiology is not clear, but it is probably the result of a number of factors.

The type and degree of damage done by *electrical injury* depend on the course of the current through the body, its voltage, and whether it is direct or alternating current. Tissue, including that of the central and peripheral nervous system, which receives a sufficient amount of current is coagulated by the heat produced and is irreversibly injured.

Cardiac arrhythmias are a common part of electrocution, and hypoxic brain damage can also result from circulatory impairment. Damage to muscle can produce myoglobinuria.

Hypoxia is produced by strangulation or suffocation. Seizures followed by coma occur, and if the hypoxia is severe and prolonged, there is death of neural tissue. Management is complicated by the development of cerebral edema. A delayed encephalopathy has been reported to have its onset within several weeks of the original insult. Mental changes, myoclonic seizures, and progressive spasticity occur.

Fat embolism following fracture of a long bone presents in the first 24 hr following injury with changes in mental status and seizures. Diffuse or focal neurological damage can occur. The diagnosis is suggested by the clinical picture, but only becomes clear when petechiae and characteristic changes on chest x-ray studies appear.

POISONING

The catalog of toxic agents ingested by children is limited only by the number of environmental poisons that exist. The majority of accidental ingestions involve the toddler age group and result from the combination of a drive to explore the environment and poor judgment. In older children, poisoning is more typically a result of the use of substances for their mind-altering effect or attempts at suicide. This discussion will be limited to some of the more common toxic agents seen in pediatric practice, and those which are unusual but are associated with serious neurological disease.

Neurological manifestations of toxic substances have one or more of the features listed in Table 29-1. The approach to the patient with metabolic coma is discussed in Chapter 27.

The general principles of treatment are the same for ingestion of all toxic substances. These are[19]

- Consider the possibility of poisoning
- Maintain vital signs
- Identify the poison
- Quantitate the poison
- Prevent continued absorption
- Enhance elimination
- Correct the pathophysiology
- Use all informational resources
- Attend to psychiatric needs

Salicylate intoxication has always been a major pediatric problem, although its frequency decreased dramatically with the introduction of child-proof containers and limitation of the amount of drug in any single container. There has been a further decline with the popularization of acetaminophen as an antipyretic. The clinical signs are hyperventilation, lethargy, and confusion. With very high salicylate levels, coma can occur.

Mercury is a component of fungicides and is found predominantly in agricultural communities. Acute poisoning with mercurials causes severe gastrointestinal and pulmonary symptoms. There is also ataxia, paresthesias, dysarthria, and an organic mental syndrome. Residual impairment of hearing and vision has been reported. Chronic mercury poisoning causes acrodynia. Systemic signs include redness and cyanosis of the hands and feet, profuse perspiration, and

TABLE 29-1
Neurological Signs in Poisoning

Depression of central nervous system function	Parasympathetic overactivity
Lethargy	Miosis
Confusion	Sialorrhea
Disorientation	Cramps and diarrhea
Apnea	Bronchial hypersecretion
Coma	Peripheral nerve function
Excitation of central nervous system function	Paresthesias
Agitation	Weakness or paralysis
Seizures	Areflexia
Hallucinations	Neuromuscular blockade
Sympathetic overactivity	Weakness or paralysis
Mydriasis	Fasciculations
Tachycardia	
Hypertension	
Pyrexia	

pruritus. Neurological involvement is widespread; the patient shows lethargy, restlessness, and a motor and sensory neuropathy.

Lead poisoning is also decreasing in frequency, since the discontinuation of the manufacture of lead-based paints for residential structures. Older residences with multiple coats of paint still contain a good deal of lead in the deeper layers, and this can be ingested by children. The classical presentation is with the onset of an acute encephalopathy following a prodromal period of abdominal symptoms. The child develops seizures and rapidly becomes comatose. There is markedly increased intracranial pressure due to cerebral edema. The diagnosis is confirmed by demonstrating an elevated blood lead level and an increased level of free erythrocyte protoporphyrin. Treatment depends on vigorous management of the cerebral edema and the use of chelating agents to bind the lead and promote its excretion. The prognosis depends on the duration and intensity of the lead ingestion and the severity of the encephalopathy. Many of the children suffer serious damage to the CNS, however, even with the best treatment. Prevention is the most important issue.

There is evidence suggesting that children who have higher-than-average blood lead concentrations are at risk for learning disabilities. These studies have a number of methodological problems, however, and replication is needed.

Organophosphate compounds are commonly present in home and agricultural insecticides. These are potent cholinesterase inhibitors, and their effects are a result of cholinergic overactivity at the neuromuscular junction (nicotinic receptors) and the parasympathetic ganglia (muscarinic receptors). Muscle weakness occurs and can be profound. In milder intoxications, there are muscle cramps, fatigability and fasciculations. Parasympathetic effects include diaphoresis, abdominal cramps, diarrhea, and salivation. Emergency treatment is based on the use of large doses of atropine to correct the parasympathetic overactivity. Pralidoxime chloride competes with the toxin at the neuromuscular junction and helps reverse the paralysis.

REFERENCES

1. Moran, J. R., and Greene, H. L., 1979, The B vitamins and vitamin C in human nutrition. I. General considerations and "obligatory" B vitamins, *Am. J. Dis. Child.* **133:**192–199.
2. Moran, J. R., and Greene, H. L., 1979, The B vitamins and vitamin KC in human nutrition. II. "Conditional" B vitamins and vitamin C, *Am. J. Dis. Child.* **133:**308–314.
3. Minns, R., 1980, Vitamin B_6 deficiency and dependency, *Dev. Med. Child. Neurol.* **22:**795–799.
4. Guggenheim, M. A., Jackson, V., Lilly, J., and Silverman, A., 1983, Vitamin E deficiency and neurologic disease in children with cholestasis, *J. Pediatr.* **102:**577–579.
5. Rosenbloom, A. L., Riley, W. J., Weber, F. T., Malone, J. I., and Donnelly, W. H., 1980, Cerebral edema complicating diabetic ketoacidosis in childhood, *J. Pediatr.* **96:**357–361.
6. White, N. H., Waltman, S. R., Krupin, T., and Santiago, J. V., 1981, Reversal of neuropathic and gastrointestinal complications related to diabetes mellitus in adolescents with improved metabolic control, *J. Pediatr.* **99:**41–45.
7. Rubin, H. M., Kramer, R., and Drash, A., 1969, Hyperosmolality complicating diabetes mellitus in childhood, *J. Pediatr.* **74:**177–186.

8. Bale, J. F., Siegler, R. L., Bray, P. F., 1980, Encephalopathy in young children with moderate renal failure, *Am. J. Dis. Child.* **134:**581–583.

9. Rasbury, W. C., Fennell, R. S., and Morris, M. K., 1983, Cognitive functioning of children with end-stage renal disease before and after successful transplantation, *J. Pediatr.* **102:**589–592.

10. Oh, S. J., Clements, R. S., Lee, Y. W., and Diethelm, A. G., 1978, Rapid improvement in nerve conduction velocity following renal transplantation, *Ann. Neurol.* **4:**369–373.

11. Lederman, R. J., and Henry, C. E., 1978, Progressive dialysis encephalopathy, *Ann. Neurol.* **4:**199–204.

12. DiGeorge, A. M., 1983, The endocrine system, in: *Textbook of Pediatrics* (R. E. Behrman and V. C. Vaughn, eds.), W.B. Saunders, Philadelphia, pp. 1432–1514.

13. O'Dougherty, M., Wright, F. S., Loewenson, R. B., and Torres, F., 1985, Cerebral dysfunction after chronic hypoxia in children, *Neurology* **35:**42–46.

15. Newburger, J. W., Silbert, A. R., Buckley, L. P., and Fyler, D. C., 1984, Cognitive function and age at repair of transposition of the great arteries in children, *N. Engl. J. Med.* **310:**1495–1499.

15. Belman, A. L., Leicher, C. R., Moshe, S. L., and Mezey, A. P., 1985, Neurologic manifestations of Schoenlein–Henoch purpura: Report of three cases and review of the literature, *Pediatrics* **75:**687–692.

16. Strauss, A. A., Modanlou, H. D., and Bosu, S. K., 1981, Neonatal manifestations of maternal phencyclidine (PCP) abuse, *Pediatrics* **68:**550–552.

17. Frates, R. C., 1981, Analysis of predictive factors in the assessment of warm-water near-drowning in children, *Am. J. Dis. Child.* **135:**1006–1008.

18. Mohnot, D., Snead, O. C., and Benton, J. W., 1982, Burn encephalopathy in children, *Ann. Neurol.* **12:**42–47.

19. Lietman, P. S., 1983, Chemical and drug poisoning, in: *Textbook of Pediatrics* (R. E. Behrman and V. C. Vaughn, eds.), W. B. Saunders, Philadelphia, pp. 1786–1788.

Index